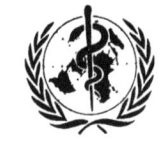

WORLD HEALTH ORGANIZATION

INTERNATIONAL AGENCY FOR RESEARCH ON CANCER

IARC MONOGRAPHS
ON THE
EVALUATION OF CARCINOGENIC RISKS TO HUMANS

Occupational Exposures in Petroleum Refining; Crude Oil and Major Petroleum Fuels

VOLUME 45

This publication represents the views and expert opinions
of an IARC Working Group on the
Evaluation of Carcinogenic Risks to Humans,
which met in Lyon,

1-8 March 1988

1989

IARC MONOGRAPHS

In 1969, the International Agency for Research on Cancer (IARC) initiated a programme on the evaluation of the carcinogenic risk of chemicals to humans involving the production of critically evaluated monographs on individual chemicals. In 1980 and 1986, the programme was expanded to include the evaluation of the carcinogenic risk associated with exposures to complex mixtures and other agents.

The objective of the programme is to elaborate and publish in the form of monographs critical reviews of data on carcinogenicity for agents to which humans are known to be exposed, and on specific exposure situations; to evaluate these data in terms of human risk with the help of international working groups of experts in chemical carcinogenesis and related fields; and to indicate where additional research efforts are needed.

This project is supported by PHS Grant No. 5 UO1 CA33193-06 awarded by the US National Cancer Institute, Department of Health and Human Services. Additional support has been provided since 1986 by the Commission of the European Communities.

©International Agency for Research on Cancer 1989

ISBN 92 832 1245 2

ISSN 0250-9555

All rights reserved. Application for rights of reproduction or translation, in part or *in toto*, should be made to the International Agency for Research on Cancer.

Distributed for the International Agency for Research on Cancer
by the Secretariat of the World Health Organization

PRINTED IN THE UK

CONTENTS

NOTE TO THE READER 5

LIST OF PARTICIPANTS 7

PREAMBLE 11
    Background 13
    Objective and Scope 13
    Selection of Topics for Monographs 14
    Data for Monographs 14
    The Working Group 15
    Working Procedures 15
    Exposure Data 16
    Biological Data Relevant to the Evaluation of Carcinogenicity to Humans ... 17
    Evidence for Carcinogenicity in Experimental Animals 18
    Other Relevant Data in Experimental Systems and Humans 20
    Evidence for Carcinogenicity in Humans 21
    Summary of Data Reported 24
    Evaluation 25
    References 28

GENERAL REMARKS 31

THE MONOGRAPHS

    Occupational Exposures in Petroleum Refining 39
    Crude Oil 119
    Gasoline 159
    Jet Fuel 203
    Diesel Fuels 219
    Fuel Oils (Heating Oils) 239

CONTENTS

SUMMARY OF FINAL EVALUATIONS 271

APPENDIX 1 273

GLOSSARY 275

CUMULATIVE CORRIGENDA TO VOLUMES 1-44 283

CUMULATIVE INDEX TO THE *MONOGRAPHS* SERIES 285

NOTE TO THE READER

The term 'carcinogenic risk' in the *IARC Monographs* series is taken to mean the probability that exposure to an agent will lead to cancer in humans.

Inclusion of an agent in the *Monographs* does not imply that it is a carcinogen, only that the published data have been examined. Equally, the fact that an agent has not yet been evaluated in a monograph does not mean that it is not carcinogenic.

The evaluations of carcinogenic risk are made by international working groups of independent scientists and are qualitative in nature. No recommendation is given for regulation or legislation.

Anyone who is aware of published data that may alter the evaluation of the carcinogenic risk of an agent to humans is encouraged to make this information available to the Unit of Carcinogen Identification and Evaluation, International Agency for Research on Cancer, 150 cours Albert Thomas, 69372 Lyon Cedex 08, France, in order that the agent may be considered for re-evaluation by a future Working Group.

Although every effort is made to prepare the monographs as accurately as possible, mistakes may occur. Readers are requested to communicate any errors to the Unit of Carcinogen Identification and Evaluation, so that corrections can be reported in future volumes.

IARC WORKING GROUP ON THE EVALUATION OF CARCINOGENIC RISKS TO HUMANS: OCCUPATIONAL EXPOSURES IN PETROLEUM REFINING; CRUDE OIL AND MAJOR PETROLEUM FUELS

Lyon, 1-8 March 1988

Members[1]

E. Dybing, Department of Toxicology, National Institute of Public Health, Geitmyrsveien 75, 0462 Oslo 4, Norway

S.L. Eustis, National Toxicology Program, National Institute of Environmental Health Sciences, PO Box 12233, Research Triangle Park, NC 27709, USA

M. Gérin, University of Montreal, Department of Occupational and Environmental Health, Faculty of Medicine, CP 6128 Station A, Montréal, Québec H3C 3J7, Canada

M. Ishidate, Jr, Biological Safety Research Center, National Institute of Hygienic Sciences, 1-18-1 Kami Yooga, Setagaya-ku, Tokyo 158, Japan

V.A. Krutovskikh, Cancer Research Centre, USSR Academy of Medical Sciences, Karshirskoye Shosse 24, 115478 Moscow, USSR

S. Langård, Telemark Central Hospital, Department of Occupational Medicine, Olavsgt 26, 39000 Porsgrunn, Norway

A.J. McMichael, Department of Community Medicine, University of Adelaide, Adelaide, SA 5000, Australia (*Chairman*)

S. Nesnow, Carcinogenesis and Metabolism Branch, US Environmental Protection Agency (MD-68), Research Triangle Park, NC 27711, USA

J.F. Payne, Research and Source Services, Department of Fisheries and Oceans, PO Box 5667, St John's, Newfoundland A1C 5X1, Canada

G. Pershagen, The National Institute of Environmental Medicine, Box 60208, 10401 Stockholm, Sweden

---

[1]Unable to attend: E.A. Emmett, National Institute of Occupational Health and Safety, GPO Box 58, Sydney, NSW 2001, Australia

A. Pinter, Department of Morphology, National Institute of Hygiene, Gyali ut 2–6, 1966 Budapest, Hungary

U. Saffiotti, Laboratory of Experimental Pathology, Division of Cancer Etiology, National Cancer Institute, Building 41, Room C–105, Bethesda, MD 20892, USA

J.T. Sanderson, Exxon Chemical Ltd, Esso Refinery, Fawley, Southampton SO4 1TX, UK

M. Sorsa, Institute of Occupational Health, Topeliuksenkatu 41 a A, 00250 Helsinki, Finland (*Vice-chairman*)

R. Stahlmann, Institute of Toxicology and Embryonal Pharmacology of the Free University of Berlin, Garystrasse 5, 1000 Berlin (West) 33, Federal Republic of Germany

G. Thériault, School of Occupational Health, McGill University, 1130 Pine Avenue West, Montréal, Québec H3A 1A3, Canada

T.L. Thomas, Department of Medicine and Surgery – 10QA1, Veterans' Administration, 810 Vermont Avenue NW, Washington DC 20420, USA

Representatives and Observers[1]

Representative of the National Cancer Institute

T.P. Cameron, Division of Cancer Etiology, National Cancer Institute, Landow Building, Room 1D–34, Bethesda, MD 20892, USA

Representative of the Commission of the European Communities

E. Krug, Commission of the European Communities, Health and Safety Directorate, Bâtiment Jean Monnet, 2920 Luxembourg, Grand Duchy of Luxembourg

Representative of Tracor Jitco, Inc.

S. Olin, Tracor Jitco, Inc., 1601 Research Boulevard, Rockville, MD 20850, USA

Representative of the American Petroleum Institute

G.K. Raabe, Corporate Medical Department, Epidemiology and Medical Information Services, Mobil Oil Corporation, 150 East 42nd Street, New York, NY 10017, USA

Representative of CONCAWE

B.J. Simpson, Health, Safety and Environment Division, Shell International Petroleum Maatschappij, van Hogenhouklaan 60, The Hague, The Netherlands

---

[1]Unable to attend: R.W. Niemeier, National Institute for Occupational Safety and Health, R.A. Taft Laboratories, 4676 Columbia Parkway, Cincinnati, OH 45226–1998, USA

PARTICIPANTS

Secretariat

A. Aitio, Unit of Carcinogen Identification and Evaluation (*Officer-in-Charge of the Programme*)

H. Bartsch, Unit of Environmental Carcinogenesis and Host Factors

J.R.P. Cabral, Unit of Mechanisms of Carcinogenesis

E. Cardis, Unit of Biostatistics Research and Informatics

M. Coleman, Unit of Descriptive Epidemiology

K. Enomoto, Unit of Mechanisms of Carcinogenesis

M. Friesen, Unit of Environmental Carcinogenesis and Host Factors

M.-J. Ghess, Unit of Carcinogen Identification and Evaluation

E. Heseltine, Lajarthe, St Léon-sur-Vézère, 24290 Montignac, France

T. Kauppinen, Unit of Carcinogen Identification and Evaluation

D. Mietton, Unit of Carcinogen Identification and Evaluation

R. Montesano, Unit of Mechanisms of Carcinogenesis

C.S. Muir, Deputy Director

I. O'Neill, Unit of Environmental Carcinogenesis and Host Factors

C. Partensky, Unit of Carcinogen Identification and Evaluation

I. Peterschmitt, Unit of Carcinogen Identification and Evaluation, Geneva

R. Saracci, Unit of Analytical Epidemiology

L. Shuker, Unit of Carcinogen Identification and Evaluation (*Secretary*)

L. Simonato, Unit of Analytical Epidemiology

E. Smith, International Programme on Chemical Safety, World Health Organization, 1211 Geneva 27, Switzerland

L. Tomatis, Director

A. Tossavainen, Institute of Occupational Health, Topeliuksenkatu 41 a A, 00250 Helsinki, Finland

J.D. Wilbourn, Unit of Carcinogen Identification and Evaluation

H. Yamasaki, Unit of Mechanisms of Carcinogenesis

Secretarial assistance

J. Cazeaux

M. Lézère

S. Reynaud

PREAMBLE

IARC MONOGRAPHS PROGRAMME ON THE EVALUATION OF CARCINOGENIC RISKS TO HUMANS[1]

PREAMBLE

1. BACKGROUND

In 1969, the International Agency for Research on Cancer (IARC) initiated a programme to evaluate the carcinogenic risk of chemicals to humans and to produce monographs on individual chemicals. The *Monographs* programme has since been expanded to include consideration of exposures to complex mixtures of chemicals (which occur, for example, in some occupations and as a result of human habits) and of exposures to other agents, such as radiation and viruses. With Supplement 6(1), the title of the series was modified from *IARC Monographs on the Evaluation of the Carcinogenic Risk of Chemicals to Humans* to *IARC Monographs on the Evaluation of Carcinogenic Risks to Humans*, in order to reflect the widened scope of the programme.

The criteria established in 1971 to evaluate carcinogenic risk to humans were adopted by the working groups whose deliberations resulted in the first 16 volumes of the *IARC Monographs* series. Those criteria were subsequently re-evaluated by working groups which met in 1977(2), 1978(3), 1979(4), 1982(5) and 1983(6). The present preamble was prepared by two working groups which met in September 1986 and January 1987, prior to the preparation of Supplement 7 to the *Monographs*(7).

2. OBJECTIVE AND SCOPE

The objective of the programme is to prepare, with the help of international working groups of experts, and to publish in the form of monographs, critical reviews and evaluations of evidence on the carcinogenicity of a wide range of agents to which humans are or may be exposed. The *Monographs* may also indicate where additional research efforts are needed.

---

[1]This project is supported by PHS Grant No. 5 UO1 CA33193-06 awarded by the US National Cancer Institute, Department of Health and Human Services, and with a subcontract to Tracor Jitco, Inc. and Technical Resources, Inc. Since 1986, this programme has also been supported by the Commission of the European Communities.

The *Monographs* represent the first step in carcinogenic risk assessment, which involves examination of all relevant information in order to assess the strength of the available evidence that, under certain conditions of exposure, an agent could alter the incidence of cancer in humans. The second step is quantitative risk estimation, which is not usually attempted in the *Monographs*. Detailed, quantitative evaluations of epidemiological data may be made in the *Monographs*, but without extrapolation beyond the range of the data available. Quantitative extrapolation from experimental data to the human situation is not undertaken.

These monographs may assist national and international authorities in making risk assessments and in formulating decisions concerning any necessary preventive measures. **No recommendation is given for regulation or legislation, since such decisions are made by individual governments and/or other international agencies.** The *IARC Monographs* are recognized as an authoritative source of information on the carcinogenicity of chemicals and complex exposures. A users' survey, made in 1984, indicated that the *Monographs* are consulted by various agencies in 45 countries. Each volume is printed in 4000 copies for distribution to governments, regulatory bodies and interested scientists. The *Monographs* are also available *via* the Distribution and Sales Service of the World Health Organization.

3. SELECTION OF TOPICS FOR MONOGRAPHS

Topics are selected on the basis of two main criteria: (a) that they concern agents for which there is evidence of human exposure, and (b) there is some evidence or suspicion of carcinogenicity. The term agent is used to include individual chemical compounds, groups of chemical compounds, physical agents (such as radiation), biological factors (such as viruses) and mixtures of agents such as occur in occupational exposures and as a result of personal and cultural habits (like smoking and dietary practices). Chemical analogues and compounds with biological or physical characteristics similar to those of suspected carcinogens may also be considered, even in the absence of data on carcinogenicity.

The scientific literature is surveyed for published data relevant to an assessment of carcinogenicity; the IARC surveys of chemicals being tested for carcinogenicity(8) and directories of on-going research in cancer epidemiology(9) often indicate those agents that may be scheduled for future meetings. An ad-hoc working group convened by IARC in 1984 gave recommendations as to which chemicals and exposures to complex mixtures should be evaluated in the *IARC Monographs* series(10).

As significant new data on subjects on which monographs have already been prepared become available, re-evaluations are made at subsequent meetings, and revised monographs are published.

4. DATA FOR MONOGRAPHS

The *Monographs* do not necessarily cite all of the literature on a particular agent. Only those data considered by the Working Group to be relevant to making an evaluation are included.

With regard to biological and epidemiological data, only reports that have been published or accepted for publication in the openly available scientific literature are reviewed by the working groups. In certain instances, government agency reports that have undergone peer review and are widely available are considered. Exceptions may be made on an ad-hoc basis to include unpublished reports that are in their final form and publicly available, if their inclusion is considered pertinent to making a final evaluation (see pp. 25 *et seq.*). In the sections on chemical and physical properties and on production, use, occurrence and analysis, unpublished sources of information may be used.

5. THE WORKING GROUP

Reviews and evaluations are formulated by a working group of experts. The tasks of this group are five-fold: (i) to ascertain that all appropriate data have been collected; (ii) to select the data relevant for the evaluation on the basis of scientific merit; (iii) to prepare accurate summaries of the data to enable the reader to follow the reasoning of the Working Group; (iv) to evaluate the results of experimental and epidemiological studies; and (v) to make an overall evaluation of the carcinogenicity of the agent to humans.

Working Group participants who contributed to the consideration and evaluation of the agents within a particular volume are listed, with their addresses, at the beginning of each publication. Each participant who is a member of a working group serves as an individual scientist and not as a representative of any organization, government or industry. In addition, representatives from national and international agencies and industrial associations are invited as observers.

6. WORKING PROCEDURES

Approximately one year in advance of a meeting of a working group, the agents to be evaluated are announced and participants are selected by IARC staff in consultation with other experts. Subsequently, relevant biological and epidemiological data are collected by IARC from recognized sources of information on carcinogenesis, including data storage and retrieval systems such as CAS ONLINE, MEDLINE and TOXLINE, including EMIC and ETIC for data on genetic and related effects and on teratogenicity, respectively.

The major collection of data and the preparation of first drafts of the sections on chemical and physical properties, on production and use, on occurrence, and on analysis are carried out under a separate contract funded by the US National Cancer Institute. Efforts are made to supplement this information with data from other national and international sources. Representatives from industrial associations may assist in the preparation of sections on production and use.

Production and trade data are obtained from governmental and trade publications and, in some cases, by direct contact with industries. Separate production data on some agents may not be available because their publication could disclose confidential information.

Information on uses is usually obtained from published sources but is often complemented by direct contact with manufacturers.

Six months before the meeting, reference material is sent to experts, or is used by IARC staff, to prepare sections for the first drafts of monographs. The complete first drafts are compiled by IARC staff and sent, prior to the meeting, to all participants of the Working Group for review.

The Working Group meets in Lyon for seven to eight days to discuss and finalize the texts of the monographs and to formulate the evaluations. After the meeting, the master copy of each monograph is verified by consulting the original literature, edited and prepared for publication. The aim is to publish monographs within nine months of the Working Group meeting.

7. EXPOSURE DATA

Sections that indicate the extent of past and present human exposure, the sources of exposure, the persons most likely to be exposed and the factors that contribute to exposure to the agent under study are included at the beginning of each monograph.

Most monographs on individual chemicals or complex mixtures include sections on chemical and physical data, and production, use, occurrence and analysis. In other monographs, for example on physical agents, biological factors, occupational exposures and cultural habits, other sections may be included, such as: historical perspectives, description of an industry or habit, exposures in the work place or chemistry of the complex mixture.

The Chemical Abstracts Services Registry Number, the latest Chemical Abstracts Primary Name and the IUPAC Systematic Name are recorded. Other synonyms and trade names are given, but the list is not necessarily comprehensive. Some of the trade names may be those of mixtures in which the agent being evaluated is only one of the ingredients.

Information on chemical and physical properties and, in particular, data relevant to identification, occurrence and biological activity are included. A separate description of technical products gives relevant specifications and includes available information on composition and impurities.

The dates of first synthesis and of first commercial production of an agent are provided; for agents which do not occur naturally, this information may allow a reasonable estimate to be made of the date before which no human exposure to the agent could have occurred. The dates of first reported occurrence of an exposure are also provided. In addition, methods of synthesis used in past and present commercial production and different methods of production which may give rise to different impurities are described.

Data on production, foreign trade and uses are obtained for representative regions, which usually include Europe, Japan and the USA. It should not, however, be inferred that those areas or nations are necessarily the sole or major sources or users of the agent being evaluated.

Some identified uses may not be current or major applications, and the coverage is not necessarily comprehensive. In the case of drugs, mention of their therapeutic uses does not necessarily represent current practice nor does it imply judgement as to their clinical efficacy.

Information on the occurrence of an agent in the environment is obtained from data derived from the monitoring and surveillance of levels in occupational environments, air, water, soil, foods and animal and human tissues. When available, data on the generation, persistence and bioaccumulation of the agent are also included.

Statements concerning regulations and guidelines (e.g., pesticide registrations, maximal levels permitted in foods, occupational exposure limits) are included for some countries as indications of potential exposures, but they may not reflect the most recent situation, since such limits are continuously reviewed and modified. The absence of information on regulatory status for a country should not be taken to imply that that country does not have regulations with regard to the agent.

The purpose of the section on analysis is to give the reader an overview of current methods cited in the literature, with emphasis on those widely used for regulatory purposes. No critical evaluation or recommendation of any of the methods is meant or implied. Methods for monitoring human exposure are also given, when available. The IARC publishes a series of volumes, *Environmental Carcinogens: Selected Methods of Analysis*(11), that describe validated methods for analysing a wide variety of agents.

8. BIOLOGICAL DATA RELEVANT TO THE EVALUATION OF CARCINOGENICITY TO HUMANS

The term 'carcinogen' is used in these monographs to denote an agent that is capable of increasing the incidence of malignant neoplasms; the induction of benign neoplasms may in some circumstances (see p. 19) contribute to the judgement that an agent is carcinogenic. The terms 'neoplasm' and 'tumour' are used interchangeably.

Some epidemiological and experimental studies indicate that different agents may act at different stages in the carcinogenic process, probably by fundamentally different mechanisms. In the present state of knowledge, the aim of the *Monographs* is to evaluate evidence of carcinogenicity at any stage in the carcinogenic process independently of the underlying mechanism involved. There is as yet insufficient information to implement a classification of agents according to their mechanism of action(6).

Definitive evidence of carcinogenicity in humans is provided by epidemiological studies. Evidence relevant to human carcinogenicity may also be provided by experimental studies of carcinogenicity in animals and by other biological data, particularly those relating to humans.

The available studies are summarized by the working groups, with particular regard to the qualitative aspects discussed below. In general, numerical findings are indicated as they appear in the original report; units are converted when necessary for easier comparison. The Working Group may conduct additional analyses of the published data and use them in their assessment of the evidence and may include them in their summary of a study; the results of such supplementary analyses are given in square brackets. Any comments are also made in square brackets; however, these are kept to a minimum, being restricted to those instances in which it is felt that an important aspect of a study, directly impinging on its interpretation, should be brought to the attention of the reader.

9. EVIDENCE FOR CARCINOGENICITY IN EXPERIMENTAL ANIMALS

For several agents (e.g., 4-aminobiphenyl, bis(chloromethyl)ether, diethylstilboestrol, melphalan, 8-methoxypsoralen (methoxsalen) plus UVR, mustard gas and vinyl chloride), evidence of carcinogenicity in experimental animals preceded evidence obtained from epidemiological studies or case reports. Information compiled from the first 41 volumes of the *IARC Monographs*(12) shows that, of the 44 agents for which there is *sufficient* or *limited evidence* of carcinogenicity to humans (see pp. 25-26), all 37 that have been tested adequately experimentally produce cancer in at least one animal species. Although this association cannot establish that all agents that cause cancer in experimental animals also cause cancer in humans, nevertheless, **in the absence of adequate data on humans, it is biologically plausible and prudent to regard agents for which there is** *sufficient evidence* **(see p. 26) of carcinogenicity in experimental animals as if they presented a carcinogenic risk to humans.**

The monographs are not intended to summarize all published studies. Those that are inadequate (e.g., too short a duration, too few animals, poor survival; see below) or are judged irrelevant to the evaluation are generally omitted. They may be mentioned briefly, particularly when the information is considered to be a useful supplement to that of other reports or when they provide the only data available. Their inclusion does not, however, imply acceptance of the adequacy of the experimental design or of the analysis and interpretation of their results. Guidelines for adequate long-term carcinogenicity experiments have been outlined (e.g., ref. 13).

The nature and extent of impurities or contaminants present in the agent being evaluated are given when available. Mention is made of all routes of exposure by which the agent has been adequately studied and of all species in which relevant experiments have been performed. Animal strain, sex, numbers per group, age at start of treatment and survival are reported.

Experiments in which the agent was administered in conjunction with known carcinogens or factors that modify carcinogenic effects are also reported. Experiments on the carcinogenicity of known metabolites and derivatives may be included.

(a) Qualitative aspects

The overall assessment of the carcinogenicity of an agent involves several considerations of qualitative importance, including (i) the experimental conditions under which the test was performed, including route and schedule of exposure, species, strain, sex, age, duration of follow-up; (ii) the consistency with which the agent has been shown to be carcinogenic, e.g., in how many species and at which target organs(s); (iii) the spectrum of neoplastic response, from benign tumours to malignant neoplasms; and (iv) the possible role of modifying factors.

Considerations of importance to the Working Group in the interpretation and evaluation of a particular study include: (i) how clearly the agent was defined; (ii) whether the dose was adequately monitored, particularly in inhalation experiments; (iii) whether the doses used were appropriate and whether the survival of treated animals was similar to that of controls; (iv) whether there were adequate numbers of animals per group; (v) whether animals of both sexes were used; (vi) whether animals were allocated randomly to groups; (vii) whether the duration of observation was adequate; and (viii) whether the data were adequately reported. If available, recent data on the incidence of specific tumours in historical controls, as well as in concurrent controls, should be taken into account in the evaluation of tumour response.

When benign tumours occur together with and originate from the same cell type in an organ or tissue as malignant tumours in a particular study and appear to represent a stage in the progression to malignancy, it may be valid to combine them in assessing tumour incidence. The occurrence of lesions presumed to be preneoplastic may in certain instances aid in assessing the biological plausibility of any neoplastic response observed.

Among the many agents that have been studied extensively, there are few instances in which the only neoplasms induced were benign. Benign tumours in experimental animals frequently represent a stage in the evolution of a malignant neoplasm, but they may be 'endpoints' that do not readily undergo transition to malignancy. However, if an agent is found to induce only benign neoplasms, it should be suspected of being a carcinogen and it requires further investigation.

(b) Quantitative aspects

The probability that tumours will occur may depend on the species and strain, the dose of the carcinogen and the route and period of exposure. Evidence of an increased incidence of neoplasms with increased exposure strengthens the inference of a causal association between exposure to the agent and the development of neoplasms.

The form of the dose-response relationship can vary widely, depending on the particular agent under study and the target organ. Since many chemicals require metabolic activation before being converted into their reactive intermediates, both metabolic and pharmacokinetic aspects are important in determining the dose-response pattern. Saturation of steps such as absorption, activation, inactivation and elimination of the carcinogen may produce nonlinearity in the dose-response relationship, as could saturation of processes such as DNA repair(14,15).

(c) Statistical analysis of long-term experiments in animals

Factors considered by the Working Group include the adequacy of the information given for each treatment group: (i) the number of animals on study and the number examined histologically, (ii) the number of animals with a given tumour type and (iii) length of survival. The statistical methods used should be clearly stated and should be the generally accepted techniques refined for this purpose(15,16). When there is no difference in survival between control and treatment groups, the Working Group usually compares the proportions of animals developing each tumour type in each of the groups. Otherwise, consideration is given as to whether or not appropriate adjustments have been made for differences in survival. These adjustments can include: comparisons of the proportions of tumour-bearing animals among the 'effective number' of animals alive at the time the first tumour is discovered, in the case where most differences in survival occur before tumours appear; life-table methods, when tumours are visible or when they may be considered 'fatal' because mortality rapidly follows tumour development; and the Mantel-Haenszel test or logistic regression, when occult tumours do not affect the animals' risk of dying but are 'incidental' findings at autopsy.

In practice, classifying tumours as fatal or incidental may be difficult. Several survival-adjusted methods have been developed that do not require this distinction(15), although they have not been fully evaluated.

10. OTHER RELEVANT DATA IN EXPERIMENTAL SYSTEMS AND HUMANS

(a) Structure-activity considerations

This section describes structure-activity correlations that are relevant to an evaluation of the carcinogenicity of an agent.

(b) Absorption, distribution, excretion and metabolism

Concise information is given on absorption, distribution (including placental transfer) and excretion. Kinetic factors that may affect the dose-reponse relationship, such as saturation of uptake, protein binding, metabolic activation, detoxification and DNA-repair processes, are mentioned. Studies that indicate the metabolic fate of the agent in experimental animals and humans are summarized briefly, and comparisons of data from animals and humans are made when possible. Comparative information on the relationship between exposure and the dose that reaches the target site may be of particular importance for extrapolation between species.

(c) Toxicity

Data are given on acute and chronic toxic effects (other than cancer), such as organ toxicity, immunotoxicity, endocrine effects and preneoplastic lesions. Effects on reproduction, teratogenicity, feto- and embryotoxicity are also summarized briefly.

(d) Genetic and related effects

Tests of genetic and related effects may indicate possible carcinogenic activity. They can also be used in detecting active metabolites of known carcinogens in human or animal body fluids, in detecting active components in complex mixtures and in the elucidation of possible mechanisms of carcinogenesis.

The available data are interpreted critically by phylogenetic group according to the endpoints detected, which may include DNA damage, gene mutation, sister chromatid exchange, micronuclei, chromosomal aberrations, aneuploidy and cell transformation. The concentrations (doses) employed are given and mention is made of whether an exogenous metabolic system was required. When appropriate, these data may be represented by bar graphs (activity profiles), with corresponding summary tables and listings of test systems, data and references. Detailed information on the preparation of these profiles is given in an appendix to those volumes in which they are used.

Positive results in tests using prokaryotes, lower eukaryotes, plants, insects and cultured mammalian cells suggest that genetic and related effects (and therefore possibly carcinogenic effects) could occur in mammals. Results from such tests may also give information about the types of genetic effects produced by an agent and about the involvement of metabolic activation. Some endpoints described are clearly genetic in nature (e.g., gene mutations and chromosomal aberrations), others are to a greater or lesser degree associated with genetic effects (e.g., unscheduled DNA synthesis). In-vitro tests for tumour-promoting activity and for cell transformation may detect changes that are not necessarily the result of genetic alterations but that may have specific relevance to the process of carcinogenesis. A critical appraisal of these tests has been published(13).

Genetic or other activity detected in the systems mentioned above is not always manifest in whole mammals. Positive indications of genetic effects in experimental mammals and in humans are regarded as being of greater relevance than those in other organisms. The demonstration that an agent can induce gene and chromosomal mutations in whole mammals indicates that it may have the potential for carcinogenic activity, although this activity may not be detectably expressed in any or all species tested. The relative potency of agents in tests for mutagenicity and related effects is not a reliable indicator of carcinogenic potency. Negative results in tests for mutagenicity in selected tissues from animals treated *in vivo* provide less weight, partly because they do not exclude the possibility of an effect in tissues other than those examined. Moreover, negative results in short-term tests with genetic endpoints cannot be considered to provide evidence to rule out carcinogenicity of agents that act through other mechanisms. Factors may arise in many tests that could give misleading results; these have been discussed in detail elsewhere(13).

The adequacy of epidemiological studies of reproductive outcomes and genetic and related effects in humans is evaluated by the same criteria as are applied to epidemiological studies of cancer.

11. EVIDENCE FOR CARCINOGENICITY IN HUMANS

(a) Types of studies considered

Three types of epidemiological studies of cancer contribute data to the assessment of carcinogenicity in humans — cohort studies, case-control studies and correlation studies. Rarely, results from randomized trials may be available. Case reports of cancer in humans exposed to particular agents are also reviewed.

Cohort and case-control studies relate individual exposure to the agent under study to the occurrence of cancer in individuals, and provide an estimate of relative risk (ratio of incidence in those exposed to incidence in those not exposed) as the main measure of association.

In correlation studies, the units of investigation are usually whole populations (e.g., in particular geographical areas or at particular times), and cancer incidence is related to a summary measure of the exposure of the population to the agent under study. Because individual exposure is not documented, however, a causal relationship is less easy to infer from correlation studies than from cohort and case-control studies.

Case reports generally arise from a suspicion, based on clinical experience, that the concurrence of two events — that is, exposure to a particular agent and occurrence of a cancer — has happened rather more frequently than would be expected by chance. Case reports usually lack complete ascertainment of cases in any population, definition or enumeration of the population at risk and estimation of the expected number of cases in the absence of exposure.

The uncertainties surrounding interpretation of case reports and correlation studies make them inadequate, except in rare instances, to form the sole basis for inferring a causal relationship. When taken together with case-control and cohort studies, however, relevant case reports or correlation studies may add materially to the judgement that a causal relationship is present.

Epidemiological studies of benign neoplasms and presumed preneoplastic lesions are also reviewed by working groups. They may, in some instances, strengthen inferences drawn from studies of cancer itself.

(b) Quality of studies considered

It is necessary to take into account the possible roles of bias, confounding and chance in the interpretation of epidemiological studies. By 'bias' is meant the operation of factors in study design or execution that lead erroneously to a stronger or weaker association between an agent and disease than in fact exists. By 'confounding' is meant a situation in which the relationship between an agent and a disease is made to appear stronger or to appear weaker than it truly is as a result of an association between the agent and another agent that is associated with either an increase or decrease in the incidence of the disease. In evaluating the extent to which these factors have been minimized in an individual study, working groups consider a number of aspects of design and analysis as described in the report of the study. Most of these considerations apply equally to case-control, cohort and correlation studies. Lack of clarity of any of these aspects in the reporting of a study can decrease its credibility and its consequent weighting in the final evaluation of the exposure.

Firstly, the study population, disease (or diseases) and exposure should have been well defined by the authors. Cases in the study population should have been identified in a way that was independent of the exposure of interest, and exposure should have been assessed in a way that was not related to disease status.

Secondly, the authors should have taken account in the study design and analysis of other variables that can influence the risk of disease and may have been related to the exposure of interest. Potential confounding by such variables should have been dealt with either in the design of the study, such as by matching, or in the analysis, by statistical adjustment. In cohort studies, comparisons with local rates of disease may be more appropriate than those with national rates. Internal comparisons of disease frequency among individuals at different levels of exposure should also have been made in the study.

Thirdly, the authors should have reported the basic data on which the conclusions are founded, even if sophisticated statistical analyses were employed. At the very least, they should have given the numbers of exposed and unexposed cases and controls in a case-control study and the numbers of cases observed and expected in a cohort study. Further tabulations by time since exposure began and other temporal factors are also important. In a cohort study, data on all cancer sites and all causes of death should have been given, to avoid the possibility of reporting bias. In a case-control study, the effects of investigated factors other than the agent of interest should have been reported.

Finally, the statistical methods used to obtain estimates of relative risk, absolute cancer rates, confidence intervals and significance tests, and to adjust for confounding should have been clearly stated by the authors. The methods used should preferably have been the generally accepted techniques that have been refined since the mid-1970s. These methods have been reviewed for case-control studies(17) and for cohort studies(18).

(c) *Quantitative considerations*

Detailed analyses of both relative and absolute risks in relation to age at first exposure and to temporal variables, such as time since first exposure, duration of exposure and time since exposure ceased, are reviewed and summarized when available. The analysis of temporal relationships can provide a useful guide in formulating models of carcinogenesis. In particular, such analyses may suggest whether a carcinogen acts early or late in the process of carcinogenesis(6), although such speculative inferences cannot be used to draw firm conclusions concerning the mechanism of action of the agent and hence the shape (linear or otherwise) of the dose-response relationship below the range of observation.

(d) *Criteria for causality*

After the quality of individual epidemiological studies has been summarized and assessed, a judgement is made concerning the strength of evidence that the agent in question is carcinogenic for humans. In making their judgement, the Working Group considers several criteria for causality. A strong association (i.e., a large relative risk) is more likely to indicate causality than a weak association, although it is recognized that relative risks of small magnitude do not imply lack of causality and may be important if the disease is common. Associations that are replicated in several studies of the same design or using different epidemiological approaches or under different circumstances of exposure are more likely to represent a causal relationship than isolated observations from single studies. If there are inconsistent results among investigations, possible reasons are sought (such as differences in amount of exposure), and results of studies judged to be of high quality are given more weight than those from studies judged to be methodologically less sound. When suspicion of carcinogenicity arises largely from a single study, these data are not combined with those from later studies in any subsequent reassessment of the strength of the evidence.

If the risk of the disease in question increases with the amount of exposure, this is considered to be a strong indication of causality, although absence of a graded response is not necessarily evidence against a causal relationship. Demonstration of a decline in risk after cessation of or reduction in exposure in individuals or in whole populations also supports a causal interpretation of the findings.

Although the same carcinogenic agent may act upon more than one target, the specificity of an association (i.e., an increased occurrence of cancer at one anatomical site or of one morphological type) adds plausibility to a causal relationship, particularly when excess cancer occurrence is limited to one morphological type within the same organ.

Although rarely available, results from randomized trials showing different rates among exposed and unexposed individuals provide particularly strong evidence for causality.

When several epidemiological studies show little or no indication of an association between an agent and cancer, the judgement may be made that, in the aggregate, they show evidence of lack of carcinogenicity. Such a judgement requires first of all that the studies giving rise to it meet, to a sufficient degree, the standards of design and analysis described above. Specifically, the possibility that bias, confounding or misclassification of exposure or outcome could explain the observed results should be considered and excluded with reasonable certainty. In addition, all studies that are judged to be methodologically sound should be consistent with a relative risk of unity for any observed level of exposure to the agent and, when considered together, should provide a pooled estimate of relative risk which is at or near unity and has a narrow confidence interval, due to sufficient population size. Moreover, no individual study nor the pooled results of all the studies should show any consistent tendency for relative risk of cancer to increase with increasing amount of exposure to the agent. It is important to note that evidence of lack of carcinogenicity obtained in this way from several epidemiological studies can apply only to the type(s) of cancer studied and to dose levels of the agent and intervals between first exposure to it and observation of disease that are the same as or less than those observed in all the studies. Experience with human cancer indicates that, for some agents, the period from first exposure to the development of clinical cancer is seldom less than 20 years; latent periods substantially shorter than 30 years cannot provide evidence for lack of carcinogenicity.

12. SUMMARY OF DATA REPORTED

In this section, the relevant experimental and epidemiological data are summarized. Only reports, other than in abstract form, that meet the criteria outlined on pp. 14-15 are considered for evaluating carcinogenicity. Inadequate studies are generally not summarized: such studies are usually identified by a square-bracketed comment in the text.

(a) Exposures

Human exposure is summarized on the basis of elements such as production, use, occurrence in the environment and determinations in human tissues and body fluids. Quantitative data are given when available.

(b) Experimental carcinogenicity data

Data relevant to the evaluation of the carcinogenicity of the agent in animals are summarized. For each animal species and route of administration, it is stated whether an increased incidence of neoplasms was observed, and the tumour sites are indicated. If the agent produced tumours after prenatal exposure or in single-dose experiments, this is also indicated. Dose-response and other quantitative data may be given when available. Negative findings are also summarized.

(c) *Human carcinogenicity data*

Results of epidemiological studies that are considered to be pertinent to an assessment of human carcinogenicity are summarized. When relevant, case reports and correlation studies are also considered.

(d) *Other relevant data*

Structure-activity correlations are mentioned when relevant.

Toxicological information and data on kinetics and metabolism in experimental animals are given when considered relevant. The results of tests for genetic and related effects are summarized for whole mammals, cultured mammalian cells and nonmammalian systems.

Data on other biological effects in humans of particular relevance are summarized. These may include kinetic and metabolic considerations and evidence of DNA binding, persistence of DNA lesions or genetic damage in humans exposed to the agent.

When available, comparisons of such data for humans and for animals, and particularly animals that have developed cancer, are described.

13. EVALUATION

Evaluations of the strength of the evidence for carcinogenicity arising from human and experimental animal data are made, using standard terms.

It is recognized that the criteria for these evaluations, described below, cannot encompass all of the factors that may be relevant to an evaluation of the carcinogenicity of an agent. In considering all of the relevant data, the Working Group may assign the agent to a higher or lower category than a strict interpretation of these criteria would indicate.

(a) *Degrees of evidence for carcinogenicity in humans and in experimental animals and supporting evidence*

It should be noted that these categories refer only to the strength of the evidence that these agents are carcinogenic and not to the extent of their carcinogenic activity (potency) nor to the mechanism involved. The classification of some agents may change as new information becomes available.

(i) *Human carcinogenicity data*

The evidence relevant to carcinogenicity from studies in humans is classified into one of the following categories:

Sufficient evidence of carcinogenicity: The Working Group considers that a causal relationship has been established between exposure to the agent and human cancer. That is, a positive relationship has been observed between exposure to the agent and cancer in studies in which chance, bias and confounding could be ruled out with reasonable confidence.

Limited evidence of carcinogenicity: A positive association has been observed between exposure to the agent and cancer for which a causal interpretation is considered by the Working Group to be credible, but chance, bias or confounding could not be ruled out with reasonable confidence.

Inadequate evidence of carcinogenicity: The available studies are of insufficient quality, consistency or statistical power to permit a conclusion regarding the presence or absence of a causal association.

Evidence suggesting lack of carcinogenicity: There are several adequate studies covering the full range of doses to which human beings are known to be exposed, which are mutually consistent in not showing a positive association between exposure to the agent and any studied cancer at any observed level of exposure. A conclusion of 'evidence suggesting lack of carcinogenicity' is inevitably limited to the cancer sites, circumstances and doses of exposure and length of observation covered by the available studies. In addition, the possibility of a very small risk at the levels of exposure studied can never be excluded.

In some instances, the above categories may be used to classify the degree of evidence for the carcinogenicity of the agent for specific organs or tissues.

(ii) *Experimental carcinogenicity data*

The evidence relevant to carcinogenicity in experimental animals is classified into one of the following categories:

Sufficient evidence of carcinogenicity: The Working Group considers that a causal relationship has been established between the agent and an increased incidence of malignant neoplasms or of an appropriate combination of benign and malignant neoplasms (as described on p. 19) in (a) two or more species of animals or (b) in two or more independent studies in one species carried out at different times or in different laboratories or under different protocols.

Exceptionally, a single study in one species might be considered to provide sufficient evidence of carcinogenicity when malignant neoplasms occur to an unusual degree with regard to incidence, site, type of tumour or age at onset.

In the absence of adequate data on humans, it is biologically plausible and prudent to regard agents for which there is *sufficient evidence* of carcinogenicity in experimental animals as if they presented a carcinogenic risk to humans.

Limited evidence of carcinogenicity: The data suggest a carcinogenic effect but are limited for making a definitive evaluation because, e.g., (a) the evidence of carcinogenicity is restricted to a single experiment; or (b) there are unresolved questions regarding the adequacy of the design, conduct or interpretation of the study; or (c) the agent increases the incidence only of benign neoplasms or lesions of uncertain neoplastic potential, or of certain neoplasms which may occur spontaneously in high incidences in certain strains.

Inadequate evidence of carcinogenicity: The studies cannot be interpreted as showing either the presence or absence of a carcinogenic effect because of major qualitative or quantitative limitations.

Evidence suggesting lack of carcinogenicity: Adequate studies involving at least two species are available which show that, within the limits of the tests used, the agent is not carcinogenic. A conclusion of evidence suggesting lack of carcinogenicity is inevitably limited to the species, tumour sites and doses of exposure studied.

(iii) *Supporting evidence of carcinogenicity*

The other relevant data judged to be of sufficient importance as to affect the making of the overall evaluation are indicated.

(b) *Overall evaluation*

Finally, the total body of evidence is taken into account; the agent is described according to the wording of one of the following categories, and the designated group is given. The categorization of an agent is a matter of scientific judgement, reflecting the strength of the evidence derived from studies in humans and in experimental animals and from other relevant data.

Group 1 — The agent is carcinogenic to humans.

This category is used only when there is *sufficient evidence* of carcinogenicity in humans.

Group 2

This category includes agents for which, at one extreme, the degree of evidence of carcinogenicity in humans is almost sufficient, as well as agents for which, at the other extreme, there are no human data but for which there is experimental evidence of carcinogenicity. Agents are assigned to either 2A (probably carcinogenic) or 2B (possibly carcinogenic) on the basis of epidemiological, experimental and other relevant data.

Group 2A — The agent is probably carcinogenic to humans.

This category is used when there is *limited evidence* of carcinogenicity in humans and *sufficient evidence* of carcinogenicity in experimental animals. Exceptionally, an agent may be classified into this category solely on the basis of *limited evidence* of carcinogenicity in humans or of *sufficient evidence* of carcinogenicity in experimental animals strengthened by supporting evidence from other relevant data.

Group 2B — The agent is possibly carcinogenic to humans.

This category is generally used for agents for which there is *limited evidence* in humans in the absence of *sufficient evidence* in experimental animals. It may also be used when there is *inadequate evidence* of carcinogenicity in humans or when human data are nonexistent but there is *sufficient evidence* of carcinogenicity in experimental animals. In some instances, an agent for which there is *inadequate evidence* or no data in humans but *limited evidence* of carcinogenicity in experimental animals together with supporting evidence from other relevant data may be placed in this group.

Group 3 — The agent is not classifiable as to its carcinogenicity to humans.

Agents are placed in this category when they do not fall into any other group.

Group 4 — The agent is probably not carcinogenic to humans.

This category is used for agents for which there is *evidence suggesting lack of carcinogenicity* in humans together with *evidence suggesting lack of carcinogenicity* in experimental animals. In some circumstances, agents for which there is *inadequate evidence* of or no data on carcinogenicity in humans but *evidence suggesting lack of carcinogenicity* in experimental animals, consistently and strongly supported by a broad range of other relevant data, may be classified in this group.

References

1. IARC (1987) *IARC Monographs on the Evaluation of Carcinogenic Risks to Humans*, Supplement 6, *Genetic and Related Effects: An Updating of Selected IARC Monographs from Volumes 1 to 42*, Lyon
2. IARC (1977) *IARC Monographs Programme on the Evaluation of the Carcinogenic Risk of Chemicals to Humans. Preamble (IARC intern. tech. Rep. No. 77/002)*, Lyon
3. IARC (1978) *Chemicals with Sufficient Evidence of Carcinogenicity in Experimental Animals — IARC Monographs Volumes 1-17 (IARC intern. tech. Rep. No. 78/003)*, Lyon
4. IARC (1979) *Criteria to Select Chemicals for IARC Monographs (IARC intern. tech. Rep. No. 79/003)*, Lyon
5. IARC (1982) *IARC Monographs on the Evaluation of the Carcinogenic Risk of Chemicals to Humans*, Supplement 4, *Chemicals, Industrial Processes and Industries Associated with Cancer in Humans (IARC Monographs, Volumes 1 to 29)*, Lyon
6. IARC (1983) *Approaches to Classifying Chemical Carcinogens According to Mechanism of Action (IARC intern. tech. Rep. No. 83/001)*, Lyon
7. IARC (1987) *IARC Monographs on the Evaluation of Carcinogenic Risks to Humans*, Supplement 7, *Overall Evaluations of Carcinogenicity: An Updating of IARC Monographs Volumes 1 to 42*, Lyon
8. IARC (1973-1986) *Information Bulletin on the Survey of Chemicals Being Tested for Carcinogenicity*, Numbers 1-12, Lyon
   Number 1 (1973) 52 pages
   Number 2 (1973) 77 pages
   Number 3 (1974) 67 pages
   Number 4 (1974) 97 pages
   Number 5 (1975) 88 pages
   Number 6 (1976) 360 pages

Number 7 (1978) 460 pages
Number 8 (1979) 604 pages
Number 9 (1981) 294 pages
Number 10 (1983) 326 pages
Number 11 (1984) 370 pages
Number 12 (1986) 385 pages
Number 13 (1988) 404 pages

9. Muir, C. & Wagner, G., eds (1977-87) *Directory of On-going Studies in Cancer Epidemiology 1977-87 (IARC Scientific Publications)*, Lyon, International Agency for Research on Cancer

10. IARC (1984) *Chemicals and Exposures to Complex Mixtures Recommended for Evaluation in* IARC Monographs *and Chemicals and Complex Mixtures Recommended for Long-term Carcinogenicity Testing (IARC intern. tech. Rep. No. 84/002)*, Lyon

11. *Environmental Carcinogens. Selected Methods of Analysis:*

    Vol. 1. *Analysis of Volatile Nitrosamines in Food (IARC Scientific Publications No. 18)*. Edited by R. Preussmann, M. Castegnaro, E.A. Walker & A.E. Wasserman (1978)

    Vol. 2. *Methods for the Measurement of Vinyl Chloride in Poly(vinyl chloride), Air, Water and Foodstuffs (IARC Scientific Publications No. 22)*. Edited by D.C.M. Squirrell & W. Thain (1978)

    Vol. 3. *Analysis of Polycyclic Aromatic Hydrocarbons in Environmental Samples (IARC Scientific Publications No. 29)*. Edited by M. Castegnaro, P. Bogovski, H. Kunte & E.A. Walker (1979)

    Vol. 4. *Some Aromatic Amines and Azo Dyes in the General and Industrial Environment (IARC Scientific Publications No. 40)*. Edited by L. Fishbein, M. Castegnaro, I.K. O'Neill & H. Bartsch (1981)

    Vol. 5. *Some Mycotoxins (IARC Scientific Publications No. 44)*. Edited by L. Stoloff, M. Castegnaro, P. Scott, I.K. O'Neill & H. Bartsch (1983)

    Vol. 6. N-*Nitroso Compounds (IARC Scientific Publications No. 45)*. Edited by R. Preussmann, I.K. O'Neill, G. Eisenbrand, B. Spiegelhalder & H. Bartsch (1983)

    Vol. 7. *Some Volatile Halogenated Hydrocarbons (IARC Scientific Publications No. 68)*. Edited by L. Fishbein & I.K. O'Neill (1985)

    Vol. 8. *Some Metals: As, Be, Cd, Cr, Ni, Pb, Se, Zn (IARC Scientific Publications No. 71)*. Edited by I.K. O'Neill, P. Schuller & L. Fishbein (1986)

    Vol. 9. *Passive Smoking (IARC Scientific Publications No. 81)*. Edited by I.K. O'Neill, K.D. Brunnemann, B. Dodet & D. Hoffmann (1987)

12. Wilbourn, J., Haroun, L., Heseltine, E., Kaldor, J., Partensky, C. & Vainio, H. (1986) Response of experimental animals to human carcinogens: an analysis based upon the IARC Monographs Programme. *Carcinogenesis*, 7, 1853-1863

13. Montesano, R., Bartsch, H., Vainio, H., Wilbourn, J. & Yamasaki, H., eds (1986) *Long-term and Short-term Assays for Carcinogenesis — A Critical Appraisal (IARC Scientific Publications No. 83)*, Lyon, International Agency for Research on Cancer
14. Hoel, D.G., Kaplan, N.L. & Anderson, M.W. (1983) Implication of nonlinear kinetics on risk estimation in carcinogenesis. *Science, 219*, 1032-1037
15. Gart, J.J., Krewski, D., Lee, P.N., Tarone, R.E. & Wahrendorf, J. (1986) *Statistical Methods in Cancer Research*, Vol. 3, *The Design and Analysis of Long-term Animal Experiments (IARC Scientific Publications No. 79)*, Lyon, International Agency for Research on Cancer
16. Peto, R., Pike, M.C., Day, N.E., Gray, R.G., Lee, P.N., Parish, S., Peto, J., Richards, S. & Wahrendorf, J. (1980) *Guidelines for simple, sensitive significance tests for carcinogenic effects in long-term animal experiments*. In: *IARC Monographs on the Evaluation of the Carcinogenic Risk of Chemicals to Humans*, Supplement 2, *Long-term and Short-term Screening Assays for Carcinogens: A Critical Appraisal*, Lyon, pp. 311-426
17. Breslow, N.E. & Day, N.E. (1980) *Statistical Methods in Cancer Research*, Vol. 1, *The Analysis of Case-control Studies (IARC Scientific Publications No. 32)*, Lyon, International Agency for Research on Cancer
18. Breslow, N.E. & Day, N.E. (1987) *Statistical Methods in Cancer Research*, Vol. 2, *The Design and Analysis of Cohort Studies (IARC Scientific Publications No. 82)*, Lyon, International Agency for Research on Cancer

GENERAL REMARKS

This forty-fifth volume of the *IARC Monographs* comprises six monographs: one on occupational exposures in petroleum refining, one on crude oil, and four monographs on the main saleable fuel products of petroleum refining. Some other products of petroleum refining — mineral oils and bitumens — were evaluated previously (IARC, 1984, 1985a, 1987a,b). Petroleum solvents and engine exhausts will be considered by future working groups.

The selection of petroleum fuels for evaluation was based on four main criteria: their origin, use, chemical composition and physical properties. Only fuels that are produced from crude petroleum oil are considered. Some products based on shale-oil and coal were evaluated previously (IARC, 1985b,c, 1987c,d). Fuels produced from natural gas, biomaterials and synthetic chemicals were excluded.

Among saleable petroleum refinery products, only those used as engine or burner fuels for power or heat production or for illumination are included. All intermediate products used in the petrochemical industry to produce plastics, monomers and other products were considered to be outside the scope of the present volume. Similarly, nonfuel products, such as lubricant oils, bitumens and petroleum solvents, which have already been or will shortly be evaluated in the *IARC Monographs* programme, were considered only as process streams to which employees carrying out certain jobs in petroleum refineries may be exposed.

All the fuels considered are complex mixtures mainly of aliphatic, alicyclic and aromatic hydrocarbons. In addition, they may contain substances that have nitrogen, sulfur or some other element, but only (except for residual fuel oils) as a minor component or as an additive in blending of the final product. Table 1 lists agents previously evaluated in the *IARC Monographs* that may occur in petroleum refining, crude oil and in some of the fuel products considered in this volume. The fuels covered were further restricted to liquids or semisolids, thus excluding liquefied petroleum gas and petroleum coke, which are fuels of minor importance compared with those considered.

On the basis of these criteria, the monograph on petroleum refining covers occupational exposures to raw materials (different crude oils), intermediate process streams, petroleum products and a variety of process chemicals, fuel additives and other substances that occur in petroleum refineries. Experimental data on the carcinogenicity or other related effects of the main process streams are reviewed and summarized because they are relevant to making an overall evaluation of carcinogenicity of occupational exposures in petroleum refineries, and in evaluating the carcinogenicity of products that contain these streams as major

Table 1. Agents previously evaluated in the *IARC Monographs* that may occur in petroleum refining, crude oil or major petroleum fuels

Monograph	Agent	Evidence of carcinogenicity[a]		
		Human	Animal	Group
Petroleum refining	*ortho*-Anisidine	ND	S	2B
	para-Anisidine	ND	I	3
	Arsenic compounds	S	L	1*
	Asbestos	S	S	1
	Benzene	S	S	1
	Bitumens	I		3
	Steam-refined and cracking residue bitumens		L	
	Air-refined bitumens		I	
	Extracts of steam-refined and air-refined bitumens		S	2B
	1,3-Butadiene	I	S	2B
	Carbazole	ND	L	3
	Chlorinated hydrocarbons	varies	varies	2B–3
	Chromium and chromium compounds			
	Chromium metal	I	I	3
	Trivalent chromium compounds	I	I	3
	Hexavalent chromium compounds	S	S	1*
	1,2-Dibromoethane (ethylene dibromide)	I	S	2A
	1,2-Dichloroethane (ethylene dichloride)	ND	S	2B
	Hydrazine	I	S	2B
	Lead and lead compounds			
	Inorganic	I	S	2B
	Organolead	I	I	3
	Mineral oils			
	Untreated and mildly treated oils	S	S	1
	Highly-refined oils	I	I	3
	Nickel and nickel compounds	S	S	1*
	para-Phenylenediamine	ND	I	3
	Polycyclic aromatic compounds	ND	varies	2A–3
	Silica			
	Crystalline silica	L	S	2A
	Amorphous silica	I	I	3
Crude oil	Arsenic compounds	S	L	1*
	Benzene	S	S	1
	Carbazole	ND	L	3
	Nickel and nickel compounds	S	S	1*
	Polycyclic aromatic compounds	ND	varies	2A–3
Gasoline	Benzene	S	S	1
	1,3-Butadiene	I	S	2B
	1,2-Dibromoethane (ethylene dibromide)	I	S	2A
	1,2-Dichloroethane (ethylene dichloride)	ND	S	2B

Table 1 (contd)

Monograph	Agent	Evidence of carcinogenicity[a]		
		Human	Animal	Group
Gasoline (contd)	Lead and lead compounds			
	Inorganic	I	S	2B
	Organolead	I	I	3
	para-Phenylenediamine	ND	I	3
Jet fuel	Benzene	S	S	1
Diesel fuels	Benzene	S	S	1
	Polycyclic aromatic compounds	ND	varies	2A–3
Fuel oils	Benzene	S	S	1
(Heating oils)	Carbazole	ND	L	3
	Nickel and nickel compounds	S	S	1*
	Polycyclic aromatic compounds	ND	varies	2A–3

[a]From Supplement 7 (IARC, 1987e); I, inadequate evidence; L, limited evidence; ND, no adequate data; S, sufficient evidence; 1, Group 1 – the agent is carcinogenic to humans; 2A, Group 2A – the agent is probably carcinogenic to humans; 2B, Group 2B – the agent is possibly carcinogenic to humans; 3, Group 3 – the agent is not classifiable as to its carcinogenicity to humans

*This evaluation applies to the group of chemicals as a whole and not necessarily to all individual chemicals within the group

components. The experimental studies summarized in the monograph on occupational exposures in petroleum refining are those in which any sample from petroleum refining processes or effluents was tested; laboratory fractions of process streams (e.g., distillates, extracts) are included but not evaluated.

The monograph on crude oil includes experimental studies in which undiluted or diluted crude petroleum oils or their composite mixtures were tested for carcinogenicity, and hygiene and epidemiological studies on persons potentially exposed to crude oil or its volatile components. Analogously to the treatment of process streams in the monograph on occupational exposures in petroleum refining, tests of laboratory-derived fractions of crude oil were included in the monograph.

The monograph on gasoline includes automotive gasoline (leaded and unleaded) used in automotive vehicles, and aviation gasoline used in aeroplanes with reciprocating engines. Aviation gasoline (boiling range, 25–170°C) differs from jet fuels (boiling range, usually 150–300°C), which are used in aeroplanes equipped with turbine engines. Automotive gasoline is manufactured by blending several process streams and additives. The principal streams used are full-range reformed naphtha, catalytically cracked and light steam-cracked naphtha, light straight-run naphtha and n-butane. One or more additional components may be used. Aviation gasoline usually contains 50–70% alkylated naphtha, as compared to 0–5% in automotive gasoline.

The fourth monograph in the present volume covers jet fuels. The basic component of most commercial and military jet fuels is the straight-run kerosene fraction produced by the atmospheric distillation of crude oil. However, wide-cut jet fuels also include lower-boiling fractions, e.g., heavy straight-run naphtha. Straight-run kerosene is a versatile process stream used, for the most part, in the production of jet fuels, but which may also be used as diesel fuel (diesel fuel No. 1), as heating oil (fuel oil No. 1), as lamp oil, as a solvent and for other purposes. Studies concerning aviation kerosene are described in the monograph on jet fuels, whereas kerosene as a refinery stream or as diesel fuel or fuel oil is considered in the corresponding monographs.

The monograph on diesel fuels considers three grades of diesel fuel. Diesel fuel No. 1 is essentially similar to kerosene except for its additives, and it is used mainly in city buses. Diesel fuel No. 2 has a similar processing history and chemical composition, with the exception of the additives, to fuel oil No. 2; it is the most widely used diesel fuel and is employed in cars, lorries, locomotives and small boats. Diesel fuel No. 4 (marine diesel fuel), used mainly in ships, is slightly less volatile than diesel fuel No. 2 and may contain up to 15% residual process streams.

The last monograph in this volume covers data on fuel oils (heating oils). Fuel oils are numbered from 1 to 6 according to the type of burner in which they may be used. The most volatile fuel oils (Nos 1 and 2) are manufactured from straight-run or processed distillates; their chemical composition is approximately the same as that of kerosene (equivalent to fuel oil No. 1) and diesel fuel No. 2 (equivalent to fuel oil No. 2). Fuel oils Nos 4–6 are also called residual fuel oils because they normally include residues from atmospheric distillation, vacuum distillation and cracking processes as major components. Also, other by-products from refinery processes, such as propane-precipitated bitumen and solvent extracts of lubricant oils may be added. Studies on bitumens and lubricant oils, which have been evaluated in previous volumes (IARC, 1984, 1985a, 1987a,b) and which are minor components of residual fuel oils, are not reported in this volume; the main results are summarized briefly when the data were considered useful for the evaluation of residual fuel oils.

It was noted that there is a paucity of data on occupational exposures to volatile hydrocarbons prior to the 1970s. Since that period, more data have been published, and it is assumed that considerably more data exist in unpublished company records. The Working Group suggests that scientists in the petroleum industry be encouraged to publish representative exposure data in the open literature, which would be useful in the design and interpretation of epidemiological studies. Such data should preferably cover the ranges encountered under both normal operating conditions and in non-routine situations such as major turn-rounds. Also noted is the fact that no standard methodology exists for the objective assessment of skin exposure to petroleum oils of biological concern. It is hoped that academic and industrial scientists can address this perceived need in order to attain objectivity in assessing skin exposures and to improve standards of surveillance.

The Working Group recognized that in many of the carcinogenicity bioassays reported there was no detailed characterization of the test materials, and the results could not necessarily be taken to be representative of all samples in a given category. In addition, most samples were tested in only one test system — mainly mouse skin painting assays.

The paucity of data on genetic and related effects in humans relevant to the evaluation of human exposures in the petroleum refining industry or to crude oil or any of the saleable fuel products was also noted.

In the few epidemiological studies available, there was little information on actual exposures to the final saleable products. In nearly all of the cohort studies reviewed in these monographs, the cancer experience of an entire occupational cohort was compared with that of the general (national) population. Because of the influence of the 'healthy worker effect', such comparisons tend to underestimate the true magnitude of any risk attributable to occupation; the extent of this underestimation, however, cannot be quantified. (This methodological consideration is discussed further on p. 81.)

In the many population- and hospital-based case-control studies reviewed in this volume, most of the positive associations with the exposures considered arose as a result of simultaneous exploration of a number of industries and occupations as risk factors for cancer. A 'positive reporting bias' may therefore have applied. (This methodological consideration is discussed further on p. 100.)

The main products of petroleum refining are evaluated in the last four monographs in this volume. The available data on the carcinogenicity in experimental animals of the component streams of these products are described and evaluated in the monograph on occupational exposures in petroleum refining. These evaluations were used in the overall evaluation of the carcinogenicity of the petroleum products in the relevant monograph, when deemed appropriate, i.e., when the refinery stream was considered to be a consistent and major component of the product. Some of the minor components of petroleum fuels were evaluated in previous monographs. These evaluations are also used as supporting evidence in some overall evaluations. When possible, process streams cited in each monograph are cross-referenced to Table 2 and Figure 1 of the monograph on occupational exposures in petroleum refining, by the use of the systematic names and the square-bracketed numbers assigned in the table and figure.

References

IARC (1984) *IARC Monographs on the Evaluation of the Carcinogenic Risk of Chemicals to Humans*, Vol. 33, *Polynuclear Aromatic Compounds, Part 2, Carbon Blacks, Mineral Oils and Some Nitroarenes*, Lyon, pp. 87–168

IARC (1985a) *IARC Monographs on the Evaluation of the Carcinogenic Risk of Chemicals to Humans*, Vol. 35, *Polynuclear Aromatic Compounds, Part 4, Bitumens, Coal-tars and Derived Products, Shale-oils and Soots*, Lyon, pp. 39–181, 243–247

IARC (1985b) *IARC Monographs on the Evaluation of the Carcinogenic Risk of Chemicals to Humans*, Vol. 35, *Polynuclear Aromatic Compounds, Part 4, Bitumens, Coal-tars and Derived Products, Shale-oils and Soots*, Lyon, pp. 161–217, 243–247

IARC (1985c) *IARC Monographs on the Evaluation of the Carcinogenic Risk of Chemicals to Humans*, Vol. 35, *Polynuclear Aromatic Compounds, Part 4, Bitumens, Coal-tars and Derived Products, Shale-oils and Soots*, Lyon, pp. 83–159, 243–247

IARC (1987a) *IARC Monographs on the Evaluation of Carcinogenic Risks to Humans*, Suppl. 7, *Overall Evaluations of Carcinogenicity: An Updating of* IARC Monographs *Volumes 1 to 42*, Lyon, pp. 252–254

IARC (1987b) *IARC Monographs on the Evaluation of Carcinogenic Risks to Humans*, Suppl. 7, *Overall Evaluations of Carcinogenicity: An Updating of* IARC Monographs *Volumes 1 to 42*, Lyon, pp. 133–134

IARC (1987c) *IARC Monographs on the Evaluation of Carcinogenic Risks to Humans*, Suppl. 7, *Overall Evaluations of Carcinogenicity: An Updating of* IARC Monographs *Volumes 1 to 42*, Lyon, pp. 339–341

IARC (1987d) *IARC Monographs on the Evaluation of Carcinogenic Risks to Humans*, Suppl. 7, *Overall Evaluations of Carcinogenicity: An Updating of* IARC Monographs *Volumes 1 to 42*, Lyon, pp. 174–176

IARC (1987e) *IARC Monographs on the Evaluation of Carcinogenic Risks to Humans*, Suppl. 7, *Overall Evaluations of Carcinogenicity: An Updating of* IARC Monographs *Volumes 1 to 42*, Lyon, pp. 56–74

THE MONOGRAPHS

OCCUPATIONAL EXPOSURES IN PETROLEUM REFINING

1. Historical Perspectives and Description of the Processes

1.1 Historical perspectives

Petroleum oil was used for many centuries in Egypt, China, Mesopotamia and Persia for heating, lighting, roadmaking and building. Small accumulations of oil were reported at Pechelbronn in Alsace in 1498 and in Poland in 1506, and Marco Polo noted 'oil springs' at Baku on the Caspian Sea in the latter part of the thirteenth century. Raleigh, in 1595, reported the existence of the Trinidad Pitch Lake, and there are accounts of Franciscan visits to 'oil springs' in New York in 1632. Similarly, in 1748, a Russian traveller to the Americas commented on sources of oil in Pennsylvania. Oil was produced in Burma from hand-dug wells in substantial quantities by the end of the eighteenth century (Royal Dutch/Shell Group of Companies, 1983).

The modern oil industry began in the USA in 1859 with the successful completion of the Drake well near Titusville, PA (Chiles, 1987). By 1886, Pennsylvania was the leading oil producing state, and total US production was 28 million barrels[1] per year, nearly 60% of the world's total. The principal refined product was kerosene, used mainly for illumination. Because of its smaller supply in relation to coal, petroleum was not used as an industrial or transportation fuel, but continued to be used mainly for lubrication and burning in stoves and lamps (Chiles, 1987).

With the discovery of new oil reserves in the early 1900s, the utilization of oil began to change rapidly as the price of oil dropped significantly. Railroads were the first to take advantage of the oversupply and low prices: between 1899 and 1919, the use of oil by railroads in the USA increased 14 fold. Development of petroleum as a marine fuel took place during the same period. The first vessels to use oil were the tankers transporting crude oil, but conversion of other commercial vessels followed, and the military advantages of oil were soon realized. Industry was also in need of cheap energy, and the switch from coal to oil occurred quickly, beginning with the use of oil as a boiler fuel. In the USA, production tripled from 1900 to 1910 as oil was discovered in Texas, California and the midwest (Chiles, 1987).

---

[1] 1 barrel = 0.136 metric tonne of crude oil of specific gravity 0.858 (or °API gravity, 33.5; British Petroleum Co., 1977); see monograph on crude oil

After about 1900, worldwide expansion was much more rapid. Mexico became a producer in 1901, followed by Argentina in 1907 and Trinidad in 1908. By 1910, world production had grown to 900 000 barrels per day, the bulk originating in the USA (560 000) and most of the remainder in Russia (200 000). Oil was found in Persia (Iran) in 1908, and exports there commenced in 1911, leading to the prominence of that region as a source of crude oil. Production in British Borneo and Venezuela began in 1911 and 1914, respectively (Royal Dutch/Shell Group of Companies, 1983).

The development of the internal combustion engine and the rapid growth of the automotive industry after the First World War provided the market needed to support this increased production and assured that the industry would continue to be a major source of transportation and industrial fuels. Gasoline consumption in the USA increased from six million barrels in 1899 — mostly for cleaning, industrial solvents and stove fuel — to 87 million barrels in 1919 (Chiles, 1987). By the mid-1960s, it had already reached 1700 million barrels yearly (Energy Information Administration, 1986). During this period, improvements in automotive engine design necessitated the manufacture of motor fuels of higher quality. Research octane ratings (see glossary) increased from about 70 in 1925 to their present levels of close to 100. The need to increase both the quantity and the quality of motor gasoline in order to meet the demands of the market required the development of new refining processes. The most important of these are shown in Table 1. All are directed towards effecting either a change in the product distribution or product quality or, less often, both.

Table 1. Important process developments in petroleum refining[a]

Year[b]	Process	Operation
1910–15	Thermal cracking	Change gas oil to gasoline
1916	Sweetening	Eliminate mercaptans
1925–29	Vacuum distillation	Produce lubricating oils, change residues to cracking stock and bitumen
1926–29	Alkyllead production	Improve octane number
1930	Thermal reforming	Improve octane number
1932	Hydrogenation	Remove sulfur
1932	Coking	Produce lighter products from residues
1933	Solvent extraction	Improve viscosity index
1935	Solvent dewaxing	Improve pour point
1935	Catalytic polymerization	Increase gasoline yield, improve octane number
1939	Catalytic cracking	Increase gasoline yield, improve octane number
1939	Visbreaking	Reduce quantity of residue
1940–43	Alkylation	Increase gasoline yield, improve octane number
1950	Propane decarbonizing (deasphalting)	Increase cracking stock
1952	Catalytic reforming	Improve octane number
1954	Hydrodesulfurization	Remove sulfur
1956	Inhibitor sweetening	Remove mercaptans
1957	Catalytic isomerization	Improve octane number

Table 1 (contd)

Year[b]	Process	Operation
1960[c]	Fluid catalytic cracking	Increase gasoline yield
1961[c]	Catalytic hydrocracking	Increase gasoline yield
1965[c]	Molecular sieve catalysts	Increase gasoline yield
1974[c]	Catalytic dewaxing	Improve pour point
1975[c]	Residue hydrocracking	Reduce quantity of residue

[a]Adapted and updated from Nelson (1960); for definitions, see glossary
[b]Dates are approximate year of commercialization of the process
[c]From Royal Dutch/Shell Group of Companies (1983)

Today, the world petroleum refining industry produces more than 2500 products, including liquefied petroleum gas, gasoline, kerosene, aviation fuels, diesel fuels, a variety of other fuel oils, lubricating oils and feedstocks for the petrochemical industry. Refineries range from those which simply produce fuels to those which include the manufacture of other products, such as lubricants and bitumens. Processes which are used solely in the manufacture of petrochemicals are specifically excluded from this monograph.

Section 1.2, which describes the major processes used in fuel manufacture, is divided into four parts describing different types of processes: (1) crude separation; (2) light hydrocarbon processing; (3) middle distillate processing; and (4) heavy hydrocarbon processing. Not all of the processes described are used in every refinery. Larger refineries do, however, use most of them. US refineries have generally been designed to maximize automotive gasoline production, while European refineries have generally maximized production of fuel oils. US refineries have therefore typically used more processes and generally produced a minimum of residual oil (Royal Dutch/Shell Group of Companies, 1983).

Most petroleum products are manufactured to specifications of performance, rather than chemistry, and hence may originate from several refinery streams. The composition of the product and the volume produced vary with location, climate and season. For example, in winter, there is a greater demand for fuel oils, and automotive gasoline must contain a larger percentage of volatile products to assure cold-weather starts. Summer weather imposes a reduction in the concentration of volatile components to minimize engine vapour lock and losses due to vaporization. Refinery operations must be sufficiently flexible to accommodate these changing demands.

1.2 Major fuel manufacturing processes

Descriptions of petroleum refining processes are available (Jahnig, 1982; Royal Dutch/Shell Group of Companies, 1983). Processes that lead to lubricant base oils and their derived products and to bitumens have been described in previous volumes of the *Monographs* series (IARC, 1984, 1985). In the present monograph, attention is given principally to processes used in the production of petroleum-based fuels.

Fig. 1. Principal refinery process streams[a]

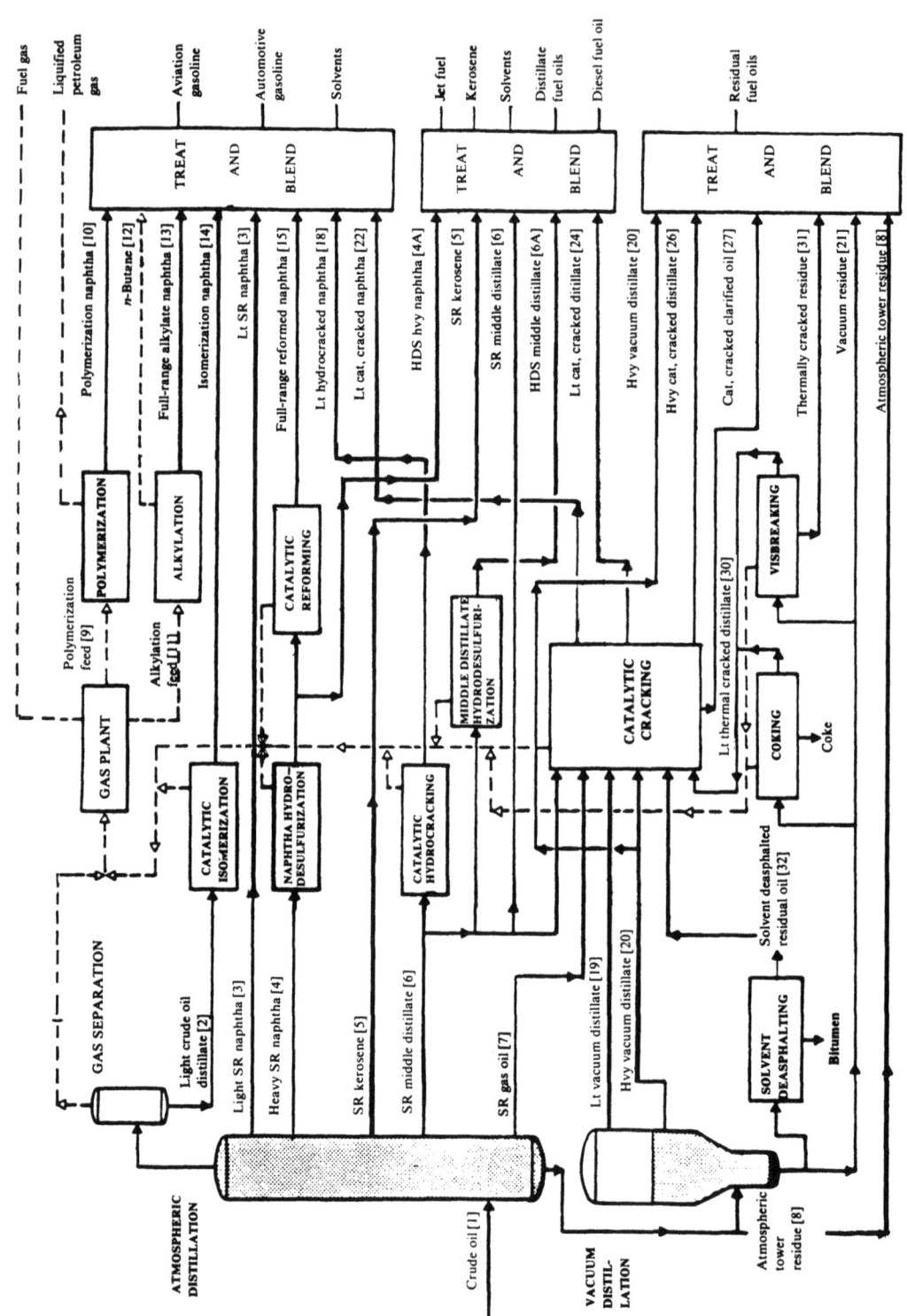

[a]Provided by the American Petroleum Institute; Cat, catalytic; HDS, hydrodesulfurized; Hvy, heavy; Lt, light; SR, straight-run

Figure 1 summarizes the major fuel manufacturing processes commonly used in petroleum refining and shows the interrelationships that exist between process units in a petroleum refining complex; it is not intended to be a diagram of an actual refinery configuration. Most of the processes discussed in detail are shown, although several that are less common or that are used for a particular type of crude oil are described only in the text. In Figure 1, the process unit feed and product streams are identified by the common designation accepted by the industry. Each name is followed by a number which also appears in Table 2, which gives the Chemical Abstracts designation for the stream, the Chemical Abstracts Service Registry Number and the broad definition of its composition adopted in 1978 under the US Toxic Substances Control Act (US Environmental Protection Agency, 1978, 1979) and, in 1981, under the Commission of the European Communities' Sixth Amendment to the Dangerous Substances Directive — European Inventory of Existing Commercial Chemical Substances (EINECS) (Commission of the European Communities, 1981). Not all of the possible feed and product streams are shown, but those of major importance to the blending of the final fuel products addressed in the monographs on gasoline, jet fuel, diesel fuels and fuel oils (heating oils) are included. The process descriptions that follow are intended to provide an understanding of their purpose and nature, to define the operating conditions and to identify the unit feedstocks and products.

(a) *Crude separation*

(i) *Atmospheric distillation*

Distillation at atmospheric pressure physically separates crude oil into fractions of a specific boiling range by distillation and steam stripping. The major processing equipment items include the heat exchanger preheat train, direct-fired furnace, atmospheric fractionator and side-stream product strippers.

Desalted crude oil is preheated in the heat exchanger train by recovering process heat. The preheated crude oil is then charged to a directly fired furnace, where additional heat is supplied to achieve partial vaporization. Both the liquid and vaporized portions are charged to the atmospheric fractionator at a temperature of about 345–370°C.

The crude charge is separated into a number of fractions. The lightest streams are taken from the tower overhead, where they are condensed, and the noncondensible light ends are treated and/or recovered in other refinery units. A number of liquid side-stream fractions are withdrawn from the fractionator at different elevations within the tower. These fractions are charged to strippers where lower-boiling hydrocarbons are removed and returned to the fractionation tower. The stripping medium is either steam, light petroleum gases or reboiler vapours. The atmospheric fractionator also has a zone for stripping bottoms, where lower-boiling hydrocarbons are steam stripped from the atmospheric residue. The fractions from the atmospheric tower are progressively higher boiling as they are withdrawn at successively lower elevations in the tower; however, the final boiling-point of the heaviest side stream generally approximates the temperature at which the crude oil is charged.

Table 2. Characteristics of principal refinery process streams[a]

Process stream[b] (synonym)	CAS No.	Unit from which produced	Unit to which fed	Carbon no. distribution	Boiling range (°C)	Remarks
Crude oil [1] (petroleum)	8002-05-9	—	Atmospheric distillation	C2—>C50	−80 − >600	As a naturally occurring substance, crude oil is not included in the TSCA/EINECS listing
Light crude oil distillate [2]	68410-05-9	Atmospheric distillation	Gas processing, isomerization	C2−C7	−88 − 99	
Light straight-run naphtha [3]	64741-46-4	Atmospheric distillation	—	C4−C10	−20 − 180	Mainly aliphatic hydrocarbons
Heavy straight-run naphtha [4]	64741-41-9	Atmospheric distillation	Naphtha hydrodesulfurization	C6−C12	65−230	
Hydrodesulfurized heavy naphtha [4A]	64742-82-1	Naphtha hydrodesulfurization	Catalytic reforming	C7−C12	90−230	
Straight-run kerosene [5]	8008-20-6	Atmospheric distillation	—	C9−C16	150−290	
Hydrotreated kerosene [5A]	64742-47-8	Kerosene hydrotreatment	—	C9−C16	150−290	
Hydrodesulfurized kerosene [5B]	64742-81-0	Kerosene hydrodesulfurization	—	C9−C16	150−290	
Chemically neutralized kerosene [5C]	64742-31-0	Kerosene neutralization	—	C9−C16	150−290	
Straight-run middle distillate [6]	64741-44-2	Atmospheric distillation	Catalytic hydrocracking, gas oil hydrodesulfurization, catalytic cracking	C11−C20	205−345	

Table 2 (contd)

Process stream[b] (synonym)	CAS No.	Unit from which produced	Unit to which fed	Carbon no. distribution	Boiling range (°C)	Remarks
Hydrodesulfurized middle distillate [6A]	64742-80-9	Middle distillate hydrodesulfurization		C11–C25	205–400	
Straight-run gas oil [7]	64741-43-1	Atmospheric distillation	Catalytic cracking	C11–C25	205–400	Likely to contain 5 wt % or more 4- to 6-ring condensed aromatic hydrocarbons
Atmospheric tower residue [8] (reduced crude oil)	64741-45-3	Atmospheric distillation	Vacuum distillation	>C20	>350	
Polymerization feed [9]	68476-54-0	Gas processing	Polymerization	C3–C5	−45 – 38	Complex mixture of predominantly unsaturated hydrocarbons
Polymerization naphtha	64741-72-6	Polymerization		C6–C12	65–270	Mainly monoolefinic hydrocarbons produced by catalytic polymerization of a mixture rich in propene or butene
Alkylation feed [11]	68477-83-8	Gas processing	Alkylation	C3–C5		Mixture of olefinic and paraffinic hydrocarbons. Ambient temperatures normally exceed the critical temperature for these combinations
n-Butane [12]	106-97-8	Alkylation	C4	−0.5		
Full-range alkylate naphtha [13]	64741-64-6	Alkylation		C7–C12	90–220	Mainly branched-chain saturated hydrocarbons produced by distillation of products of catalytic reaction of isobutane with C3-C5 monoolefins

Table 2 (contd)

Process stream[b] (synonym)	CAS No.	Unit from which produced	Unit to which fed	Carbon no. distribution	Boiling range (°C)	Remarks
Isomerization naphtha [14]	64741-70-4	Catalytic isomerization		C4–C6		Mainly saturated hydrocarbons obtained from catalytic isomerization of straight-chain paraffinic hydrocarbons such as isobutane, isopentane, 2,2-dimethylbutane, 2-methylbutane, 2-methylpentane and 3-methylpentane
Full-range reformed naphtha [15]	68919-37-9	Catalytic reforming		C5–C12	35–230	
Light reformed naphtha [16]	64741-63-5	Catalytic reforming		C5–C11	35–190	May contain 10% or more benzene
Heavy reformed naphtha [17]	64741-68-0	Catalytic reforming		C7–C12	90–230	Contains predominantly aromatic hydrocarbons
Light hydrocracked naphtha [18]	64741-69-1	Catalytic hydrocracking	C4–C10	−20 – 180		
Light vacuum distillate [19] (light vacuum gas oil)	64741-58-8	Vacuum distillation	Catalytic cracking	C13–C30	230–450	Contains a relatively large proportion of saturated aliphatic hydrocarbons
Light paraffinic distillate [19A]	64741-50-0	Vacuum distillation	Lubricant oil manufacture	C15–C30	>350	Contains relatively few normal paraffins
Light naphthenic distillate [19B]	64741-52-2	Vacuum distillation	Lubricant oil manufacture	C15–C30	>350	
Heavy vacuum distillate [20] (heavy vacuum gas oil)	64741-57-7	Vacuum distillation	Catalytic cracking	C20–C50	350–600	Likely to contain 5 wt % or more 4- to 6-ring condensed aromatic hydrocarbons
Heavy paraffinic distillate [20A]	64741-51-1	Vacuum distillation	Lubricant oil manufacture	C20–C50	>350	Contains a relatively low proportion of saturated aliphatic hydrocarbons

Table 2 (contd)

Process stream[b] (synonym)	CAS No.	Unit from which produced	Unit to which fed	Carbon no. distribution	Boiling range (°C)	Remarks
Heavy naphthenic distillate [20B]	64741-53-3	Vacuum distillate	Lubricant oil manufacture	C20–C50	>350	Contains relatively few normal paraffins
Chemically neutralized heavy naphthenic distillate [20C]	64742-34-3	Vacuum distillation	Lubricant oil manufacture	C20–C50	>350	Contains relatively few normal paraffins
Hydrotreated heavy naphthenic distillate [20D]	64742-52-5	Vacuum distillation	Lubricant oil manufacture	C20–C50	>350	Contains relatively few normal paraffins
Vacuum residue [21]	64741-56-6	Vacuum distillation	Solvent deasphalting, coking, visbreaking	>C34	>495	
Light catalytically cracked naphtha [22]	64741-55-5	Catalytic cracking		C4–C11	−20 – 190	Contains a relatively large proportion of unsaturated hydrocarbons
Heavy catalytically cracked naphtha [23]	64741-54-4	Catalytic cracking		C6–C12	65–230	Contains a relatively large proportion of unsaturated hydrocarbons
Light catalytically cracked distillate [24]	64741-59-9	Catalytic cracking		C9–C25	150–400	Contains a relatively large proportion of bicyclic aromatic hydrocarbons
Intermediate catalytically cracked distillate [25]	64741-60-2	Catalytic cracking		C11–C30	205–450	Contains a relatively large proportion of tricyclic aromatic hydrocarbons
Heavy catalytically cracked distillate [26]	64741-61-3	Catalytic cracking		C15–C35	260–500	Likely to contain 5 wt % or more 4- to 6-ring condensed aromatic hydrocarbons

Table 2 (contd)

Process stream[b] (synonym)	CAS No.	Unit from which produced	Unit to which fed	Carbon no. distribution	Boiling range (°C)	Remarks
Catalytically cracked clarified oil [27]	64741-62-4	Catalytic cracking		>C20	>350	Likely to contain 5 wt % or more 4- to 6-ring condensed aromatic hydrocarbons
Light thermally cracked naphtha [28]	64741-74-8	Coking, visbreaking		C4–C8	−10 – 130	Consists predominantly of unsaturated hydrocarbons
Heavy thermally cracked naphtha [29]	64741-83-9	Coking, visbreaking		C6–C12	65–220	Consists predominantly of unsaturated hydrocarbons
Light thermally cracked distillate [30]	64741-82-8	Coking, visbreaking	Catalytic cracking	C10–C22	160–370	
Thermally cracked residue [31]	64741-80-6	Visbreaking		>C20	>350	Likely to contain 5 wt % or more 4- to 6-ring condensed aromatic hydrocarbons
Solvent deasphalted residual oil [32]	64741-95-3	Solvent deasphalting	Catalytic cracking	>C25	>400	Obtained as the solvent-soluble fraction from C3–C4 solvent deasphalting of a residue
Light steam-cracked naphtha [33]	64742-83-2	Steam cracking		C4–C11	−20 – 190	Consists predominantly of unsaturated hydrocarbons; likely to contain 10% or more benzene
Steam-cracked residue [34]	64742-90-1	Steam cracking		≥C14	>260	Consists predominantly of unsaturated hydrocarbons likely to contain 5% or more of 4- to 6-ring polycyclic aromatic hydrocarbons

[a]From US Environmental Protection Agency (1978); Commission of the European Communities (1981)
[b]Number in brackets is the identifying number for the process stream in Figure 1

Atmospheric tower residue [8] (reduced crude oil) is the highest-boiling fraction and is the charge to the vacuum distillation unit. The products of atmospheric distillation are generally light crude oil distillate [2], light and heavy straight-run naphthas [3 and 4, respectively], straight-run kerosene [5], straight-run middle distillate [6], straight-run gas oil [7] and reduced crude oil. The naphtha streams may be blended into motor fuels or other refinery products or further processed to improve octane rating and reduce sulfur content. The straight-run kerosene [5] may be chemically sweetened or hydrogen-treated and sold directly or sent to blending. The straight-run middle distillate [6] may be sold for diesel or fuel oil, or may be hydrogen-treated, hydrocracked, catalytically cracked or blended. Straight-run gas oil [7] may be sold as fuel oil, or may be hydrogen-treated, hydrocracked, catalytically cracked or blended. Reduced crude oil is usually fed to the vacuum tower, although it may be sold for fuel, blended into fuels, or be hydrogen treated or catalytically cracked. As its name implies, the fractionator operates at atmospheric pressure; temperatures range from 120°C at the top to about 370°C at the bottom.

(ii) *Gas processing*

The purpose of gas processing is to stabilize (i.e., reduce the volatility of) the lightest process stream by removing gaseous hydrocarbons and then to separate the various fractions of hydrocarbon gases. Separation is accomplished by a series of distillation and absorption operations. The particular recovery scheme applied depends primarily on the desired purity. Gas processing can be a simple operation producing fuel gases composed of *n*-butane [12], more volatile hydrocarbons and a light naphtha or a complex one that produces a wide range of individual gaseous and light hydrocarbon products. The feed is a light, sweet gas that comes from various processing units. Units which can directly or indirectly provide the feed gas are: crude distillation, hydrodesulfurization, catalytic cracking, catalytic reforming, thermal cracking and hydrocracking. The operating conditions depend on the products being recovered. Temperatures as low as −73°C are required to obtain an ethane fraction, and high pressures, about 360 psi [24 atm], are used in absorbing propane.

(iii) *Vacuum distillation*

Vacuum distillation separates the residue from the atmospheric fractionator into a vacuum residue [21] and one or more distillate streams. The distillate streams include light and heavy vacuum distillates [19 and 20, respectively] as well as light and heavy distillates of paraffinic or naphthenic crude oils. Light and heavy distillates are used in the production of lubricant oils, the processing of which was described in a previous volume of *Monographs* (IARC, 1984). Vacuum fractionators are maintained at approximately 100 mm Hg [0.13 atm] absolute pressure by either steam ejectors or mechanical vacuum pumps. Distillation temperatures of up to 400°C are not uncommon. Vacuum distillation can be carried out in one or two fractionation stages. Atmospheric tower residue [8] is heated in a directly fired furnace and charged to a preflash tower where a small quantity of distillate is produced as an overhead product. The preflash tower bottoms are charged to the vacuum fractionator for separation of additional distillate. Vacuum residue [21] is recovered as the bottoms product. Steam stripping may or may not be applied to the distillates. The production of well fractionated distillates, such as lubricant oil stocks, requires steam stripping, whereas the production of heavy catalytic cracking feedstocks, such as vacuum distillate, does not. Depending mainly upon the crude feedstock and the nature of the refinery, the vacuum residue [21] may be converted to bitumen, coked to make gasoline, cracked in a visbreaker to make distillate fuel oils or blended into residual fuel oils. With suitable feedstocks, the vacuum residue [21] may be used to manufacture heavy lubricant oils. Similarly, the heavy distillate from a suitable paraffinic crude oil feed may be used as a charge stock for lubricant oil manufacture. Other distillates are treated much like the gas oil stream from the atmospheric fractionator and are catalytically hydrocracked, catalytically cracked or used as fuel oil.

(b) *Light hydrocarbon processing*

(i) *Polymerization*

Polymerization is used to produce high-octane gasoline or a petrochemical feedstock from gaseous olefins. The feedstock may be a relatively pure olefin stream or any combination of olefins, such as ethylene, propylene and butenes. Polymerization naphtha [10] and other liquid products are formed when the olefin gases are passed over an acid catalyst. The most common catalyst used is phosphoric acid, usually dispersed on an inert support. The reaction is exothermic. After reaction, the gaseous product passes through a heat exchanger which heats the incoming feed. The reactor effluent is then fractionated by distillation to produce the product or products required. Reactor temperatures are generally in the range of 135–190°C, at a pressure of about 500 psi [34 atm].

(ii) *Alkylation*

The term alkylation, as commonly used in the petroleum industry, refers to the chemical reaction of a low molecular weight olefin and an isoparaffin to form multiply branched paraffins of high octane rating. Typically, butene and isobutane are reacted to produce the high octane components known as alkylate. The reaction is catalysed by either anhydrous sulfuric or anhydrous hydrofluoric acid. A dry olefinic feed is mixed with excess isobutane and added to the liquid catalyst in the reaction vessel. The reactor effluent is separated into hydrocarbon and acid phases in a settler, and the acid is returned to the reactor. If hydrofluoric acid is used, the alkylate and excess isobutane from the settler are sent to a stripping tower for separation. The stripper yields an isobutane, which is recycled to the feed stream, an *n*-butane side stream and an alkylate bottoms stream which is charged to a fired heater to decompose any organic fluorides. The effluent from the fired heater is the finished alkylate. If sulfuric acid is used as the catalyst, the hydrocarbon liquid from the settler is washed with caustic and water before fractionation. The operating temperature depends upon the catalyst system used. Sulfuric acid alkylation is generally carried out at about 7°C; when hydrofluoric acid is used, the temperature is about 27°C. Pressures are in the range of 100–150 psi [7–10 atm], regardless of the catalyst.

(iii) *Naphtha hydrodesulfurization*

Hydrodesulfurization is used to remove sulfur and nitrogen compounds from the naphtha streams. Both must be reduced to very low levels when naphtha is used as a feed for reforming or for other processes which are susceptible to catalyst poisoning by sulfur and nitrogen compounds. The naphthas are vaporized, mixed with a hydrogen-rich gas, heated to reaction temperature and passed through a fixed bed of non-noble metal catalyst — generally cobalt-molybdenum. The organic sulfur and nitrogen are converted to hydrogen sulfide and ammonia. Some cracking of hydrocarbons also occurs. The hot effluent from the reactor is cooled and sent to a high-pressure separator, where hydrogen flashes off and is recycled to the feed stream. The liquid from the separator is sent to a fractionator, where hydrogen sulfide, ammonia and any low-boiling hydrocarbons are removed, and the remaining naphtha is distilled into fractions of the desired boiling range. The feed to hydrodesulfurization is a sour naphtha from the crude fractionator with a boiling-point range of about 65–230°C. Operating conditions vary with the composition of the feed, but generally temperatures in the range of 315–430°C and pressures of 300–1000 psi [20–68 atm] are used.

Hydrodesulfurization is applied to other process streams (e.g., kerosene, gas oil, residual oil) under conditions of varying severity.

(iv) *Catalytic isomerization*

Isomerization is used to convert n-butane, n-pentane and n-hexane into their respective isoparaffins. The isobutane is used as a feedstock for alkylation; isopentanes and isohexanes are of sufficiently high octane quality to be used directly as gasoline blending stocks. The feedstock to the isomerization unit must be both dehydrated and desulfurized. Sweet, dry feedstock is mixed with hydrogen, heated to reaction temperature and catalytically hydrogenated to remove any benzene and olefins. It is then mixed with hydrogen chloride (or organic chloride) and passed over a fixed bed of chlorinated platinum-aluminium oxide isomerization catalyst, where straight-chain hydrocarbons are converted to isoparaffins. The effluent product is cooled and passes into a high-pressure separator where recycled hydrogen flashes off. The liquid from the separator is sent to a stripper column where hydrogen chloride is removed. The resulting isoparaffins are neutralized and sent to storage. Isomerization units are operated at temperatures of 240–255°C and at pressures of 300–400 psi [20–27 atm].

(v) *Catalytic reforming*

Catalytic reforming is used to convert low-octane naphthas into high-octane gasoline blending stocks; it may also be done to produce aromatic hydrocarbons such as benzene and toluene for use as solvents and chemical feedstocks. In reforming, cycloparaffins are converted to aromatic compounds by a combination of dehydrogenation and dehydroisomerization. Some paraffins also form aromatic compounds by dehydrocyclization. Hydrogen is a net product of reforming, which can be used in the hydrotreating and hydrodesulfurization units of a refinery. The naphtha feedstock is mixed with hydrogen and heated by exchangers almost to reaction temperatures. The mixture then passes through a series of alternating furnaces and fixed-bed reactors (usually three or four) containing a platinum or platinum-rhenium on alumina catalyst. The furnaces maintain the reaction temperatures between the catalyst beds. The reactor effluent is cooled by heat exchange and sent through a separator where hydrogen is flashed off. The liquid from the separator is taken to a stripping tower where light ends are removed. The stabilized reformate is sent to storage or is further refractionated in a second tower. Since platinum catalysts are subject to poisoning by sulfur and nitrogen, reforming units require prior hydrodesulfurization of the naphtha feed or contain a pretreater containing a non-noble metal catalyst through which the feedstock and hydrogen pass before entering the main reaction vessels. Reformers are generally operated at temperatures of 427–482°C and at pressures of 100–200 psi [7–14 atm]. The operating conditions depend somewhat upon the boiling range of the feedstock and the activity of the catalyst.

(iv) *Steam cracking*

Steam cracking is used to produce olefinic raw materials which, in turn, are employed in the manufacture of petrochemicals. Although this is essentially a petrochemical operation, the facility is often integrated into larger refinery complexes.

The process involves the thermal cracking of feedstock ranging from ethane to vacuum distillate and utilizes temperatures of around 800–850°C at slightly greater than atmospheric pressure. Heavier feeds produce higher yields of by-products such as naphtha, which, when blended into gasoline, has been called 'pyrolysis gasoline'. Naphtha from steam cracking typically has very high concentrations of benzene (see IARC, 1982, 1987b), and, since approximately the early 1960s, benzene has normally been extracted from naphtha for its commercial value. After mild hydrotreating to saturate olefins and polyolefins that cause instability and gum formation, naphtha from which the benzene has been removed may be blended with other streams to produce gasoline with the required performance specification.

Depending on the nature of the feedstock, the steam cracking process generates residual tars which may sometimes be blended in small quantities into residual heavy fuels.

(c) *Middle distillate processing*

(i) *Chemical sweetening*

Chemical sweetening, often referred to as 'doctoring', is used to oxidize low concentrations of mercaptans to disulfides to reduce the odour of products containing mercaptans. This is a frequent practice in refineries that utilize relatively low-sulfur crude oils. With such crude oils, it is more economical to eliminate the odour problem by chemical means than by removing the sulfur in a hydrodesulfurization unit. In all sweetening processes, the stream to be treated is put into contact with an oxidizing agent, with or without a catalyst. Caustics or hypochlorites are commonly used, and a variety of processes can be used to treat mercaptans in virgin streams.

Inhibitor and air–cresylate sweetening are frequently used in combination for catalytically cracked naphthas. In inhibitor sweetening, mercaptans are oxidized in the presence of a phenylenediamine (see IARC, 1978, 1987b) inhibitor, trace amounts of caustic and olefin. The requirement that olefins be present makes the process well suited for the treating of catalytic naphthas; however, the reaction is relatively slow and the process is therefore usually used in combination with air–cresylate sweetening which uses the cresols present in catalytic naphthas as both solvents and oxidation catalysts. Although still in use in many refineries, this process is gradually being replaced by Merox sweetening. In the liquid–liquid Merox process, the stream to be treated is brought into contact with air and 10% caustic solution containing an oxidation catalyst in a mixing vessel. It then passes to a settler where caustic and excess air are removed and the caustic is recirculated back to the mixer. Any caustic which remains dispersed in the treated product is removed in a sand coalescer. Chemical sweetening is generally carried out at temperatures from ambient to 65°C and at pressures of about 20 psi [1.4 atm].

(ii) *Kerosene hydrodesulfurization*

Hydrodesulfurization can be used to remove sulfur, saturate any olefins and reduce the aromatic content and gum-forming tendency of kerosene. The sour straight-run kerosene [5] feed is mixed with hydrogen, heated in a fired heater and then passed through a fixed-bed reactor containing a nickel- (see IARC, 1976, 1987b) or cobalt-molybdenum catalyst. Organic sulfur is removed as hydrogen sulfide. The reactor effluent is cooled, usually by heat exchange with the feed, and the excess hydrogen is separated and recycled. It is then reheated and steam-stripped to remove dissolved hydrogen sulfide. Operating temperatures are generally in the range of 205–410°C with pressures of 500–800 psi [34–54 atm].

(iii) *Gas oil hydrodesulfurization*

Hydrodesulfurization is used to improve the quality of straight-run gas oil [7] by removing sulfur, nitrogen and metallic contaminants. Any olefins are also saturated. Some cracking into lighter components will occur. The feed to the hydrodesulfurization unit is a sour gas oil from the crude distillation tower. The boiling range varies widely, from 205°C to 400°C. The feed is vaporized, mixed with a hydrogen-rich gas stream, heated to reaction temperature and passed through a fixed-bed reactor containing a non-noble metal catalyst, where nitrogen and sulfur are removed as ammonia and hydrogen sulfide. The hot reactor effluent is cooled and condensed by heat exchange with the feed, and the liquid is sent to a high-pressure separator where the hydrogen flashes off and is recycled. The liquid from the high-pressure separator then flows to a low-pressure separator where the hydrogen sulfide, ammonia and gaseous hydrocarbons are removed. The effluent product is a stabilized, hydrodesulfurized gas oil of improved colour and odour which is sent to storage for later blending or cracking. Operating temperatures are in the range of 260–415°C and pressures 500–800 psi [34–54 atm].

(iv) *Fluid-bed catalytic cracking*

Fluid-bed catalytic cracking is used to convert distillate oil streams into a product commonly described as synthetic crude oil. Synthetic crude oil is a wide boiling-range material from which gaseous hydrocarbons, catalytically cracked naphthas [22, 23] and light and heavy catalytically cracked distillates [24, 26, respectively] are fractionated by distillation. The feed to a fluid-bed catalytic cracker may be any hydrocarbon stock from straight-run kerosene [5] to heavy vacuum distillate [20] or solvent-deasphalted residual oil [32]. It is usually a heavy distillate, with the wide boiling range of 205–400°C. A fluid catalytic cracking unit consists of a catalyst section and a fractionating section which operate together as an integrated processing unit. The catalyst section contains the reactor and regenerator, which, together with the standpipe and riser, form the catalyst circulation unit. The catalyst moves up the riser to the reactor, down through a stripper to the regenerator, across to the regenerator standpipe and back to the riser. The catalyst is in the form of very small spherical particles which behave like a fluid when aerated with a vapour. Fresh feed and recycling gas oil enter the unit at the base of the riser, where they are vaporized and raised to reaction temperature by the hot catalyst. The mixture of oil vapour and catalyst travels up the riser into the reactor. Cracking commences in the riser and continues until the oil vapours are disengaged from the catalyst in the reactor. The cracked products travel through the reactor vapour line to the fractionator. The spent catalyst flows from the reactor to the regenerator where carbon deposits are burned off. In the fractionation section, the reactor effluent is separated from the catalyst and travels to the fractionation section, where it is separated by distillation into a recycling gas oil which is returned to the riser for further cracking into catalytically cracked clarified oil [27], light catalytically cracked distillate [24], catalytically cracked naphthas [22, 23] and wet gas. Between 50% and 80% of the feed is cracked in a single pass. Typical reactor temperatures and pressures are 475–550°C and 10–30 psi [0.7–2 atm]. A variety of acid-function catalysts are used, including natural clays, silica-aluminas and synthetic zeolites (see IARC, 1987a,b).

(v) *Moving-bed catalytic cracking*

The function of moving-bed catalytic cracking is the same as that of fluidized catalytic cracking. Moving-bed catalytic crackers use the same type of catalyst as fluid units but in the form of extruded pellets about 0.25 [0.6 cm] in diameter by about 0.5 [1.3 cm] in length. They are usually smaller than fluid-bed crackers and generally consist of a catalyst section, contained in a single, tall vessel comprising the reactor and generator, and an associated fractionation section. The catalyst is moved continuously to the top of the unit by bucket elevator or pneumatic lift pipes and flows downwards at a rate of about 4 ft [1.2 m] per min through the surge hopper, which acts as a temporary storage ahead of the reactor, through the reactor where it comes into contact with the feedstocks and into the regenerator where carbon deposits are burned off. The reactor is isolated from the surge hopper and regenerator by steam seals. The products of cracking are separated by distillation into a recycling gas oil, catalytically cracked clarified oil [27], light catalytically cracked distillate [24], catalytically cracked naphthas [22, 23] and wet gas. The feedstocks and operating conditions are essentially the same as those used for fluid-bed catalytic cracking.

(vi) *Catalytic hydrocracking*

Hydrocracking is used to convert heavy feedstocks into lower-boiling, more valuable products. The process employs high pressure, high temperatures, a cobalt- or nickel-molybdenum catalyst and hydrogen. The reaction section is usually divided into two stages: the first is designed to remove sulfur and nitrogen compounds, while actual cracking takes place in the second stage in the presence of excess hydrogen. The effluent from the second-stage reactor is fractionated by distillation into the desired products. The usual feed is a straight-run gas oil [7] or other distillate from the crude fractionator. Temperatures and pressures in the first stage are generally 370°C and 3000 psi [200 atm], and those in the second stage are about 315°C and 1500 psi [100 atm].

(d) *Heavy hydrocarbon processing*

(i) *Deasphalting*

Deasphalting is used to separate asphaltic materials from heavy oil fractions. This separation (sometimes referred to as decarbonizing) produces an oil for use as a feed to catalytic cracking or for the manufacture of heavy lubricants, and as a raw bitumen (see IARC, 1985). Deasphalting is usually accomplished by solvent extraction with propane. The feed to a deasphalting unit is usually a vacuum residue [21], reduced crude oil [8] or any other heavy crude fraction containing bitumen. The feed and liquid propane are pumped to an extraction tower in a controlled ratio and at a controlled temperature. The extraction unit is often a rotating-disc contactor. A separation based on the differences in solubility is effected, producing a solution of deasphalted residual oil and one of bitumen. The effluents are processed by evaporation and steam stripping to recover the propane from the oil and the bitumen. Temperatures are usually in the range of 70–105°C and pressures range from 450–600 psi [30–40 atm].

(ii) *Visbreaking*

The purpose of visbreaking (viscosity breaking) is to crack residual oils thermally into lower-boiling and less viscous materials under mild conditions. The charge to the unit, which is typically a waxy reduced crude oil [8], is heated and slightly cracked in the visbreaker furnace. The furnace effluent is quenched with a light gas oil and is fed to the lower or evaporator section of a fractionation tower where it is flashed. A tar, thermally cracked residue [31], accumulates in the base of the tower, while in the upper part the vapours are fractionated into gas, thermally cracked naphthas [28, 29] and thermally cracked distillates [30]. The tower bottoms are withdrawn and vacuum-flashed in a stripping tower and the vacuum distillate returned to the fractionator. Visbreaker furnaces generally operate at temperatures of 450–480°C and at atmospheric pressure.

(iii) *Coking*

Coking is a thermal cracking process in which crude oil residues, catalytically cracked clarified oil [27] and refinery tars are cracked at high temperature and low pressure to produce thermally cracked distillates [30] and petroleum coke. There are two principal coking processes: the fluid coking process and the delayed coking process. Delayed coking is used most widely; in this process, the charge stock is fed to the bottom section of a fractionation tower where material lighter than the desired end-point of the heavy thermal distillate is removed. The remaining material is pumped from the bottom of the fractionator to a coking heater, where its temperature is raised rapidly. The vaporized liquid leaving the coking heater enters a coke drum where coke is formed. The coke is recovered by cutting it out of the drum with a high-pressure water stream. The coker tower is generally operated at a temperature of about 380°C and at pressures of 25–30 psi [1.7–2 atm]. Coking heater temperatures are about 480–580°C.

(iv) *Residual oil hydrodesulfurization*

The function of a residual oil hydrodesulfurization unit is to reduce the sulfur and metal contents of atmospheric tower residues. Reduced crude oil [8] is mixed with hydrogen, heated in a fired heater and then passed through a fixed bed of catalyst where the reactions occur. The active components of the catalyst are typically chromium (see IARC, 1980, 1987b), molybdenum, iron, cobalt or nickel. Organic sulfur and nitrogen compounds are converted to hydrogen sulfide and ammonia. The products from the reactor are cooled, usually by heat exchange with the feed, the excess hydrogen flashed off in a high-pressure separator and recycled, and the bulk of the ammonia and hydrogen sulfide removed in a low-pressure separator. The products are then reheated and steam stripped to remove any residual hydrogen sulfide or ammonia. The desulfurized residue can be blended into fuel or be processed further to recover gas oil. Residual oil hydrodesulfurization units are generally operated at temperatures of 340–450°C and at pressures of about 1000 psi [68 atm].

1.3 Worldwide distribution of petroleum refinery operations

A general picture of the extent of petroleum refinery operations in various regions of the world can be obtained from data on refinery throughputs (Table 3). Between 1976 and 1986, the total petroleum throughput of refineries in the developed countries of the western world declined, while in other countries refinery throughput has generally increased.

Table 3. Refinery throughputs (thousands of barrels daily)[a], 1976-87

Geographical region	1976[b]	1981[b]	1987[c]		
			Through-put	% of total	Refinery capacity
USA	13 435	12 470	12 855	22.6	15 695
Canada	1 710	1 945	1 605	2.8	2 050
Latin America	5 670	6 575	5 530	9.7	7 420
Western Europe	13 625	11 890	9 795	17.2	14 010
Middle East	2 300	2 205	2 970	5.2	4 120
Africa	1 055	1 525	2 170	3.8	2 630
Japan	4 230	3 630	2 910	5.1	4 505
South-east Asia	1 865	2 480	2 750	4.8	3 745
South Asia	550	795	1 145	2.0	1 295
Australia and New Zealand	655	655	570	1.0	730
Centrally planned economies[d]	11 575	13 420	14 700	25.8	17 880
Total world	56 670	57 590	57 000	–	74 080

[a]1 barrel = 0.136 metric tonne of crude oil (specific gravity, 0.858)

[b]From British Petroleum Company (1986)

[c]From British Petroleum Company (1988)

[d]Albania, Bulgaria, China, Cuba, Czechoslovakia, Democratic Kampuchea, the Democratic People's Republic of Korea, the German Democratic Republic, Hungary, the Lao People's Democratic Republic, Mongolia, Poland, Romania, the USSR, Viet Nam and Yugoslavia

The importance of the various refinery process streams varies somewhat from region to region and even from season to season for individual refineries. Although detailed data are not available to compare the throughput of various process streams in different geographic regions, regional consumption data for different product groups generally parallel local refinery product distribution, since, historically, refined products are mostly used in the same geographic region in which they are produced. While there are many exceptions to this generalization (e.g., in the Middle East increasing quantities of crude oil are being converted into finished products for export), production and consumption patterns still correlate fairly well at the regional level. Table 4 shows the consumption of gasolines, middle distillates, fuel oils and other petroleum products in several regions of the world from 1976 to 1986. The data reflect the fact that refinery process streams feeding the gasoline pool are most important in the USA, Canada and Australia/New Zealand, whereas middle distillates predominate in European refineries. The most notable trends are the worldwide decline in fuel oil production and consumption and the steady growth in production of all products (except fuel oil) in the lesser developed countries. In Albania, Bulgaria, China, Cuba, Czechoslovakia, Democratic Kampuchea, the Democratic People's Republic of Korea, the German Democratic Republic, Hungary, the Lao People's Democratic Republic, Mongolia, Poland, Romania, the USSR, Viet Nam and Yugoslavia, overall consumption increased from 580.5 million tonnes in 1976 (British Petroleum Co., 1986) to 670.3 million tonnes in 1986 (British Petroleum Co., 1988).

Table 4. Consumption of petroleum products[a] by geographical region (millions of tonnes per year)

Region and product	1976[b]	1981[c]	1987[c] Consumption	% of total
USA				
Gasolines	320.4	297.9	324.1	42.5
Middle distillates	206.3	199.2	216.1	28.3
Fuel oil	146.8	110.6	68.6	9.0
Others	148.9	138.3	154.6	20.2
Total	822.4	746.0	763.4	–
Canada				
Gasolines	29.6	31.3	27.5	39.6
Middle distillates	27.3	25.0	21.8	31.5
Fuel oil	17.1	11.2	6.7	9.6
Others	11.9	14.2	13.4	19.3
Total	85.9	81.7	69.4	–
Western Europe				
Gasolines	131.8	131.1	144.5	24.7
Middle distillates	238.3	220.7	236.3	40.4
Fuel oil	238.3	179.3	111.5	19.1
Others	87.4	87.3	92.9	15.8
Total	695.8	618.4	585.2	–

Table 4 (contd)

Region and product	1976[b]	1981[c]	1987[c] Consumption	% of total
Japan				
Gasolines	43.6	39.8	44.0	21.1
Middle distillates	54.2	60.6	69.0	33.2
Fuel oil	125.7	91.2	57.0	27.4
Others	30.0	32.3	38.1	18.3
Total	253.5	223.9	208.1	–
Australia and New Zealand				
Gasolines	12.2	13.1	13.6	41.5
Middle distillates	9.9	9.8	11.3	34.4
Fuel oil	7.3	5.6	2.4	7.3
Others	4.9	4.7	5.5	16.8
Total	34.3	33.2	32.8	–
Rest of world[d]				
Gasolines	72.7	96.0	110.2	18.3
Middle distillates	139.3	178.1	216.6	35.9
Fuel oil	150.8	190.8	188.0	31.2
Others	59.4	74.5	88.0	14.6
Total	422.2	539.4	602.8	–
Total				
Gasolines	610.3	609.2	663.9	29.4
Middle distillates	675.3	693.4	771.1	34.1
Fuel oil	686.0	588.7	434.2	19.2
Others	342.5	351.3	382.5	17.3
TOTAL	2314.1	2242.6	2260.7	–

[a]'Gasolines' consists of aviation and motor gasolines and light distillate feedstock; 'middle distillates' consists of jet and burning kerosenes, and gas and diesel oils (including marine bunkers); 'fuel oil' includes marine bunkers; 'others' consists of refinery gas, liquified petroleum gases, solvents, petroleum coke, lubricants, bitumen, wax, refinery fuel and loss

[b]From British Petroleum Company (1986)

[c]From British Petroleum Company (1988)

[d]Excluding centrally planned economies (see footnote d to Table 3)

2. Exposures in the Workplace

Those compounds that occur in the working environment of petroleum refineries that have been evaluated in previous *IARC Monographs* are listed in Table 1 of the 'General Remarks', p. 32.

2.1 Workers and working conditions

It has been estimated that the world petroleum refining industry employs from 400 000 to 500 000 persons (International Labour Office, 1986) in approximately 700 refineries (American Petroleum Institute, 1987).

A wide range of potential occupational health hazards is present in petroleum refineries. Exposures result from skin contact and the inhalation of gases and vapours, mainly hydrocarbons either naturally present in crude oil and emitted during its refining or formed and emitted during one of the many transformations of the various process streams. Gaseous sulfur compounds such as hydrogen sulfide, sulfur dioxide and mercaptans are emitted during removal and treatment of sulfur. Exposure to dusts and fumes results mostly from maintenance operations such as abrasive blasting, the use of catalysts and the handling of viscous or solid products such as bitumen and coke.

In general, it is considered that exposures to hydrocarbons have not been subject to major reductions over the past two or three decades. Nevertheless, useful reductions have resulted from the gradual introduction of controls over fugitive emissions, increased attention to the control of benzene exposures (CONCAWE, 1986) and greater automation of refinery operations, including sampling and analysis of streams. Over the last 30 years or so, since a large conference in 1951 (Page, 1951) created a much greater awareness of the potential skin hazards from some mineral oil streams, there has been a significant reduction in skin exposure as a result of more effective use of personal protective clothing, improved personal hygiene and safer operating procedures.

The petroleum industry has reached a stage of high automatization, with a concurrent reduction of the work force during the last two decades. It is not known whether such automatization has occurred in all countries to the same extent. Due to the intrinsic risks of fire and explosion from many refinery streams, operations take place in closed systems, and refinery operators spend most of their time in control rooms with little potential exposure to hazardous agents. Ubiquitous exposure exists mainly to hydrocarbon gases and vapours at usually very low levels resulting from constant and fugitive emissions from seals and valves in the complex network of pipes and columns; there is also potential dermal exposure during sampling (Darby *et al.*, 1978). Heavier exposures may be encountered, however, during routine maintenance and turn-round operations (Dynamac Corp., 1985) from episodic or periodic emissions resulting from opening the system or performing specific tasks such as repair, overhaul and construction. Outside contractors are often brought in for major turn-round operations. [The Working Group noted that no data were available on the numbers of outside contractor workers involved in such operations.] During these operations, cutaneous exposure to a number of chemicals is also a possibility. Other groups with potential heavy exposure to such hazards are those in bulk handling of final products and in laboratories (Clayton Environmental Consultants, Inc., 1982).

The overall distribution of employees in ten US refineries by exposure-based job type has been reported as follows: administration, 21%; maintenance, 36%; operations, 40%; and unknown, 3% (Nelson et al., 1983). A job code classification system for oil refineries has been developed (American Petroleum Institute, 1985) in which workers can be classified using two standardized variables: process and task. This scheme was devised in order to allow better regroupment of workers who share a set of qualitatively common exposures. Other exposure-based work category classifications have been devised for both epidemiological purposes (Nelson et al., 1983; Thomas et al., 1984) and for planning industrial hygiene studies (Futagaki, 1983).

The main substances to which workers may be exposed in petroleum refineries are given in Table 5. The main occupational agents for which airborne exposure levels are available are presented in Tables 6–8. [The Working Group noted the paucity of exposure data available for the period prior to the mid-1970s and for refineries in developing countries, and the lack of any data on skin exposures.]

Table 5. Main substances (and classes of substances) to which workers may be exposed in petroleum refineries[a]

Material	Principal uses or sources of emission
Alumina	Catalyst support, catalyst (sulfur recovery)
Aluminium chloride	Catalyst (isomerization)
Amines, aliphatic (e.g., methylamine) and alkanolamines (e.g. monoethanolamine)	Hydrodesulfurization, acid gas adsorbents
Amines, aromatic (e.g., anisidines* and phenylenediamines*)	Catalytic cracking, residual processing, gasoline antioxidants
Ammonia	Atmospheric distillation, catalytic cracking, sulfur recovery, residual processing, lubricant oil processing, waste waters
Antimony trichloride	Inhibitor (isomerization)
Arsenic compounds*	Crude oil, gas scrubbing
Asbestos*	Pipe insulation, gaskets (formerly), valve seals
Bitumen (asphalt) fumes*	Solvent deasphalting, tanker loading, tank cleaning
tert-Butyl alcohol	Unleaded gasoline blending
Carbon monoxide	Catalyst regeneration (catalytic cracking), use of inert gases, boilers, flares
Chlorine	Rejuvenation of platinum catalyst, cooling water treatment
Chromium and chromium compounds*	Catalyst (catalytic reforming), welding
Clays (e.g., bentonite)	Catalyst supports, grease fillers

Table 5 (contd)

Material	Principal uses or sources of emission
Cobalt and cobalt compounds (including cobalt carbonyl, cobalt molybdate, oxides)	Catalyst (catalytic reforming, hydrocracking, hydrotreating)
Coke	Coking units*
Copper and copper compounds (e.g. copper chloride, copper alloys)	Desulfurization, sweetening operations, catalyst (catalytic reforming)
Crude oil	Crude oil distillation and processing unit
1,2-Dibromoethane (ethylene dibromide)*	Leaded gasoline blending
1,2-Dichloroethane (ethylene dichloride)*	Leaded gasoline blending
Earth, diatomaceous (amorphous silica*)	Crude oil filtration, catalyst support, lubricant oil filtration
Fuels (e.g., gasoline, diesel oil, jet fuel, heating oil)	Fuel blending, storage, loading
Furfural	Oil and grease manufacture, desulfurization
Graphite	Grease filler
Hydrazine*	Boiler-water additive
Hydrocarbons, aliphatic (e.g., propane, n-hexane)	Most process units
Hydrocarbons, aromatic (e.g., benzene*, toluene)	Most process units, catalytic cracking and reforming, gasoline blending and loading, wax preparation unit
Hydrocarbons, chlorinated*	Rejuvenation of catalyst (catalytic reforming), solvents
Hydrogen chloride	Isomerization
Hydrogen fluoride (hydrofluoric acid)	Catalyst (alkylation)
Hydrogen sulfide and sulfur compounds (e.g., mercaptans, carbon disulfide)	Atmospheric distillation, catalytic cracking and reforming, hydrocracking, hydrotreating, sulfur recovery, residual processing, lubricant oil processing, waste waters
Iron and iron compounds*	Catalyst (hydrocracking), welding
Ketones (e.g., methyl ethyl ketone)	Lubricant oil solvent dewaxing, atmospheric distillation, residual processing
Lead, inorganic compounds (e.g., lead oxide)*	Desulfurization, removal, sweetening operations
Manganese compounds, organic	Unleaded gasoline blending
Methyl-*tert*-butyl ether	Unleaded gasoline blending
N-Methyl-2-pyrrolidone	Lubricant oil manufacture
Mineral oils (e.g., lubricating oils)*	Oil and grease units
Molybdenum and molybdenum compounds	Catalyst (catalytic reforming, hydrocracking, isomerization, hydrotreating)
Nickel and nickel compounds (e.g., nickel sulfides, nickel carbonyl, nickel oxide)*	Catalyst (isomerization, hydrotreating, hydrocracking, catalytic reforming), welding, cleaning residual fuel oils, combustion products
Nitrogen oxides	Flares, furnaces

Table 5 (contd)

Material	Principal uses or sources of emission
Palladium	Catalyst (catalytic reforming, hydrocracking)
Phenol	Crude distillation, catalytic cracking, residual processing, waste waters, desulfurization, lubricant oil, solvent dewaxing
Phosgene	Catalyst rejuvenation by chlorination (catalytic reforming)
Pitch (petroleum)	Bitumen department, loading operations
Phosphoric acid	Catalyst (polymerization)
Platinum	Catalyst (catalytic reforming, isomerization, hydrotreating)
Polynuclear aromatic compounds*	Atmospheric distillation, catalytic cracking, residual fuel oil, lubricant oil processing, bitumen processing and loading, coking, waste-water treatment
Refined petroleum solvents (e.g., petroleum ether, rubber solvent, varnish makers' and painters' naphtha, Stoddard solvent)	Petroleum solvent manufacturing
Rhenium	Catalyst (catalytic reforming)
Silica, crystalline*	Abrasive blasting, demolition and rebuilding, cracking (catalyst)
Sodium hydroxide	Caustic wash of acid catalysts or acid-treated streams, sweetening operations
Sulfur	Sulfur recovery
Sulfur dioxide	Sulfur recovery, furnaces, flares
Sulfuric acid	Catalyst (alkylation, polymerization), acid treating of lubricant oils
Tetraethyllead and tetramethyllead*	Gasoline blending operations, gasoline storage tank cleaning
Tungsten sulfide	Catalyst (hydrocracking)
Vanadium compounds (e.g., vanadium pentoxide)	Residual fuel oils, cleaning of combustion deposits, flue cleaning

*Compounds marked with an asterisk have been evaluated by the IARC (see IARC, 1987; see also Table 1 of 'General Remarks', p. 32)

[a]From Darby *et al.* (1978); Burgess (1981); Clayton Environmental Consultants, Inc. (1982); Hobson (1982); Futagaki (1983); CONCAWE (1985); Dynamac Corp. (1985); Suess *et al.* (1985)

Table 6. Airborne concentrations of total hydrocarbons and selected aliphatic hydrocarbons in petroleum refineries in mg/m^3; 8-h TWA[a] on personal samples (range)

Operation or job description[b] (no. of samples)	Total hydrocarbons	n-Butane	n-Hexane	Reference
Production on-site (62)	53 (0.7–1820)	10.3 (0–460)	3.0 (0–154)	CONCAWE (1987)
Production off-site (27)	66 (3.7–923)	11.2 (0–221)	2.8 (0–14)	CONCAWE (1987)
Drumming of gasoline (9)	858 (61–1750)	120 (0–301)	52 (2.4–297)	CONCAWE (1987)
Laboratory technician (9)	31 (7–83)	3.7 (0.1–29.5)	4.5 (0.4–8.5)	Viau et al. (1987)
Bulk plant operator (4)	66 (13–73)	4.0 (0.5–11.8)	1.4 (0.5–3.2)	Viau et al. (1987)
Refinery operator on-site (11)	4 (1–8)	0.4 (ND–1.7)	0.3 (ND–1.8)	Viau et al. (1987)
Refinery operator off-site (13)	16 (2–96)	2.8 (0.1–20.5)	0.4 (ND–1.7)	Viau et al. (1987)
Refinery, clerical or administration employee (69)	0.2–2.1[c]	–	–	Viau et al. (1987)
Process unit operator[d] (56, 54, 54, respect.)	18.9 (10.7–27.2)[e]	3.4 (1.8–5.1)[e]	0.47 (0.32–0.63)[e]	Rappaport et al. (1987)

[a]TWA, time-weighted average

[b]On-site involves operators controlling refining process units; operator time is spent in control room, inspection tours of units and specific activities ranging from routine maintenance to collection of samples, opening and closing of valves, etc. Off-site involves operators conducting ancillary operations, such as laboratory technicians, control of bulk storage facilities, tank dipping and sampling, and water-effluent treatment operations.

[c]Range of area samples

[d]Work is primarily outside of the control room, taking readings, obtaining samples, inspecting facilities, etc.

[e]Approximate 95% confidence interval

ND, not detected; –, not measured

Table 7. Airborne concentrations of selected aromatic hydrocarbons in petroleum refineries in mg/m³; 8-h TWA[a] on personal samples (range)

Operation or job description (no. of samples)	Benzene	Toluene	Reference
Production on-site (62)	0.9 (0–23.8)	2.0 (0–67)	CONCAWE (1987)
Production off-site (27)	1.0 (0–14.1)	2.2 (0–19.6)	CONCAWE (1987)
Drumming of gasoline (9)	27.2 (0–116)	41.3 (3.1–195)	CONCAWE (1987)
Maintenance worker (4 studies)	0.3–1.2 (0.03–24)	–	CONCAWE (1986)
Laboratory technician (9)	–	0.8 (ND–3.5)	Viau et al. (1987)
Bulk plant operator (4)	–	3.1 (0.7–8.0)	Viau et al. (1987)
Refinery operator, on-site (11)	–	0.3 (ND–0.7)	Viau et al. (1987)
Refinery operator, off-site (13)	–	0.6 (0.2–2.4)	Viau et al. (1987)
Atmospheric distillation of crude oil	0.8	–	Holmberg & Lundberg (1985)
Catalytic reforming	0.2	–	Holmberg & Lundberg (1985)
Laboratory personnel	1.0	–	Holmberg & Lundberg (1985)
Product analysis	0.2	–	Holmberg & Lundberg (1985)
Other refinery workers	0.1	–	Holmberg & Lundberg (1985)
Refining (in general) (14 824)[b]	0.7 ± 2.2 (SD)	–	Runion & Scott (1985)
Lubricant-dewaxing process (66 and 82)	0.1 ± 0.06 (SD)	3.2 ± 9.7 (SD)	Wen et al. (1985)
Lubricant oil extraction	–	<0.1–77 ppm	CONCAWE

[a]TWA, time-weighted average

[b]Estimated TWA >4 h

ND, not detected; –, not measured

Table 8. Airborne concentrations of polynuclear aromatic compounds (PAC)[a] in petroleum refineries

Unit	Job description or process	Sample type[b] (no. of measurements)	Results[c] ($\mu g/m^3$)	Reference
Fluid catalytic cracker units	Supervisor	Personal samples TWA, 7–8 h (4)	GM: 8.8 GSD: 2.6	Futagaki (1983)
	Inside operator	Personal samples TWA, 7–8 h (22)	GM: 11.9 GSD: 3.3	Futagaki (1983)
	Outside operator	Personal samples TWA, 7–8 h (61)	GM: 11.4 GSD: 3.7	Futagaki (1983)
Delayed coker units	Operators	Personal samples TWA, 7–8 h (40)	GM: 7.8 GSD: 8.4	Futagaki (1983)
	Coke handlers	Personal samples TWA, 7–8 h (50)	GM: 14.6 GSD: 4.1	Futagaki (1983)
Bitumen processing units	Bitumen blowing	Area samples TWA, 7–8 h (5)	Range: 1.6–30.6	Futagaki (1983)
	Deasphalting	Area samples TWA, 7–8 h (4)	Range: 1.4–41.2	Futagaki (1983)
	Vacuum distillation	Area samples TWA, 7–8 h (11)	Range of GM: 2.8–18.0	Futagaki (1983)
Bulk handling of bitumen	Road tanker loading	Personal samples[d] TWA, 8 h (4)	Average: 0.033 Range: 0.004–0.095	Brandt & Molyneux (1985)
Turn-round activity on reaction and fractionator towers	Chipping coke	Personal samples[e] TWA, 8 h	120–320	Dynamac Corp. (1985)
	Cutting steel liner	Personal samples TWA, 8 h	210–470	Dynamac Corp. (1985)
	Cutting out distillation trays	Personal samples TWA, 8 h	70	Dynamac Corp. (1985)

[a]23 individual or groups of PAC and azo heterocyclics with 2–7 rings

[b]TWA, time-weighted average

[c]GM, geometric mean; GSD, geometric standard deviation

[d]11 individual PAC

[e]Six individual or groups of PAC

2.2 Aliphatic hydrocarbons

Nearly all workers in petroleum refineries are exposed to aliphatic hydrocarbons. The principal individual aliphatic hydrocarbon compounds found in petroleum refinery air samples are butanes, pentanes and hexanes, which account for an overwhelming part of the total hydrocarbons measured. Concentrations of up to 150 hydrocarbons, mostly aliphatic, have been reported in gasoline vapour in gasoline manufacture and distribution operations in Europe (CONCAWE, 1987).

Average exposure levels to hydrocarbons for various categories of workers are summarized in Table 6. These range from fractions of 1 mg/m^3 for administrative or clerical employees to above 1000 mg/m^3 in drumming operations. The latter operation corresponds to a 'worst case' situation, in which operators fill drums with gasoline without good local exhaust ventilation (CONCAWE, 1987). A mean exposure level of 5.4 ppm with a standard deviation of 16.5 ppm, covering a wide number of refinery workers in the USA (1201 full-exposure samples), has been reported (Wen *et al.*, 1984a). In general, gasoline loading operations represent the highest potential for exposure to hydrocarbons. Various short-term and 8-h time-weighted average (TWA) exposure levels for these operations are summarized in the monograph on gasoline. Average exposure of refinery production operators, both on-site and off-site, is well below 100 mg/m^3, with potential short-term extremes above 1000 mg/m^3, which varies according to specific tasks and the relative amount of time spent on the process units and in the control rooms (CONCAWE, 1987). Data on exposure to 1,3-butadiene are given in the monograph on gasoline.

2.3 Aromatic hydrocarbons

In petroleum refineries, exposure to aromatic hydrocarbons originates from their presence in crude oils and the conversion of naphthenes and paraffins during the catalytic reforming process. Exposure levels to benzene and toluene in various work situations are summarized in Table 7.

Group average exposures of production and maintenance workers to benzene vary from about 0.3 to 1 mg/m^3, with higher individual values of above 10 mg/m^3. The highest values have been observed during gasoline drumming operations without good local exhaust ventilation. Gasoline loading operations, in general, give rise to average 8-h levels of about 1–5 mg/m^3, depending on the type of operation (road tanker, railcar, marine) and loading technique. Various short-term and 8-h TWA exposure levels for these operations are summarized in the monograph on gasoline.

Data on exposure to benzene derived from personal sampling of employees of a large refinery in Texas, USA, have been compiled for the period 1973–82 (benzene concentration range in mg/m^3, % of samples): <0.3, 52; 0.3–3, 37; 3–16, 9; 16–30, 1; >30, 0 (727 samples covering 4 h or more). The refinery under investigation included benzene petrochemical units (Tsai *et al.*, 1983). Full-shift personal exposure measurements have also been obtained for 29 work categories in two French refineries, including work in catalytic cracking and reforming units. In only six work categories were the levels of benzene near or above

1 mg/m³; in two work categories (cracker operator and rail car top-loading), maximum concentrations exceeded 10 mg/m³ (Cicolella & Vincent, 1987). In Canada, exposure to benzene in a typical non-benzene producing facility was reported to be usually well below 1 ppm (3 mg/m³). In refineries where pure benzene is produced, exposures can exceed 10 ppm (30 mg/m³) on occasion, with a range of 1–4 ppm (3–13 mg/m³) observed in the laboratory (Petroleum Association for Conservation of the Canadian Environment, 1979). At one US refinery, of 75 samples taken around a catalytic cracking unit, 61 contained less than 0.1 ppm (0.3 mg/m³), 12 had 0.1–0.5 ppm (0.3–1.6 mg/m³) and two exceeded 10 ppm (32 mg/m³; Weaver et al., 1983).

In 1984, the American Petroleum Institute commissioned a study of exposure to benzene in petroleum companies over the period 1978–84 (Spear et al., 1987). Personal exposure data submitted by nine refining companies were analysed in detail to characterize the distribution of exposures within work operations and job categories; the data covered 123 location- and unit-specific job categories. Most 8-h TWA exposures were reported to be below 1.0 ppm (3 mg/m³); however, for some groups, 10% or more of exposures exceeded 1.0 ppm, although only about 5% of measurements reported for maintenance workers exceeded that level. Some short-term exposure data (15-min TWA) were also submitted; most showed levels below 1.0 ppm, although certain groups had very variable exposures with some measurements in excess of 5 ppm (16 mg/m³). These situations frequently involved loading and unloading of barges or tanker trucks.

Several other mononuclear aromatic hydrocarbons were monitored in the CONCAWE (1987) study on gasoline and refineries, including toluene, the xylenes, the trimethylbenzenes and isopropylbenzene (cumene). Mean exposure levels were 6 mg/m³ for toluene, 4.2 mg/³ for the trimethylbenzenes and below 1 mg/m³ for the other hydrocarbons. Worker exposure to aromatic hydrocarbons has also been measured during the performance of various maintenance turn-round activities (Dynamac Corp., 1985). Median 8-h TWA concentrations of benzene, toluene, xylene and cumene were well below 1 mg 34m³ for all jobs. Higher exposure levels (maximum, 7 mg/m³ for benzene) were observed for a pipe fitter and a machinist.

Biological monitoring data on benzene exposure of gasoline-exposed workers are summarized in the monograph on gasoline.

2.4 Polynuclear aromatic compounds

Polynuclear aromatic compounds (PAC) are present in crude oil in various concentrations depending on its source. They are further concentrated in the high-boiling fractions and modified in structure by the various fractionation and cracking operations that yield PAC-containing intermediate or final products, such as gas oils, residual fuel oils, bitumen and coke. PAC are also present in solvent extracts of mineral oils and in waste waters.

Few data have been reported on exposure to PAC in petroleum refineries (Table 8). Three types of processing units have been investigated systematically in nine refineries in the USA (Futagaki, 1983). Personal samples taken in the fluid catalytic cracking unit and in the delayed coker unit both showed total PAC concentrations of 10 μg/m³. Area samples taken in bitumen processing units indicated levels ranging from about 1 to 40 µg/m³. In one refinery where personal samples were taken at the deasphalting unit, total PAC levels varied from 2.5 to 49.8 µg/m³. Of the 23 individual or groups of PAC that contributed to the total, including vapour phase and particulate matter, 10 or 11 were found on average in each sample. The average distribution of PAC indicated that at least 85% of the total PAC concentration was constituted by two-ring compounds (naphthalene and its derivatives) and 94% by two- or three-ring compounds. Compounds with five rings or more contributed from less than 0.1% at the catalytic cracker unit and 0.3% at the bitumen processing unit to 1.5% at the delayed coker unit. As an example, the highest concentration of benzo[a]pyrene plus benzo[e]pyrene was 9.3 µg/m³ in a personal sample from a coke cutter. In most samples, however, these two compounds were not detected (<0.01 µg/m³).

Loading of road tankers with bitumen in refineries has been associated with levels of <0.1 µg/m³ four- to six-ring PAC. Only particulate matter was collected. Concentrations of total particulate matter and benzene-soluble matter were not found to be reliable indices of exposure to these PAC in bitumen fumes (Brandt & Molyneux, 1985).

Personal exposure to several PAC has been evaluated during performance of turn-round operations on reaction and fractionator towers. Potential sources of PAC were residual coke and heavy distillate (Dynamac Corp., 1985). Naphthalene and its methyl derivatives accounted for more than 99% of the total concentration of PAC measured; exposure to anthracene, pyrene, chrysene and benzo[a]pyrene was either too low to be detected or ≤1 µg/m³. Area monitoring for the six PAC during normal activities as well as during shut-down, leak testing and start-up operations following turn-rounds has also been reported. Total concentrations at the various sites monitored (pumps, compressors) ranged up to 400 µg/m³, with the majority of measurements below 100 µg/m³. The distribution pattern of individual PAC was the same as that reported above.

2.5 Other exposures

(a) Aromatic amines and nitrosamines

Area samples taken at fluid catalytic cracking units, bitumen processing units and coker units in US refineries contained very low concentrations (<0.1 ppm (0.6 mg/m³) TWA) of *para*-anisidine in four of 17 samples and of *ortho*-anisidine and aniline in one of the four samples. No N,N-dimethylaniline, *ortho*-toluidine, 2,4-xylidine or *para*-nitroaniline was detected in any sample, and none of seven N-nitrosamines monitored (N-nitrosodimethylamine, N-nitrosodiethylamine, N-nitrosodi-n-propylamine, N-nitrosodibutylamine, N-nitrosopiperidine, N-nitrosopyrrolidine and N-nitrosomorpholine) was found in any sample at levels above the detection limit of 0.1 µg/m³ for a 20–30-l air sample (Futagaki, 1983).

(b) Asbestos

Asbestos has been used extensively in petroleum refineries, mainly as a thermal insulator and gasket material and for protective screens around welding operations on site. TWA (8 h) concentrations for employees working with pipe insulation have been estimated to range from 0.1–0.9 fibres less than 5 μm in length per ml of air on the basis of various measurements in one refinery (Darby et al., 1978). Measurements taken during turn-round activities in two refineries involving the removal of lagging, gaskets and insulation indicated 8-h TWA concentrations ranging from 0.01 to 0.15 fibres per ml of air. Lagging from a pipe on a flash tower was found to contain 50–60% amosite asbestos (Dynamac Corp., 1985). CONCAWE reported typical airborne levels of asbestos in the breathing zone of <0.01–0.02 fibres/cm^3 in insulation stripping, valve and joint repacking and overcladding asbestos insulation. Since the mid-to-late 1960s, most refineries have begen to replace asbestos with other materials.

(c) tert-*Butyl alcohol and methyl*-tert-*butyl ether*

A few groups of workers involved in the loading of gasoline have been found to be exposed to low average concentrations of these two gasoline additives. Mean 8-h TWA exposure levels, derived from 540 personal measurements of gasoline-exposed workers both inside and outside refineries, were: *tert*-butyl alcohol, 0.26 mg/m^3 (range, 0–30) and methyl-*tert*-butyl ether, 1.8 mg/m^3 (0–170; CONCAWE, 1987).

(d) *Coke dust*

Respirable dust concentrations measured while chipping petroleum coke at various locations during turn-round operations in two refineries were found to range from 1.04 to 8.19 mg/m^3 (four personal samples; 8-h TWA), while two measurements of total dust obtained during chipping coke operations inside a regenerator showed a very high level of 166 mg/m^3. Area samples taken during similar operations in one of the two refineries showed that there was potentially substantial worker exposure to coke dust (Dynamac Corp., 1985).

(e) *1,2-Dibromoethane (ethylene dibromide) and 1,2-dichloroethane (ethylene dichloride)*

These two substances are used as lead scavengers in leaded gasolines. Concentrations of 1,2-dibromoethane ranging from 0.23 to 1.65 μg/m^3 have been measured at two locations 50–400 ft [15–120 m] down wind of a bulk transfer and a tank truck loading operation. Since service station attendants have an 8-h TWA exposure of about 40 μg/m^3, it may be expected that refinery workers involved in the loading of gasoline are exposed to similar or higher levels (National Institute for Occupational Safety and Health, 1977).

1,2-Dichloroethane, which was used as an extraction solvent, was measured at four locations within one refinery at concentrations ranging from 40 to 800 mg/m^3 (National Institute for Occupational Safety and Health, 1976).

(f) *Furfural*

Some refineries utilize furfural to extract lubricant base stocks. According to CONCAWE, the 8-h TWA exposure for maintenance personnel is in the range <0.1–11.4 ppm (0.4–45 mg/m^3).

(g) Hydrazine

Solutions of hydrazine are sometimes used to scavenge oxygen in boiler feed-water. Normally, these would be handled in a closed system; however, relatively crude systems involving transfer of liquid from drums to the boiler feed-water have been used. According to CONCAWE, breathing-zone concentrations of hydrazine are usually 0.5 mg/m^3 or less for operators wearing respiratory protection. The operation typically lasts only several minutes and is carried out infrequently.

(h) Hydrogen fluoride

Hydrofluoric acid is used as a catalyst in alkylation units. In such a unit, exposure of plant operators and maintenance men to gaseous hydrogen fluoride has been found to range from below the detection limit of 0.005 mg/m^3 up to 0.18 mg/m^3. Changes in fluoride levels in the urine of workers over a shift were found only in subgroups of workers with higher routine exposures (Brown, 1985). According to CONCAWE, exposure values (8-h TWA) for a press operator are typically 0.1 mg/m^3 or less.

(i) Hydrogen sulfide

According to CONCAWE, levels of hydrogen sulfide to which workers are exposed are usually 2 ppm (3 mg/m^3) or less during normal operations. Specific tasks may involve a potential for significantly higher exposures.

(j) Ketones

Lubricating-dewaxing workers were found in one study to be exposed to methylethylketone at 8-h TWA levels of 1.03 ppm (3 mg/m^3; SD, 2.94; 82 personal samples); less than 5% of these samples contained >5 ppm (15 mg/m^3; Wen et al., 1985). Exposures of <0.1–132 ppm (<0.3–400 mg/m^3; 8-h TWA) were measured by CONCAWE in lubricating oil extraction facilities and of 0.1–162 ppm (0.3–480 mg/m^3; 8-h TWA) for maintenance personnel.

(k) Metal welding fumes

Personal 8-h TWA measurements of iron oxide, chromium, nickel, lead and manganese fumes have been reported covering 15 cutting and welding activities during turn-round operations. In only one location was a high chromium level found, to a maximum of 1.61 mg/m^3 (Dynamac Corp., 1985).

(l) Oil mists

Airborne concentrations of oil mists in the range of 0.1–0.34 mg/m^3 (8-h TWA) have been reported by CONCAWE in a lubricating oil blending plant, while area concentrations recorded in a crude oil distillation unit ranged from <0.1 to 23 mg/m^3.

(m) *Silica*

Measurements of respirable dust containing free crystalline silica were made in one refinery during various turn-round operations, and TWA (8-h) concentrations were compared with permissible exposure limits, taking into account the percentage of free silica. All ratios of TWA concentrations to permissible exposure limits were at one or above: removing firebricks on heater for thermal cracking unit, 1–1.6; installing refractory bricks on same heater, 5.4; sandblasting fractionator, 30–60 (Dynamac Corp., 1985).

(n) *Sodium hydroxide and phosphoric acid*

Area samples taken during turn-round operations in the sulfur treating process in one refinery indicated levels of about 0.1 mg/m^3 sodium hydroxide, while none was detected near caustic circulating pumps. Personal samples taken on workers at the polymerization column during removal and replacement of phosphoric acid-containing catalyst indicated 8-h TWA exposures to phosphoric acid of 0.07–0.1 mg/m^3 for loading fresh catalyst (Dynamac Corp., 1985).

(o) *Tetraalkyllead*

CONCAWE reported typical airborne concentrations of tetraalkyllead (predominantly tetraethyllead) corresponding to various tasks: handling tanker delivery — 0.03–0.11 mg/m^3 (breathing zone, short-term monitoring); cutting/welding on tanks which had contained leaded gasoline — 0.004–0.11 mg/m^3 (breathing zone, short-term monitoring), 0.003-0.004 mg/m^3 (breathing zone, 8-h TWA). General airborne concentrations (>1 h) of 0.005–5.7 mg/m^3 have been reported in a variety of areas, including operator changing rooms, tank welding/cutting, proximity to tank valves, dip pipes and vacuum pumps.

(p) *Vanadium pentoxide and nickel oxides*

The combustion of heavy fuel oils in boilers and furnaces in refinery process units results in the deposition of oxides of vanadium and nickel in furnace boxes, associated ducting and tubes. Cleaning and maintenance of this equipment can result in exposure to the dust from these metal oxides. CONCAWE reported typical breathing-zone concentrations for these tasks as <2 mg/m^3 vanadium oxide and <0.01 mg/m^3 nickel oxides for preparatory work and removal of furnace fire bricks; <0.5 mg/m^3 vanadium oxide and <0.01 mg nickel oxides for furnace inspection; and 0.3–14 mg/m^3 vanadium oxide and 0.1–7.5 mg/m^3 nickel oxides for removal of scaffolding. These values are reported as 8-h TWAs, except for removal of scaffolding. [No data were available to the Working Group regarding exposures to nickel compounds during the loading and unloading of nickel catalyst. However, it is known that this is a short-term operation carried out infrequently.]

3. Biological Data Relevant to the Evaluation of Carcinogenic Risk to Humans

3.1 Carcinogenicity studies in animals[1]

(a) Skin application

(i) *Uncracked distillates and residues of crude oils*

Some studies on the carcinogenicity of untreated vacuum distillates (light or heavy paraffinic or naphthenic distillates [19A, 19B, 20A, 20B] (Bingham & Barkley, 1979; Kane *et al.*, 1984) were reported in a previous volume (IARC, 1984).

Mouse: In a series of experiments, Blackburn *et al.* (1984, 1986) tested a number of undiluted samples derived from the refining of crude oil. In each experiment, groups of 50 male C3H/HeJ mice, six to eight weeks old, were given twice weekly applications of 50 mg of the samples on shaven interscapular skin for 80 weeks or until a papilloma larger than 1 mm^3 appeared. Skin tumour incidence [histologically unspecified] was evaluated in mice surviving at the time at which one-half of the tumour-bearing animals had developed their tumour (or at 60 weeks, whichever came first). The controls consisted of seven groups of 50 mice treated similarly with toluene and four groups of 50 mice that were only shaven. Three skin tumours were seen in the toluene-treated controls and none in the others. The results are shown in Table 9. [The Working Group noted that treatment was suspended in mice that developed a papilloma larger than 1 mm^3 and that details were not given about time of killing or survival of treated and control mice.]

(ii) *Cracked distillates and residues*

Some studies on the carcinogenicity of certain catalytically cracked oils and residues (light and heavy catalytically cracked distillates [24, 26] and catalytically cracked clarified oil [27]; Smith *et al.*, 1951; Shubik & Saffiotti, 1955; Saffiotti & Shubik, 1963; Bingham & Barkley, 1979) were reported in a previous volume (IARC, 1984). Experiments by Blackburn *et al.* (1984, 1986), with the same experimental design as outlined above, are summarized in Table 10.

Mouse: Groups of 30 mice [strain, sex and age unspecified] received thrice weekly skin applications of cracking residues from crude oils (type of cracking unspecified [27 or 31]) of different origins [dose unspecified] for ten months. In one group treated with a cracking residue from Dolinsk crude oil (11.6% paraffins), 12/28 mice developed skin tumours (eight

---

[1]The Working Group was aware of several skin-painting studies in progress in mice using various petroleum distillates (straight-run middle distillate [6], light paraffinic distillate [19A], light catalytically cracked distillate [24], hydrotreated heavy naphthenic distillate [20D], hydrotreated light naphthenic distillate [19B], hydrodesulfurized middle distillate [6A]), naphthas (heavy catalytically cracked naphtha [23], alkylate naphtha [13], heavy reformed naphtha [17], straight-run kerosene [5], hydrodesulfurized kerosene [5B], heavy thermally cracked naphtha [29], sweetened naphtha), catalytically cracked clarified oil [27] and vacuum residue [21] (IARC, 1986). Numbers correspond to streams described in Table 2 and Figure 1 of this monograph.

Table 9. Results of experiments by Blackburn et al. (1986) on undiluted uncracked distillates and residues of crude oils

No. of groups	Sample	No. of survivors	No. with skin tumours	Average latent period (weeks)
One	Light paraffinic distillate (CAS No. 64741-50-0) [19]	42	27	35
One	Heavy paraffinic distillate (CAS No. 64741-51-1) [20A]	34	31	34
Four	Heavy naphthenic distillate (CAS No. 64741-53-3) [20B]	38 34 27 29	31 25 16 21	50 48 38 42
Two	Straight-run kerosene (CAS No. 8008-20-6) [5]	30 27	9 4	70 62
One	Hydrotreated kerosene (CAS No. 64742-47-8) [5A]	38	24	79
One	Light straight-run naphtha (CAS No. 64741-46-4) [3]	44	11	85
One	Vacuum residue (CAS No. 64741-56-6) [21]	43	1	70
Two	Hydrotreated heavy naphthenic distillate (CAS No. 64742-52-5) [20D]	41 25	36 21	51 57
One	Chemically neutralized/hydrotreated heavy naphthenic distillate (CAS No. 64742-34-3/64742-52-5) [20C/20D]	20	12	52

carcinomas). In a further group treated with a cracking residue from Bitkovsk crude oil (14% paraffins), eight papillomas developed in 13 survivors. In another group, no tumour developed after treatment with a cracking residue from Tuimazinsk crude oil (5.9% paraffins) [number of survivors unspecified] (Shapiro & Getmanets, 1962). [The Working Group noted the inadequate reporting of the data and the lack of information on the nature of the cracking process.]

Three groups of albino mice [strain, sex and age unspecified] received thrice weekly skin applications of residues from thermal cracking [31] from two crude oils [dose unspecified] for ten months. One group of 30 mice was treated with fresh residue from Dolinsk crude (11.6% paraffins) and developed 11 skin tumours (five carcinomas). A second group of 30 mice treated with the same residue after it had been stored for three years developed seven skin tumours (one carcinoma). A third group of 60 mice treated with a residue from Grozny crude oil ('low' in paraffins) developed three small papillomas (Getmanets, 1967). [The Working Group noted the inadequate reporting of the data and the lack of controls.]

Table 10. Experiments by Blackburn et al. (1984, 1986) on distillates and residues from cracking

No. of groups	Sample	Dose (mg)	No. of survivors	No. with skin tumours	Average latent period (weeks)	Controls
One	Intermediate cataly-cracked distillate (CAS No. 64741-60-2) [25]	50	43	42	16	No skin tumour in 200 sham-treated controls (shaving only)
One	50% mixture of heavy catalytically cracked distillate (CAS No. 64741-61-3) [26] and catalytically cracked clarified oil (CAS No. 64741-62-4) [27] in toluene	25	37	34	21	Three skin tumours in 300 toluene-treated controls

In a series of experiments, Lewis (1983) tested different samples derived from the refining of crude oil. Groups of 10–30 male C3H mice [age unspecified] received weekly, twice weekly or thrice weekly [exact details not given] skin applications of 50 or 100 mg of the samples at a weekly dose of 100–300 mg for 18 months or until a cancer was observed grossly. No control was available. The substances tested were ten samples of higher-boiling fractions from noncatalytic cracking [presumably thermal cracking] residues [31], seven lower-boiling distillate fractions from catalytically cracked oils [24, 26] [sources unspecified] and 19 higher-boiling residual fractions from catalytically cracked oils [27] [sources unspecified]. The samples (characterized by the percentage of distillation yields of <400°C or 400–500°C and benzo[a]pyrene content) produced high numbers of skin tumours [proportions of benign and malignant not given]. No correlation between distillation range, benzo[a]pyrene content, tumour incidence or time to appearance of the first tumour could be demonstrated for the higher-boiling fractions. A correlation between benzo[a]pyrene content and tumour yield was found for the distillates and between benzo[a]pyrene content and average tumour latency for the residues. [The Working Group noted that the author was not the original investigator of the study, which was conducted in the 1950s, the inadequate reporting and the lack of controls.]

A group of 120 female white outbred mice, three months old, received thrice weekly skin applications of about 30–40 mg of a heavy catalytic gas oil (heavy catalytically cracked distillate [26]; maximal number of paintings, 105) and were then observed for life. A group of 120 untreated mice from the same colony served as controls. Survival of treated animals was 24–334 days (average, 213 days) and 365 days (average) for controls. The first skin papilloma appeared at 15 days, after six applications; after eight applications, seven mice had papillomas. Treatment was discontinued for 22 days because of episodic disease, during which time all papillomas regressed. On resumption of treatment, the first papillomas appeared after nine subsequent applications. A total of 97 animals had skin tumours (effective number of mice at time of appearance of the first tumour, 106); of these, 76 had malignant tumours. No skin tumour was observed in controls (effective number, 70). Precancerous lesions, including leukoplakia, dysplasia and papillomas, sometimes in combination, occurred in the oesophagus and forestomach of 55/106 treated animals. Tumours of the oesophagus were found in two treated animals and in none of the controls; forestomach tumours were found in 55 treated animals (51.8%) and in one (1.4%) control. An increased incidence of leukaemia was reported in treated animals (Karimov et al., 1984, 1986). [The Working Group noted the high loss of a number of control animals and the lack of detailed histology, particularly of the leukaemias.]

Three groups of 25 male and 25 female C3H/Bd$_f$ mice, six to eight weeks of age, received thrice weekly applications of 50 μl of a sample of light catalytically cracked naphtha (API-976) [22], either undiluted or diluted 1:1 or 1:3 in acetone, on a 1-cm^2 area of dorsal skin for life or until a tumour persisted for two weeks, at which time the animal was killed. Results for the pooled sexes and three dose levels showed that, of 150 mice, 15 developed skin tumours (11 carcinomas, four papillomas). All but one of the tumours developed between 85 and 115 weeks. No tumour was observed in 100 untreated or in 100 acetone-treated controls of either sex (Witschi et al., 1987). [The Working Group noted that the distribution of tumours among the various groups was not reported.]

A group of 40 C3H/HeJ mice [sex unspecified], seven weeks of age, received skin applications of undiluted samples of 'water-quench' or 'oil-quench' pyrolysis fuel oil (steam-cracked residues [34]) [dose unspecified] thrice weekly for life (19 months). Benzo[a]pyrene, the only component measured, was found in the samples at concentrations of 300—500 ppm (mg/l). Two concurrent control groups received skin applications of benzene (solvent controls for other concurrent experiments) or distilled water. In mice treated with water-quench pyrolysis fuel oil, 36 papillomas and 35 squamous-cell carcinomas of the skin developed in 37 effective[1] animals, and, in mice treated with oil-quench pyrolysis fuel oil, 34 papillomas and 34 carcinomas were observed in 39 effective animals. The mean latent period for papilloma development was 10.2—10.3 months and that for carcinoma development was 12.2—12.1 months for both samples. No skin tumour developed among the benzene- or distilled water-treated controls (Weil & Condra, 1977).

Rabbit: Two groups of ten rabbits [strain, sex and age unspecified] received thrice weekly skin applications of residues from thermal cracking [31] of two crude oils [dose unspecified] for 10—17 months. The group treated with fresh residue from Dolinsk crude oil (11.6% paraffins) developed skin tumours [number unspecified]. The group treated with residue from Grozny crude oil ('low' in paraffins) developed 'fewer' tumours than those treated with Dolinsk residue (Shapiro & Getmanets, 1962). [The Working Group noted the inadequate reporting of the data.]

---

[1]The 'effective group' was defined by the authors as the number of mice given adequate exposure, calculated from the original number of mice started minus the number that died without a tumour. It is therefore a variable number that decreases by one with each non tumour death and is arbitrarily held constant after the time of the appearance of a tumour in the median tumour-bearing mouse.

(iii) *Effluents*

Mouse: Groups of male C57Bl mice, eight to ten weeks of age, received twice-weekly applications of a drop of test material on a 1-cm² area of upper dorsal skin for a total of 17 months, with a one-month interval after the first six months, due to toxicity. Group 1 (40 mice) was treated with undiluted extract of the effluent from a gravity oil separator at an oil refinery [source unspecified], containing 75% aliphatic and 20% aromatic hydrocarbons, collected through carbon for approximately one month in winter. Group 2 (40 mice) was treated for five months with the same sample diluted 1:1 with methyl ethyl ketone, then with undiluted sample as Group 1. The combined results showed an average survival of 13 months, an effective number of 59 mice at the time of the first tumour and a total of four papillomas and one carcinoma in 38 mice examined histologically. A control group of 25 mice was treated with methyl ethyl ketone for four months (treatment was discontinued due to high toxicity) and observed for a further 14 months. Average survival was five months, and no tumour was observed (Hueper & Ruchhoft, 1954). [The Working Group noted that the controls were inadequate and that the test samples were toxic.]

(b) *Other routes of administration*

Fish: Soxhlet (particulates) and XAD-2 resin (water) extracts of an oil refinery effluent, dissolved in acetone, were injected into eggs of rainbow trout (*Salmo gairdneri*, Kamloops strain), and trout that hatched from the injected eggs were necropsied at 12 or 24 months of age. Single injections of 6 μg Soxhlet extract or of 4 μg XAD-2 resin extract (equivalent to 200 μl effluent) from a sample taken in 1981, with or without preincubation with rat-liver S9 mix, yielded no tumour at necropsy [time unspecified] in groups of 30 trout; no tumour was found in two groups of 25 trout derived from eggs injected with 4.5 μg of Soxhlet extract from a sample taken in 1982 (Metcalfe & Sonstegard, 1985).

3.2 Other relevant data

(a) *Experimental systems*

Absorption, distribution, excretion and metabolism

Dermal absorption studies were performed with clarified slurry oil (catalytically cracked clarified oil [27]) containing radiolabelled surrogates representative of key chemical classes (carbazole, benzo[*a*]pyrene and phenanthrene) at a dose of 20 mg/cm² in four female Sprague-Dawley rats. Of the applied radioactivity, 48% of ^{14}C-carbazole, 5% of ^{3}H-benzo[*a*]pyrene and 21% of ^{14}C-phenanthrene added to the clarified oil were recovered in urine and faeces within four days or remained in the carcass, excluding the pelt (Cruzan *et al.*, 1986).

Toxic effects

In a 13-week dermal toxicity study, groups of ten male and ten female Sprague-Dawley rats received applications of clarified slurry oil (catalytically cracked clarified oil [27]) on their clipped backs on five consecutive days per week at doses of 0, 8, 30, 125, 500 or 2000 mg/kg bw per day. Primary targets of this treatment were found to be the liver, thymus and bone marrow. Liver enlargement, increases in plasma enzymes and liver-cell degeneration, necrosis and fibrosis were observed; some effects were evident at the lowest dose. The thymus was atrophic, and bone marrow showed erythroid hypoplasia at doses of ⩾30 mg/kg bw per day, with accompanying anaemia (Cruzan *et al.*, 1986).

Twenty-one-day inhalation studies were performed with seven petroleum naphtha streams in groups of ten male and ten female or 20 male Sprague-Dawley rats. The treatment groups were exposed to vapours of the test materials for 6 h per day on five days per week for a total of 15 exposures. Three of the naphthas — light straight-run naphtha [3] (1.50, 5.13 or 14.56 mg/l analytical TWA), full-range alkylate naphtha [13] (vapour concentrations, 1.54, 4.92 or 15.31 mg/l) and thermally cracked naphtha [28, 29] (1.13, 3.48 or 9.88 mg/l analytical TWA) — produced severe renal toxicity, degenerative changes and tubular dilatation in male rats, but not in female rats. The lesions consisted of excessive hyaline droplet formation in the epithelium of the proximal convoluted tubules, degenerative changes in the proximal convoluted tubules of the renal cortex and tubular dilatation and necrosis at the cortico-medullary junction. Two of the naphthas — light reformed naphtha [16] (2.00, 5.85 or 20.30 mg/l analytical TWA) and polymerization naphtha [10] (1.04, 3.05 or 9.89 mg/l analytical TWA) — produced a small, dose-related incidence of renal tubular necrosis at the cortico-medullary junction in male rats. Treatment with light catalytically cracked naphtha [22] (0.20, 2.04 or 13.06 mg/l analytical TWA) produced mild nephrotoxicity in males; heavy reformed naphtha [17] (1.03, 2.81 or 10.20 mg/l analytical TWA) did not induce any adverse renal effect (Halder *et al.*, 1984).

Aromatic-rich C_9–C_{10} and C_{11}–C_{12} fractions from reformed naphtha [15] samples were studied in rats, monkeys and mice. Rats exposed by inhalation to 616 ppm of the C_9–C_{10} fraction for 18 h per day on seven days per week for 19 weeks developed cataracts after an additional two months without exposure. Rats exposed to the same concentrations for 18 h on three alternate days and set aside nine months for observation did not develop such ocular changes. Groups of three monkeys were exposed by inhalation to 50 or 200 ppm of the C_9–C_{10} fraction for 7 h per day on five days per week for a total of 90 exposures; no significant gross or microscopic change was observed. [The Working Group noted that details were not given as to which organs and tissues were examined.] Application of 0.10–0.15 g of the C_9–C_{10} fraction on the skin of male C3H mice three times per week for 50 weeks led to skin changes (inflammation, hyperkeratosis, atrophy) and kidney damage (cortical scarring, sclerosis, papillary necrosis). Similar treatment with the C_{11}–C_{12} fraction induced similar skin changes, but microscopic examination revealed no renal change (Nau *et al.*, 1966).

Effects on reproduction and prenatal toxicity

No data were available to the Working Group.

Genetic and related effects

Some studies on the mutagenicity in *Salmonella typhimurium* of vacuum distillates [19, 20] and hydrotreated oil (CAS 64742-57-0) were reported in a previous volume (IARC, 1984).

Dimethyl sulfoxide (DMSO) extracts of six petroleum hydrocarbon samples with boiling-points in the range of 260–538°C were examined for mutagenic activity by preincubation in *S. typhimurium* TA98 in the presence of an exogenous metabolic system from Aroclor 1254-induced rat-liver S9. A mixture of heavy catalytically cracked distillate [26] and catalytically cracked clarified oil [27] produced the highest (280 revertants/μl) response. Mutagenic effects were also seen with five other samples: light paraffinic distillate [19A]; intermediate catalytically cracked distillate [25]; two samples described as a hydrotreated heavy naphthenic distillate [20D]; and a mixture of chemically neutralized heavy naphthenic distillate [20C] and hydrotreated heavy naphthenic distillate [20D] (Blackburn *et al.*, 1984).

Using modified procedures, including DMSO extraction of petroleum oils dissolved in cyclohexane, the activity of 15 petroleum oil samples in *S. typhimurium* TA98 in the presence of an exogenous metabolic system from Aroclor 1254-induced Syrian golden hamster liver S9 was seemingly dependent on the refining process and the boiling range of the mixtures. At 5 μl/plate, the active samples were intermediate catalytically cracked distillate [25] and a mixture of heavy catalytically cracked distillate [26] and catalytically cracked clarified oil [27]. Some activity was also observed at 50 μl/plate of heavy paraffinic distillate [20A]; light paraffinic distillate [19A]; two samples described as hydrotreated heavy naphthenic distillates [20D]; chemically neutralized/hydrotreated heavy naphthenic distillate [20C, 20D], which was used as a positive control; four samples described as heavy naphthenic distillate [20B]; and two samples of straight-run kerosene [5]. No activity was observed with light straight-run naphtha [3], hydrotreated kerosene [5A] or vacuum residue [21] (Blackburn *et al.*, 1986). As reported in an abstract, hydrogenated pyrolysis gasoline [near 33] induced transformed foci in both BALBc/3T3 and C3H/10T1/2 cells (Butala *et al.*, 1985).

Methanol extracts of suspended particulates in effluents from three refineries in Ontario, Canada, were weakly active in *S. typhimurium* TA100 in the presence of an exogenous metabolic system from Aroclor 1254-induced rat-liver S9 but not in *S. typhimurium* TA98 or in either strain in the absence of S9. A methanol extract from one of the three refineries induced sister chromatid exchange in cultured Chinese hamster ovary cells in the presence of an exogenous metabolic system from Aroclor 1254-induced rat-liver S9 (Metcalfe *et al.*, 1985).

Elevated mutation rates were observed in *Zea mays* (waxy system) planted in native soil and in pots of clear artificial soil placed in the vicinity of a petroleum refinery in Illinois, USA (Lower *et al.*, 1983).

(b) Humans

Absorption, distribution, excretion and metabolism

No data were available to the Working Group.

Toxic effects

In an early study, workers engaged in paraffin refining at the beginning of the century were reported to have an acute acneform, papular skin eruption, often with severely inflamed nodules and furuncles; a chronic stage with patchy dryness, hyperkeratosis, scaling and fissuring progressing to multiple warty growths was also reported (Davis, 1914). Several other studies have shown adverse skin effects (dermatosis, acne-like changes) among petroleum refinery workers (Žuškin & Žuškin, 1964; Bruevich, 1971; Ruszczak et al., 1981a,b).

Sensitive biochemical and immunological markers of nephrotoxicity were compared in 53 male petroleum refinery workers and 61 age-matched unexposed males. In petroleum refinery workers employed for an average of 11 years (8-h personal TWA hydrocarbon exposure at the time of the study, $1-156$ mg/m^3), no change was seen in urinary β-N-acetyl-D-glucosaminidase, β_2-microglobulin or retinol-binding protein, in glomerular filtration or in levels of serum circulating immune complexes. There were slight elevations in albuminuria and in mean urinary excretion of a renal antigen (BB-50) in the exposed group and slightly higher titres of antilaminin antibodies in five exposed workers, but no clinically significant renal abnormality was seen (Viau et al., 1987).

Effects on reproduction and prenatal toxicity

Of 408 women employed in petroleum processing plants in the USSR, 27.7% reported disruption of menstrual function, compared to 10.9% of 302 women employed in a garment factory (Sukhanova & Melnikova, 1974). Frequency of menstrual dysfunction increased with increasing duration of employment and was highest among women who worked in the technological laboratories and were continuously exposed to petroleum products at high concentrations. The most common forms of menstrual dysfunction reported by the petroleum processing workers were hypomenorrhoea and premenstrual syndrome. [The Working Group noted that the methods were not well described, and that the ages of all subjects were not given.]

Menstrual and child-bearing functions of 894 women employed in three petroleum processing plants in the USSR were compared with those of 500 women who worked in a machine building plant (Shamsadinskaya et al., 1976). The age distribution was reported to be comparable in the two groups. At the time of interview, 29.7% of the women employed in petroleum processing and 16.7% of the machine factory workers reported gynaecological problems. The most common disturbances reported were 'inflammatory disease' and disturbances of the menstrual cycle. A higher proportion of those employed in petroleum processing were reported to be sterile, and they had a greater rate of spontaneous abortion. [The Working Group noted that the methods were not well described.]

In a study of fetal loss among 89 wives of workers employed in a waste-water treatment plant at a petroleum refinery in Louisiana, USA (Anon., 1985), pregnancy histories were obtained by interviewing the wives, and employment histories for the men were obtained from company records (Morgan et al., 1984). Each pregnancy was classified by the exposure of the father to the waste-water treatment process during the pregnancy (unexposed; E1, any time prior to conception; E2, within four months prior to conception; and E3, three months after conception). The three 'exposed' categories overlapped; thus, a pregnancy could be classified into all three on the basis of the paternal work history. For each category, rates of fetal loss (miscarriage or stillbirth) were calculated. Odds ratios were calculated by dividing fetal loss rates among the exposed pregnancies by the fetal loss rate for unexposed pregnancies. The odds ratios for E1, E2 and E3 (95% confidence interval) were 2.1 (0.9–4.5), 2.9 (1.3–6.3) and 2.9 (1.4–6.4), respectively. The wives of crafts (maintenance) workers in waste-water treatment experienced a higher risk (odds ratio, 4.9) of fetal loss than did those of production workers (odds ratio, 0.85). [The Working Group noted that caution should be exercised in interpreting the results of this study, since the authors were uncertain about whether their data represented statistical artefact, reporting bias or biological reality.]

A cross-sectional evaluation of sperm concentration and abnormal morphology was conducted among men who had worked in the same waste-water treatment plant described above during the six months prior to the beginning of the study (Rosenberg et al., 1985). A total of 68% of the exposed workers participated in the study (n = 42). Refinery workers who did not work in waste-water treatment were chosen as controls, and the participation rate was 44% (n = 74). A stepwise regression model was used to compare outcomes controlling for age, sexual abstinence, other occupational exposures, use of prescribed drugs, smoking, marijuana use, alcohol consumption and other factors. No significant difference between sperm concentration or the proportion of abnormal morphology was found between the exposed and unexposed workers. [The Working Group noted that slightly over half of the 'unexposed' group (n = 38) were process or mechanical workers in the refinery and could have had other significant occupational exposures that were not taken into account in the analyses.]

Genetic and related effects

As reported in an abstract, an increase in the incidence of sister chromatid exchange was observed in about half of 22 workers with at least ten years of employment in petroleum refining as compared to 18 unexposed individuals controlled for smoking habits and use of medications (Carrano et al., 1980).

In an extensive cytogenetic study in China, both chromosomal aberrations and sister chromatid exchange were examined in peripheral blood lymphocytes of 180 workers in a petrochemical plant and 180 matched controls. Among 30 persons working in a catalytic cracking unit, there was no significant difference in either of the two parameters studied; however, a group of 30 persons working in the sewage-treatment unit of this catalytic cracking unit showed significantly higher mean sister chromatid exchange levels ($p < 0.01$) and increased prevalences of chromatid-type aberrations ($p < 0.001$) and of gaps ($p < 0.001$), as compared to the control group. [The Working Group noted that the increase in the frequency of chromatid-type aberrations was also significant ($p < 0.01$) for workers in the sewage-treatment unit of the phenolacetone plastic unit of the petrochemical plant.] A significant effect on the frequency of sister chromatid exchange was observed among smokers in both the control and worker groups (Zhou et al., 1986). [The Working Group noted that the analysis of chromosomal aberrations was performed in 72-h cultures.]

3.3 Epidemiological studies and case reports of carcinogenicity to humans

(a) Cohort studies

The cohorts of refinery workers reviewed below had mortality rates for all cancers combined that were consistently lower (10-20%) than those in the general population. It is well recognized that occupational cohorts tend to have below-average mortality, both from all causes and from various major categories of specific causes. These deficits are, typically, manifestations of a health status-related selection process, referred to as the 'healthy worker effect'. The consistent deficit in cancer mortality in refinery workers, when compared with the general population, is compatible with this effect.

In view of this overall deficit in cancer mortality in refinery workers, conventional statistical evaluation of site-specific standardized mortality ratios (SMRs) may be conservative. That is, comparison of the SMR with an 'expected' value of 1.0 derived from the general population — rather than with the underlying SMR for all cancers — may underestimate the true magnitude of any occupation-related increase in risk for specific cancers.

The Working Group also noted the limitations inherent in proportionate mortality analyses in which an over- or underrepresentation of some causes of death influences the magnitude of the proportionate mortality ratio (PMR) for other causes.

The available cohort studies are summarized in Table 11.

(i) *USA*

A series of studies of employees of the Exxon (also known as Humble and Esso) Company in the USA began with a report published in 1940 describing cancer mortality and incidence among male employees of a petroleum refining company who were enrolled in a sickness benefit plan between 1933 and 1938 (Gafafer & Sitgreaves, 1940). A total of 70 cases of cancer were observed among men who contributed about 60 000 person-years of risk during the study period. There were 46 deaths from cancer; 19 were stomach cancer and 13 were cancers of other abdominal organs. The authors noted that the proportion of digestive cancer deaths observed in the study group (69.6%) was higher than that observed in the general US population (57.8%); however, this comparison was not adjusted for age.

Cancer mortality among 15 437 employees of the Humble Oil Company in the Gulf Coast states was examined for a 29-year period ending in 1963 (Baird, 1967). This study included plants previously studied by Gafafer and Sitgreaves (1940), Hendricks *et al.* (1959) and Wade (1963) and consisted of workers in exploration, pipeline, production, refining and sales operations. The proportion of cancer deaths for the period 1935-55 among Humble Oil employees was 12.1% compared with 13.8% for the USA in 1945, unadjusted for age. The proportion of cancer deaths among the 6239 company employees who had worked in petroleum refining was 11.2%. The author concluded that there was no relative excess of cancer deaths among Humble Oil Company employees. [The Working Group noted that there was no adjustment for age, sex or race, and that cancer mortality was not presented by site, length of service or work category (e.g., production, maintenance, office workers).]

Table 11. Cohort studies of petroleum refinery workers

Reference	Study subjects[a]	Comparison population	Period of follow-up	Occupation/ exposure	Cancer site (cause of death)	Number of deaths observed	SMR[b]	Comments
USA[c]								
Hendricks et al. (1959)	82 wax pressmen, Exxon, Baton Rouge, LA	US men	1937–56	Wax pressmen	Scrotum (skin)	11		Incidence rate of 806/100 000 observed vs 0.15/100 000 expected
Hanis et al. (1982)	8666 workers at Exxon, Baton Rouge, LA (refinery and chemical plant)	US general population	1970–77		All causes	1199	0.92*	
					All cancer	249	0.92	
					Pancreas	23	1.5	
					Kidney	9	1.6	
				Operators, mechanics, labourers	Kidney	9	2.1	
				Men hired before 1956	Kidney	9	1.6	
					Pancreas	23	1.5	
Hanis et al. (1985a)	15 437 employees of Exxon, Baton Rouge, LA, Bayway/Bayonne, NJ, & Baytown, TX	US general population	1970–77	Refinery and chemical plant workers	All causes	3198	0.91*	Cancer death rates were higher among 'potentially exposed' than 'unexposed' workers (Hanis et al., 1985b)
					All cancer	666	0.94	
					Liver/gallbladder/ bile duct	15	1.3	
					Kidney	22	1.4	
					Brain	15	1.2	
				Baytown, TX	Bone	7	1.6	
					Kidney	6	1.2	
					Brain	6	1.3	
				Bayway/Bayonne, NJ	Stomach	16	1.4	
					Large intestine	32	1.4	
					Lung	77	1.2	
					Kidney	7	1.5	
				Baton Rouge, LA	Pancreas	23	1.5	
					Kidney	9	1.6	

Table 11 (contd)

Reference	Study subjects[a]	Comparison population	Period of follow-up	Occupation/ exposure	Cancer site (cause of death)	Number of deaths observed	SMR[b]	Comments
Thomas et al. (1980)	1722 white male OCAW members in TX	US men	1947–77	Petroleum refinery chemical plant workers	All cancer	394	1.3*	Proportionate mortality study including deaths only among active Union members
					Digestive tract	111	1.2*	
					Respiratory tract	134	1.3*	
					Skin	14	1.9*	
					Brain	25	1.8*	
Thomas et al. (1982a,b)	2509 male OCAW members employed by 3 TX oil refineries	US men	1943–79		All cancer	553	1.2*	Proportionate mortality study including deaths among active and retired Union members
					Stomach	48	1.5*	
					Pancreas	37	1.4*	
					Lung	157	1.1	
					Skin	13	1.8*	
					Prostate	46	1.4*	
					Kidney	15	1.4	
					Brain	28	2.2*	
					Leukaemia	33	1.8*	
					Multiple myeloma	9	2.0	
Thomas et al. (1984)	Male OCAW members employed by 3 TX oil refineries	Internal comparison	1943–79	Intraplant pumping and transport of bulk liquids	Brain	7	2.8	Odds ratios from nested case-control study (Thomas et al., 1982a,b)
				Lubricating oil	Stomach	19	1.7	
				Maintenance work	Stomach	47	4.5	
				Treating	Leukaemia	6	1.6	
				Boiler makers	Leukaemia	5	1.5	
Divine et al. (1985)	19 077 white men employed 5+ years by Texaco	US white men	1947–77	Refinery, petrochemical, research	All causes	4024	0.75*	[Includes workers from refinery A (Thomas et al., 1980, 1982a,b, 1984)] Significant deficits of cancers of the stomach, large intestine, lung and bladder
					All cancer	767	0.75*	
					Pancreas	62	1.1	
					Brain	31	1.1	
					Leukaemia	48	1.2	
					Other lymphatic cancer	25	1.2	
					Benign neoplasms	20	1.5	

Table 11 (contd)

Reference	Study subjects[a]	Comparison population	Period of follow-up	Occupation/ exposure	Cancer site (cause of death)	Number of deaths observed	SMR[b]	Comments
Divine & Barron (1986)	18 798 white men employed 5+ years by Texaco	US white men	1947–77	Refinery operators, >1 year	Brain	19	1.2	Includes all men studied by Divine et al. (1985) for whom work histories were available
					Leukaemia	31	1.4	
					Other lymphatic cancer	16	1.3	
					Benign neoplasms	9	1.2	
				Maintenance work, >5 years	Pancreas	30	1.4	
					Kidney	12	1.3	
					Skin	8	1.3	
					Brain	13	1.3	
					Hodgkin's disease	6	1.4	
					Other lymphatic cancer	13	1.6	
					Benign neoplasms	8	1.6	
				Laboratory worker, >5 years	Brain	6	2.2	
					Benign neoplasms	3	2.6	
				Pipe fitters and boiler makers, >5 years	Leukaemia	12	2.9*	
Wen et al. (1983)	15 095 men employed at least 1 day at Gulf, Port Arthur, TX	US men	1937–78		All causes	4269	0.84*	[Includes workers from Refinery B (Thomas et al., 1980, 1982a,b, 1984)] Significant deficits of cancers of the oesophagus, liver, bladder and rectum and of lymphosarcoma and reticulosarcoma
					All cancer	839	0.96	
					Bone	11	2.1*	
					Skin	16	1.2	
					Kidney	22	1.1	
					Hodgkin's disease	16	1.5	
					Leukaemia	38	1.1	
					Other lymphatic cancer	20	1.2	

Table 11 (contd)

Reference	Study subjects[a]	Comparison population	Period of follow-up	Occupation/ exposure	Cancer site (cause of death)	Number of deaths observed	SMR[b]	Comments
				White blue-collar workers	Pancreas	37	1.1	
					Lung	185	1.1	
					Skin	13	1.2	
					Prostate	54	1.2	
					Kidney	18	1.2	
					Eye	2	3.4	
					Leukaemia	32	1.3	
					Hodgkin's disease	9	1.1	
					Bone	9	2.3*	
Wen et al. (1984b)	12 526 white men employed at least 1 day at Gulf, Port Arthur, TX	US white men	1937–78	Actively employed workers	Bone	3	1.6	Includes white men studied by Wen et al. (1983)
					Kidney	8	1.4	
					Leukaemia	14	1.6	
				Terminated workers before retirement	Lung	87	1.2	
					Bone	3	2.2	
					Skin	7	1.6	
					Prostate	16	1.3	
					Hodgkin's disease	6	1.6	
				Retirees	Lung	77	1.2	
					Bone	3	2.5	
					Skin	4	1.2	
					Prostate	37	1.1	
					Kidney	7	1.3	
					Brain	5	1.2	
					Leukaemia	16	1.6	
					Other lymphatic cancer	8	1.6	
Wen et al. (1982)	17 251 male and female workers employed at least 1 day at Gulf, Port Arthur, TX	US general population	1935–79	Men employed 20+ years	Brain	20	1.4	Includes all men studied by Wen et al. (1983, 1984b)

Table 11 (contd)

Reference	Study subjects[a]	Comparison population	Period of follow-up	Occupation/ exposure	Cancer site (cause of death)	Number of deaths observed	SMR[b]	Comments
Wen et al. (1985)	1008 men who worked in the lubricating department of Gulf, Port Arthur TX, refinery	US men	1935–78		Bone	3	10.3*	SMR for prostate cancer increased with duration employed
					Stomach	5	1.2	
					Pancreas	5	1.7	
					Prostate	8	1.8	
					All lymphopoietic cancer	6	1.3	
				Not exposed to solvent dewaxing	Prostate	7	1.9	
Wong & Raabe (1989)	6139 employees of Mobil, Beaumont, TX, refinery	US general population	1945–79		All causes	1582	NR	[Includes workers from refinery C (Thomas et al., 1980, 1982a,b, 1984)] SMR for lymphatic and haematopoietic malignancies increased with duration of employment; significant deficit of digestive tract cancer
					All cancer	346	0.96	
					Pancreas	23	1.1	
					Skin	7	1.4	
					Prostate	36	1.1	
					Brain	9	1.1	
					Lympho- and reticulosarcoma	10	1.5	
					Leukaemia	23	1.7*	
					Other lymphatic cancer	12	1.6	
				Men employed >30 yrs	Leukaemia	NR	2.4*	
				20–39 yrs since first employment	Leukaemia	NR	2.1*	
	4263 employees of Mobil, Paulsboro, NJ, refinery	US general population	1946–79		All causes	1164	NR	SMR for prostate cancer increased with duration employed
					All cancer	243	0.91	
					Prostate	28	1.4	
					Other lymphatic cancer	8	1.4	
				Men employed 20+ yrs	Prostate	NR	1.6*	
	1621 employees of Mobil, Torrance CA, refinery	US general population	1959–78		All causes	250	NR	
					All cancer	56	0.80	

Table 11 (contd)

Reference	Study subjects[a]	Comparison population	Period of follow-up	Occupation/exposure	Cancer site (cause of death)	Number of deaths observed	SMR[b]	Comments
McCraw et al. (1985)	3976 white male employees of Shell Oil, Wood River, IL	US white men	1973–82		All causes	640	0.76*	
					All cancer	161	0.91	
					Leukaemia (acute myeloid)	14(8)	2.1*(3.9*)	
					Other lymphatic cancer	6	1.3	
Wong et al. (1986)	14 179 workers at Chevron, Richmond, CA & El Segundo, CA	US general population	1950–80		All causes	2292	0.72*	Significant deficits of cancers of the buccal cavity and pharynx, digestive system (large intestine and pancreas) and lung
					All cancer	462	0.76*	
					Brain	22	1.3	
					Lympho- and reticulosarcoma	17	1.3	
					Other lymphatic cancer	20	1.4	
				Maintenance workers	Brain	14	1.4	
				Operators	Brain	7	1.3	
Nelson et al. (1987)	9192 white male Amoco employees	US white men	1970–82		All causes	921	0.73*	Significant deficits of respiratory tract cancer and lymphopoietic cancer
					All cancer	259	0.84*	
					Digestive tract	92	1.2	
					Skin	11	2.0*	
				Operators	Stomach	9	2.1	
					Large intestine	12	1.2	
					Rectum	5	1.8	
					Skin	8	3.8*	
				Maintenance workers	Rectum	5	1.7	
				Routine refinery	Skin	10	2.7*	
Decouflé et al. (1983)	259 men employed in a Conoco refinery then petrochemical plant	US white men	1947–77		All causes	63	0.97	
					All cancer	10	0.81	
					Lymphopoietic system	4	[3.8]*	

Table 11 (contd)

Reference	Study subjects[a]	Comparison population	Period of follow-up	Occupation/exposure	Cancer site (cause of death)	Number of deaths observed	SMR[b]	Comments
Kaplan (1986)	19 991 men employed in 17 US refineries	US men	1962–80		All causes	3349	0.78*	Study could overlap with any of the other US studies; significant deficits of cancers of buccal cavity and pharynx, lung and bladder
					All cancer	793	0.87*	
					Other lymphatic cancer	30	1.3	
Schottenfeld et al. (1981)	55 007 white male employees of 19 US refineries	US white men	1977–79		All causes	393	0.56*	Study could overlap with any of the other US studies
					All cancer	127	0.75*	
					Brain	8	1.6	
					Lymphocytic leukaemia	7	2.7*	
					Larynx	12	1.3	Incidence
					Brain	9	1.3	
					Melanoma	13	1.3	

Canada

Reference	Study subjects[a]	Comparison population	Period of follow-up	Occupation/exposure	Cancer site (cause of death)	Number of deaths observed	SMR[b]	Comments
Thériault & Provencher (1987)	1207 men employed 5+ yrs in a Shell Oil refinery in Québec	Québec men	1928–81	<20 years' employment	All causes	175	0.86*	Significant deficit of lung cancer
					All cancer	39	0.80	
					Brain	4	2.1	
					Stomach	7	1.6	
					Brain	4	5.2*	
Hanis et al. (1979)	5731 male active and retired refinery employees of Imperial Oil Ltd employed 5+ years	9301 non-refinery workers employed 5+ years	1964–73		Oesophagus and stomach	18	1.2	Standardized mortality ratios
					Intestine and rectum	28	2.0	
					Other digestive tract	21	1.8*	
					Trachea, bronchus and lung	43	1.2	
					Prostate	15	1.3	
					Bladder and kidney	10	1.2	

Table 11 (contd)

Reference	Study subjects[a]	Comparison population	Period of follow-up	Occupation/ exposure	Cancer site (cause of death)	Number of deaths observed	SMR[b]	Comments
	8612 exposed, 2202 moderately exposed to petroleum or its products	4218 unexposed	1964–73	Moderately exposed	Lymphopoietic system	4	1.9	Standardized mortality ratios; age-adjusted mortality rates for cancers of lung and of oesophagus and stomach increased with duration of employment
				Exposed	Oesophagus and stomach	28	3.3*	
				Exposed	Lung	67	1.9*	
UK								
Rushton & Alderson (1980, 1981a); Alderson & Rushton (1982)	34 781 workers at 8 UK petroleum refineries	Men in England, Wales and Scotland	1950–75		All causes	4406	0.84*	Significant deficit overall of lung cancer mortality
					All cancer	1147	0.89**	
					Nasal cavity and sinus	7	2.2*	
				Operators	Melanoma	14	2.2*	
				Operators refin. B	Oesophagus	13	[1.7]	
				Operators refin. F	Intestine	6	[2.3]	
				Labourers	Rectum	5	[2.2]	
				Labourers refin. F	Stomach	56	[1.4]*	
				Labourers refin. J	Stomach	21	[1.7]*	
				Riggers refin. J	Stomach	20	[1.7]*	
				Fire and safety workers refin. J	Stomach	7	[3.9]*	
				Scientists	Stomach	6	[2.4]*	
				Scientists refin. J	Intestine	6	[3.1]*	
					Intestine	3	[4.9]*	
Rushton & Alderson (1981b)	Employees of 8 UK oil refineries who died from leukaemia	Men in England, Wales and Scotland	1950–75		Leukaemia	30	0.95	Leukaemia cases from Rushton & Alderson (1980, 1981a); Alderson & Rushton (1982)
					Lymphatic leukaemia	2	3.0	
					Myeloid leukaemia	5	11.9	
					Acute monocytic leukaemia	4	4.3	

Table 11 (contd)

Reference	Study subjects[a]	Comparison population	Period of follow-up	Occupation/ exposure	Cancer site (cause of death)	Number of deaths observed	SMR[b]	Comments
Alderson & Rattan (1980)	446 men employed in de-waxing plants in 2 refineries	Men in England, Wales and Scotland	1950–75		Buccal cavity and pharynx	2	15.4*	
					Digestive tract	4	1.3	
Sweden								
Malker et al. (1986)	Men employed in petroleum refineries from Swedish census	Swedish men	1961–79		Gall-bladder	6	3.8*	Incidence
Norell et al., (1986)	Men employed in petroleum refineries from Swedish census	Swedish men	1961–79		Pancreas	10	1.3	Incidence

[a]OCAW, Oil, Chemical and Atomic Workers' Union

[b]*, statistically significant at the 5% level; NR, not reported

[c]Several studies covered the same US company: Exxon is described by Hendricks et al. (1959) and Hanis et al. (1982, 1985a,b); Texaco by Divine et al. (1985), Divine and Barron (1986) and part of Thomas' studies; Gulf by Wen et al. (1982, 1983, 1984a,b, 1985, 1986) and part of Thomas' studies; Mobil (Beaumont) by Wong and Raabe (1989) and part of Thomas' studies; Mobil (Paulsboro) by Wong and Raabe (1989); Mobil (Torrance) by Wong and Raabe (1989); Shell by McCraw et al. (1985); Chevron by Wong et al. (1986); Amoco by Nelson et al. (1987); and Conoco by Decouflé et al. (1983)

An elevated risk for cancer of the scrotum was observed among wax pressmen who had been employed for ten years or more during the period 1 January 1937 through 31 December 1956 in an Esso oil refinery (Exxon) in Baton Rouge, LA, where paraffin wax was manufactured (Hendricks et al., 1959; Lione & Denholm, 1959). Cancer incidence among all workers in the refinery was compared with that for the US general white male population at the midpoint of the 20-year study period (Hendricks et al., 1959). Although the overall cancer incidence rate for the refinery workers in general did not exceed that for the USA, wax pressmen who had worked for ten or more years had an overall cancer incidence rate that was more than four times that of US men. Among the 82 pressmen, the rate of scrotal cancer was 806/100 000 (11 cases) compared to a rate of 0.15/100 000 expected on the basis of the experience of US white men. In addition, three cases of stomach cancer and three of cancers at other digestive sites were observed among the wax pressmen; however, expected numbers were not calculated. The scrotal cancer cases occurred only among men who had had skin contact with crude wax saturated with aromatic oils.

A cohort of 8666 workers at the Exxon Baton Rouge, LA, petroleum refinery and chemical plant, some of whom may have been included in the study of Baird (1967), comprised workers who had been employed for at least one month between 1 January 1970 and 31 December 1977 and retirees who were alive on 1 January 1970 (Hanis et al., 1982). About 24% of the employees had begun work at the refinery prior to 1940, and another 24% in 1940-44; however, no information was presented on duration of employment. The mortality experience of the cohort from 1970 to 1977 was compared with that of the total US population, and SMRs adjusted for sex, age, calendar period and race were calculated; 835 employees (9.6%) were lost to follow-up; 85% of those lost were under 40 years of age. There was a significant deficit of all causes of death. The SMRs for pancreatic and renal cancers were elevated, but not significantly so. The renal cancer cases were seen only among employees who had worked as operators, mechanics or labourers and had been hired before 1956. [The Working Group noted the short follow-up period, and that there was no analysis by duration of employment. All of the persons studied are included in the following report.]

A cohort mortality study of employees of three Exxon refineries and chemical plants in Baton Rouge, LA, Bayway/Bayonne, NJ and Baytown, TX, included 15 437 employees who had worked for at least one month during the period 1 January 1970 to 31 December 1977 and followed through 1977, and 6261 retired employees who were alive on 1 January 1970 (Hanis et al., 1985a). More than 50% of the workers had first been employed in 1949 or earlier; 98.7% of workers were followed up. The mortality experience of the Exxon employees was compared with that of the total US population, adjusting for age, sex, race and calendar period. The SMR for all causes of death was significantly less than 1.0. Slight excess mortality was reported for cancers of the liver/gall-bladder/bile ducts, kidney and brain (ICD8 191, 192), primarily among employees hired prior to 1956. At the Baytown, TX, plant, there were elevated SMRs for cancers of the bone, kidney and brain, but none was significant. Among workers at the Bayway/Bayonne, NJ, plant, SMRs were elevated for cancers of the stomach, large intestine, lung and kidney. No analysis was shown by job class (blue-collar, white-collar) or job title. [The Working Group noted the short period of follow-up for many of the employees.]

In further analyses of the Exxon refineries and chemical plants in Baton Rouge, LA, Baytown, TX, and Bayway/Bayonne, NJ, mortality was examined by occupation and work site (Hanis et al., 1985b). Directly adjusted death rates for each subgroup of interest and for the total US population were calculated using the age, sex, race and calendar year distribution of the total cohort as a standard; thus, direct comparisons could be made between mortality rates in cohort subgroups and in the US population by calculating ratios of the directly adjusted rates. Workers were classified as having been 'potentially exposed' or 'unexposed' on the basis of their longest-held job. The 'exposed' category included those who had worked as process operators, mechanical workers and labourers (75% of the study population); while the 'unexposed' category included primarily white-collar office workers (22% of the population). Cause-specific cancer rates were higher among potentially exposed workers than among the unexposed for every cancer site except brain, but none of the site-specific rate ratios was significantly different from 1.0. Directly adjusted death rates were consistently greater than those for the total US population only for renal cancer in each of the three plants. The death rates for pancreatic cancer were higher than the US rates among employees at the Baton Rouge and Baytown plants only, and elevated rates of large intestinal cancer occurred at the Baytown and Bayway/Bayonne plants.

A series of investigations of mortality has been performed among members of the Oil, Chemical and Atomic Workers international union (OCAW) in Texas (Thomas et al., 1980, 1982a,b, 1984). In all of these reports, proportionate mortality among male members of the OCAW was compared with that among US men, adjusting for age, race and calendar period.

The first report concerned 3105 Union members in Texas whose deaths in 1947–77 while actively employed were reported to OCAW and whose death certificates could be located (90%; Thomas et al., 1980). Of the white OCAW members, 1722 had held blue-collar jobs in petroleum refineries and petrochemical plants, primarily in maintenance and production (Thomas et al., 1982a), and had significant excess frequencies of deaths from cancers of the digestive and respiratory systems, skin and brain (ICD8 191, 192).

Subsequent analyses were limited to three petroleum refineries located in the Beaumont/Port Arthur area of the Texas Gulf Coast (Thomas et al., 1982a,b, 1984) and included 1194 retired workers as well as those who had died while actively employed between 1943 and 1979. Among 2509 deceased men who had been employed by the three refineries combined (Thomas et al., 1982a,b), the adjusted PMRs using national rates for all causes of death were significantly elevated for all cancers as well as for cancers of the stomach, pancreas, skin (ICD8 172, 173), prostate and brain (ICD8 191, 192) and for leukaemia. Nine deaths from multiple myeloma were observed and 4.6 were expected, but the PMR was not significant. When national cancer rates were used to calculate proportionate cancer mortality ratios (PCMRs), these ratios were also elevated but significantly so only for brain and leukaemia in whites. When county cancer mortality rates were used, none of the PCMRs was significantly raised. A detailed examination of brain tumour mortality in whites indicated that OCAW members had had elevated frequencies of mortality from benign and unspecified tumours of the brain as well as those specified on death certificates as malignant. [The Working Group noted that, of the 2509 deaths studied,

1161 had also been included in the previous study (Thomas et al., 1980) and that the completeness of records for retired workers is unknown.]

In a nested case-control study, complete work histories of decedents with brain cancer, stomach cancer and leukaemia (31, 52 and 34 cases, respectively) were compared with those of a (1:3) control series of decedents matched by age, sex, date of death, date of first union membership and refinery (Thomas et al., 1984). Cancer-specific relative risks by occupational category were estimated by calculating maximum likelihood estimates of odds ratios using a procedure for matched data. An elevated risk for brain cancer was seen among men who had been involved in intraplant pumping and transport of bulk liquids; however, the median duration of employment in these jobs was shorter for the cases than for the controls. The risk for stomach cancer mortality was elevated among men who had worked in the manufacture of lubricating oils and in refinery maintenance work. Mortality from leukaemia was slightly elevated among men who had worked in operations that involved alkylation, polymerization, the reduction of sulfur constituents of petroleum products and the blending of additives (treating category) and among men who had worked as boiler makers. There was no significant trend by duration of employment for any work category.

In a retrospective cohort study (Divine et al., 1985), standardized mortality among 19 077 white men who had been employed for a minimum of five years by the Texaco company in refinery, petrochemical or research facilities was determined for the period 1 January 1947 to 31 December 1977. Of these, 14 609 (76.6%) were alive on 31 December 1977, and 4024 (21.1%) were dead, and for 444 (2.3%) vital status was unknown. Death certificates were not obtained for 152 (3.8%) of the decedents. Expected mortality was calculated using rates for US white men, adjusting for age and calendar period. There was no significant excess of mortality for any cancer site; however, SMRs were slightly elevated for cancers of the pancreas and brain, leukaemia, cancer of 'other lymphatic tissues' and a category of benign neoplasms which included brain tumours. [The Working Group noted that the cohort included workers in refinery, petrochemical and research facilities; that data were not shown by duration of employment or time since first employment; and that 1008 workers at refinery A in the study of Thomas et al. (1980, 1982a,b, 1984) who had died between 1947 and 1977 were included in this study.]

A second investigation of mortality among Texaco employees included 18 798 white men from the earlier analyses for whom complete work histories were available (Divine & Barron, 1986). The cohort was followed for an average of 19 years. Among men who had worked as refinery operators for more than one year, there were nonsignificant excesses of brain cancer, leukaemia, cancer of other lymphatic tissues (ICD7 202, 203, 205) and benign neoplasms; these excesses were smaller in men with five or more years' employment as an operator. Men who had been employed as maintenance workers for at least five years had elevated SMRs for cancer at the following sites: pancreas, kidney, skin (ICD7 190), brain (ICD7 193), Hodgkin's disease, cancer of other lymphatic tissues and benign neoplasms. Among subjects who had worked as laboratory workers for at least five years, there was a slight excess of mortality from brain cancer (ICD7 193) and benign neoplasms (ICD7 210–239). The only significant cancer excess noted in this study was for leukaemia among men employed as pipe fitters and boiler makers for more than five years. No consistent pattern of increasing mortality was seen by time since first employment or duration of employment for brain tumours among laboratory workers or leukaemia among pipe fitters and boiler makers.

In a cohort study at the Gulf Port Arthur, TX, refinery, all 15 095 men employed for more than one day between 1 January 1937 and 1 January 1978 were followed for vital status on 1 January 1978. Of these, 972 (6.4%) were lost to follow-up; death certificates were not available for 277 (6.5%) of the 4269 male decedents. The average follow-up was 24.7 years. Expected mortality was determined from rates in the US general population, adjusted for age, race and calendar period. Excesses were seen for cancers of the bone, skin, kidney, Hodgkin's disease, leukaemia and cancer of 'other lymphatic tissue'. Only the result for cancer of the bone was significant. When white, blue-collar employees were evaluated separately, SMRs greater than 1 were observed for cancers of the pancreas, lung, bone, skin, prostate, eye and kidney, and for Hodgkin's disease and leukaemia; however, only the SMR for cancer of the bone was significant (Wen *et al.*, 1983). [The Working Group noted that the ICD8 code cited to describe the category 'cancer of other lymphatic tissue' is probably in error and should have been reported as 202-203, 208.]

SMRs for kidney cancer were examined in a separate publication by time since first employment and duration employed; no trend was observed (Wen *et al.*, 1984a).

A separate analysis with regard to employment status (retired, terminated before retirement age, actively employed) was performed on the white men in this cohort. The number of such employees was 12 526; 730 (5.8%) were lost to follow-up, 724 of whom were in the terminated group in which 88% were followed-up successfully (Wen *et al.*, 1984b). Among those who had been actively employed, nonsignificant excess mortality was observed for cancers of bone and kidney and for leukaemia. Among white men who had terminated their employment at the refinery prior to retirement, there was excess mortality from cancers of the lung, bone, skin (ICD8 172, 173) and prostate and from Hodgkin's disease. Mortality among retired men was elevated for cancers of the lung, bone, skin (ICD8 172, 173), prostate, kidney and brain, leukaemia and cancer of 'other lymphatic tissues' (ICD8 202-203, 208). None of the results was significant. Data were not shown by duration of employment, but retirees were assumed to have worked a minimum of 15 years.

In an interim report on 15 698 male and 1823 female workers employed on 15 June 1935 and followed until 31 December 1979 (4766 deaths; 87% follow-up), nonsignificant excess mortality from brain tumours (malignant, benign and unspecified combined) was observed among men who had been employed for 20 or more years (Wen *et al.*, 1982). No variation in SMR was reported for specific cancer sites by calendar period of employment (Wen *et al.*, 1986). [The Working Group noted that the 882 employees at refinery B in the study of Thomas *et al.* (1980, 1982a,b, 1984) who had died between 1947 and 1977 were included in the studies of Wen *et al.*]

Mortality among 1008 men who had worked at any time between 15 June 1935 and 1 January 1978 in the lubricating oil department at the Gulf Port Arthur, TX, refinery was examined separately (Wen *et al.*, 1985). In this department, lubricating oil was manufactured, and wax was separated from the product using a solvent dewaxing process. A mixture of benzene and methyl ethyl ketone was used in the dewaxing process until 1945, when toluene replaced the benzene. There was a significant excess of bone cancer (SMR, 10.3) based on three deaths; nonsignificant excesses were seen for cancers of the stomach, pancreas and prostate and for all lymphopoietic cancer. Mortality for cancer of the prostate increased with duration employed and was excessive only after 20 years of employment. Seven of the eight prostatic cancer deaths occurred among men who had worked in the lubricating oil department but had not been involved in the solvent dewaxing process.

Refinery C studied by Thomas et al. (1980, 1982a,b, 1984) was included in a report by Wong and Raabe (1989). A cohort of all individuals employed at the Mobil Beaumont, TX, petroleum refinery for at least one year between 1 January 1945 and 1 January 1979 was comprised of 6139 employees (1582 deaths; 123 354 person-years). Also included in this report were the Mobil refineries in Paulsboro, NJ (1946-79: number of employees, 4263; number of deaths, 1164) and Torrance, CA (1959-78: number of employees, 1621; number of deaths, 250). Observed mortality in the study cohorts was compared with that expected on the basis of rates for the general US population, adjusted for age, calendar period, sex and race. At the Beaumont, TX, refinery, SMRs were elevated for cancers of the pancreas, skin (ICD8 172, 173), prostate and brain, but were not significant; mortality from lymphatic and haematopoeitic cancer was significantly elevated, due to excess mortality from lymphosarcoma, reticulosarcoma, leukaemia and cancer of 'other lymphatic tissues' (ICD8 202-203, 208). Mortality from lymphatic and haematopoietic cancers increased with duration of employment at the Beaumont, TX, refinery. Mortality from leukaemia was significantly elevated among white men with 30 years' service or more and with 20-39 years' latency. A nonsignificant excess of prostatic cancer was reported at the Paulsboro refinery, and the SMR was significantly elevated among white male employees who had worked for at least 20 years (SMR, 1.6). The SMR for cancer of 'other lymphatic tissues' (ICD8 202-203, 208) was also slightly elevated at the Paulsboro refinery but was not significant. Slight excesses of mortality from stomach and brain cancer were reported at the Torrance refinery.

White male employees (blue-collar and white-collar) of the Shell Oil Wood River refinery in southern Illinois who had worked for at least one day during the period 1 January 1973 to 31 December 1982 and retirees who were alive on 1 January 1973 comprised a cohort of 3976 men, 8% of whom had left employment for reasons other than retirement and were lost to follow-up (McCraw et al., 1985). Using mortality rates for US white men as a comparison, the SMR for all causes of death was 0.76 (640 observed). SMRs were shown separately only for lymphatic and haematopoietic neoplasms; all other cancers were grouped. The SMR for leukaemia was significantly elevated. Mortality from cancer of 'other lymphatic tissues' (ICD8 202-203, 208) was slightly, but not significantly, elevated. There was no excess of other cancers combined. The expected number of deaths from acute myeloid leukaemia was estimated from data on cell-type-specific mortality from US cancer registries, and a significant excess was seen. The authors determined that none of the 14 men who had died from leukaemia were known to have worked in jobs with potentially high exposure to benzene; however, five of the men had been maintenance employees who had worked in numerous plant locations, and their potential exposure to benzene was unknown.

No analysis was shown by duration of employment or job category. A nested case-control study was conducted to evaluate the work histories of the 14 leukaemia deaths observed in this study (Austin *et al.*, 1986), which were compared with those of 50 controls matched on year of birth. Cases did not appear to be clustered in any particular job or work area, and there was no evidence that the cases had had greater opportunity for exposure to benzene than had the controls. [The Working Group noted the short period of follow-up and the small size of the cohort.]

All employees who had worked for at least one year between 1 January 1950 and 31 December 1980 at the Chevron refineries in Richmond and El Segundo, CA, comprised a cohort of 14 179 workers (Wong *et al.*, 1986). In all, 2292 deaths were identified; death certificates were obtained for 98%. Cause-specific SMRs adjusted for age, race, sex and calendar year were calculated using the US general population rates as standard. The SMRs for all causes of death were significantly low for both refineries, individually and combined. The only site-specific cancer excesses noted were for cancer of the brain (ICD8 191, 192), for lymphosarcoma and reticulosarcoma and for cancer of 'other lymphatic tissues' (ICD8 202–203, 208), none of which was significant. SMRs for these cancer sites were elevated among people who had been employees at the Richmond refinery, but not among those at the El Segundo refinery. Employees were classified into three work categories — laboratory, maintenance, operating — on the basis of their first and last jobs. Excess mortality from brain cancer occurred only among employees who had worked in maintenance or as operators. Mortality from cancers of 'other lymphatic tissues' was elevated among cohort members who had worked in any of the three subcategories of blue-collar workers. None of the results by work category was significant. SMRs for cancer of the brain and of 'other lymphatic tissues' were highest ten to 19 years after first employment and decreased after 20 years since first employment. The SMR for brain cancer was highest among workers who had been employed for five to 14 years, but decreased after 15 years of employment. The SMR for lymphosarcoma and reticulosarcoma increased with duration of employment to 1.6 (14 observed) among employees who had worked for 15 or more years.

A cohort mortality study of all Amoco Oil Company employees who had worked for at least six months between 1 January 1970 and 31 December 1980 in any of ten refineries included 9192 white male workers, followed until 31 December 1982 (Nelson *et al.*, 1987). Approximately 2% were lost to follow-up. The mortality experience of refinery workers was compared with that of US white men, adjusting for age and calendar period. The SMR for all causes of death was significantly less than 1. The SMR for all digestive cancers was slightly, but not significantly, elevated. SMRs for cancers at several digestive sites including stomach, large intestine and rectum were elevated among men who had worked as operators; the SMR for rectal cancer was also elevated in maintenance workers. Mortality from skin cancer (ICD8 172, 173) was significantly elevated, and the excess occurred almost exclusively among men who had worked in maintenance jobs. There was also significant excess mortality from skin cancer among men whose exposure to refinery processes was considered to have been routine.

A Conoco plant in the USA which began as a small petroleum refinery in 1915 and was converted to a petrochemical plant between 1947 and 1949 was the subject of a report by

Decouflé et al. (1983). During the period that the plant was a petroleum refinery, the products were gasolines, light oils, bunker oils, lubricating oils and wax. After conversion to a petrochemical plant, the primary products were alkyl benzene compounds. The study cohort included 259 men (blue-collar and white-collar) employed between 1 January 1947 and 31 December 1960. The cohort was followed for vital status through 31 December 1977, and observed mortality was compared with the expected rates of US white men, adjusting for age and calendar period. Mortality from lymphatic and haematopoietic cancers among the 194 subjects who had been employed for at least one year at the plant was significantly elevated; one of the cases had multiple myeloma, one had acute monocytic leukaemia, one had chronic lymphocytic leukaemia, and the fourth had multiple myeloma (treated with radiotherapy and melphalan) followed by acute myelomonocytic leukaemia two years later. The first three cases had begun their employment at the plant prior to 1947, and, thus, had worked there during both the refinery and petrochemical phases.

A cohort of 19 991 male workers who had worked for at least one year between 1 January 1962 and 1 December 1980 in one of 17 US refineries (Wong & Raabe, 1988), 51.3% of whom had been hired between 1940 and 1954 and 17.2% before 1940, was followed for vital status through 31 December 1980, and the mortality experience of the cohort was compared with that of US men, adjusting for race, age and calendar period (Kaplan, 1986). Altogether, 3349 deaths were observed; 707 (3.5%) persons were lost to follow-up. The only site-specific cancer for which excess mortality was noted was that of 'other lymphatic tissues' (ICD 202–203, 208), but this was not significant; 16 of the 30 deaths in this category were due to multiple myeloma. [The Working Group noted that no analysis was shown by duration of employment or latency.]

A prospective cohort study conducted by Schottenfeld et al. (1981) gave morbidity and mortality among men who had been petroleum industry employees in 19 US companies. A total of 55 007 white male petroleum refinery workers who had been working at any time between 1 January 1977 and 31 December 1979 were included in the analyses; 30 769 were first employed in 1960 or after. Mortality rates during the study period were compared with those of US white men in 1977. Standardized incidence ratios (SIRs) for cancer were calculated using rates for US white men obtained from cancer registry data. Among refinery workers, the SMR for all causes of death was significantly less than 1, and significant deficits were noted for many individual causes of death. There was a slight, nonsignificant excess of mortality from brain tumours. There was a significantly elevated incidence of lymphocytic leukaemia, and incidence was slightly elevated for cancers of the larynx and brain and for melanoma. The authors noted that there was underreporting of deaths. [The Working Group noted the short follow-up period (average, 1.6 years), which can result in either higher or lower figures. No analysis by duration of employment was shown.]

[The Working Group noted that the populations in many of the US studies overlapped (see footnote c to Table 11). The two industry-wide studies (Schottenfeld et al., 1981; Kaplan, 1986) included many of the same refineries studied individually.]

(ii) *Canada*

A cohort of workers in a Shell Oil refinery located in east Montréal, Québec, consisting of men who had been employed for more than five years between the start of operations in 1928 and 31 December 1975 was studied twice, at a five-year interval (Thériault & Goulet, 1979; Thériault & Provencher, 1987). Of the 1207 men in the cohort, 175 had died by 31 December 1981 and 78 (6.5%) were lost to follow-up. Cause-specific observed mortality in the cohort was compared with that expected on the basis of mortality rates for men in the province of Québec, adjusting for age and calendar period. The SMRs for all causes and for all cancer were low (0.86 and 0.80, respectively). Site-specific excess mortality was noted for stomach cancer and brain cancer, but neither of the SMRs was significantly greater than 1. The deaths from brain cancer were clustered among workers with fewer than 20 years' employment since their date of hire (four observed; SMR, 5.2), and this SMR was significant. A fifth case of brain cancer, still alive at the end of the study, was also reported. Three of the cases had worked as operators (two in light oils, one in heavy oils). One was a boiler maker working in maintenance, and one was a stationary engineer in the thermal station. SMRs for digestive system cancers increased with time since first employment, but the numbers were small. The SMR for lung cancer showed a significant deficit.

Mortality during the period 1964–73 among 15 032 male current and past employees of Imperial Oil Limited, who had had at least five years of employment, was examined using age-adjusted direct standardization techniques (Hanis *et al.*, 1979). Cause-specific mortality rates among the 5731 refinery workers (821 deaths; 2.2% lost to follow-up) in the cohort were compared with those among the 9301 non-refinery company employees (690 deaths; 7.9% lost to follow-up). The total study cohort was also divided into 'exposed' (8612), 'moderately exposed' (2202) and 'unexposed' (4218) on the basis of their likelihood of daily contact with petroleum or its products at some time during the follow-up period. Workers classified as exposed had mortality rate ratios that were significantly elevated for cancers of the oesophagus and stomach and of the trachea, bronchus and lung. Among moderately exposed workers, there was nonsignificant excess mortality from lymphatic and haematopoietic system malignancies when they were compared to unexposed workers. Mortality rates among refinery workers were higher than those for non-refinery employees for cancers of the oesophagus and stomach, intestine and rectum, other digestive organs, trachea, bronchus and lung, prostate and bladder and kidney. Excess mortality from digestive cancer occurred primarily among men who had been employed in services, maintenance, refinery operation and garage work. There was no significantly elevated rate ratio associated with any particular job. The lung cancer rate ratios were highest among men who had worked in office jobs, plant clerk jobs and building trades. Age-adjusted mortality rates for cancers of the oesophagus and stomach and trachea, bronchus and lung increased with duration of employment among 'exposed' workers.

(iii) *UK*

A cohort of 34 781 workers at eight oil refineries in the UK included all men who had worked continuously for one year between 1 January 1950 and 31 December 1975 (Rushton & Alderson, 1980, 1981a; Alderson & Rushton, 1982). Observed mortality (4406 deaths) in the study group was compared with that expected on the basis of mortality rates among men in England and Wales for the English and Welsh refineries and among men in Scotland for the Scottish refineries, adjusted for age and calendar period; 73 men (0.2%) could not be traced. The SMR for all causes of death was significantly less than 1. The only significant excesses of site-specific cancer mortality noted were for cancer of the nasal cavities and sinuses and for melanoma (Rushton & Alderson, 1980). Among the 9589 men who had worked as operators, excess mortality was seen for oesophageal cancer when results for all the refineries were combined, for intestinal cancer at refinery B and for rectal cancer at refinery F. Labourers experienced elevated mortality from stomach cancer at all refineries combined, at refinery F and at refinery J; riggers and fire and safety workers at refinery J also had elevated risks for stomach cancer. Scientists experienced higher than expected mortality from intestinal cancer at all refineries combined and at refinery J. Stomach cancer mortality decreased with duration of employment overall and at refinery J, but increased with duration of employment at refinery F. Intestinal cancer mortality increased with duration of employment overall and at refineries B and F (Rushton & Alderson, 1981a).

Men who had been employed in methyl ethyl ketone dewaxing plants in two of the refineries included in the study described above were the subject of a separate report (Alderson & Rattan, 1980). Among the 446 men who had worked in these plants, site-specific excess mortality was noted for cancers of the buccal cavity and pharynx and of the digestive tract.

In a nested case-control study, Rushton and Alderson (1981b) compared exposure to benzene among men who had died from leukaemia and among controls selected from the study population of the eight UK oil refineries described above. Two control groups were used: one matched by refinery and year of birth, and a second matched by refinery, year of birth and length of service. There was no excess of leukaemia overall when observed mortality in the refinery population was compared with national rates; however, there were excesses for specific categories: unspecified lymphatic leukaemia, unspecified myeloid leukaemia and acute monocytic leukaemia. The SMRs for all lymphatic leukaemia combined and for all myeloid leukaemia combined were not significantly elevated. A nested case-control analysis suggested a relationship between elevated risk for leukaemia and exposure to benzene, which the authors suggested was confounded by length of service. The odds ratio for leukaemia among men with medium or high exposure to benzene relative to those with low exposure was 2.0, and risk increased with duration of service in the refinery. None of these results was significant.

(iv) *Sweden*

An investigation of occupational risk factors for histologically confirmed biliary tract cancer in Sweden was conducted by linking 1960 census information on occupation with cancer incidence data from the National Swedish Cancer Registry for 1961–79 (Malker *et al.*, 1986). SIRs among workers in specific industries and occupations were calculated by dividing the observed number of cases in each occupational group by the number expected on the basis of national rates among all employed persons, adjusting for birth cohort and sex. Men employed in petroleum refining had significantly elevated SIRs for gall-bladder and other biliary tract cancer.

In a similar analysis of the same cohort, a nonsignificant increase in SIR was noted for cancer of the pancreas (Norell *et al.*, 1986).

[The Working Group noted that these two studies were primarily of an exploratory nature to investigate occupational hazards.]

(b) Case-control studies

The case-control studies reviewed in this section were conducted within the general population setting and examined relationships between the specific cancer at issue and occupational history — either by industry or by broad categories of jobs. Often, no specific hypothesis was being tested. The Working Group presumes that, in addition to the studies reviewed here, in which positive relationships were found, there will have been an indeterminate number of other case-control studies in which no such relationship with a history of working in the petroleum refining industry was found but for which the findings were not reported.

It is unlikely that an equivalent problem exists for the other category of case-control study, conducted ('nested') within a population of petroleum refinery workers and examining the relationship of a specific cancer to specific jobs or exposures within the industry. Such nested case-control studies are included in the preceding section.

(i) *Urinary tract*

A population-based case-control study of bladder cancer conducted in three provinces of Canada included 480 male and 152 female adult case-control pairs (Howe *et al.*, 1980). Newly-diagnosed cases identified from cancer registries between April 1974 and June 1976 were matched by age and sex to neighbourhood controls. Lifetime occupational histories were obtained from personal interviews. Men who had ever worked in the petroleum industry had a significantly elevated risk for bladder cancer (odds ratio, 5.3; 95% confidence interval (CI), 1.5–28.6), which was unchanged after controlling for cigarette smoking. [The Working Group noted that no information on duration of employment was given.]

Histologically confirmed cases of bladder cancer were ascertained among white persons treated in two community hospitals in northern New Jersey, USA, in 1978 and were matched on age, sex, place of birth, hospital and census tract of current residence with patients treated for other conditions in the same hospitals, excluding those with a history of neoplasm or of tobacco-related heart disease (Najem *et al.*, 1982). The relative risk for bladder cancer was estimated by calculating odds ratios stratified by potential confounders. Lifetime occupational histories were obtained for the 75 cases and 142 controls. There was a significantly elevated risk for bladder cancer among study subjects who reported having worked in the petroleum industry (22 cases; odds ratio, 2.5; 95% CI, 1.2–5.4). Risk was highest among subjects who had never smoked (six cases; odds ratio, 5.6) and among current smokers (eight cases; odds ratio, 2.6) and was only slightly elevated among ex-smokers (eight cases; odds ratio, 1.4). [The Working Group noted that no analysis was shown by duration of employment.]

Data from the Detroit, MI, component of the population-based US National Bladder Cancer Study included 420 histologically confirmed, newly diagnosed cases of carcinoma (or papilloma not specified as benign) of the bladder, renal pelvis, ureter and urethra among adult men between 1 December 1977 and 30 November 1978; 95% were carcinoma of the urinary bladder (Silverman *et al.*, 1983). These analyses were limited to the 303 white male cases and 296 white male, randomly-selected adult population controls, matched for age and sex, who were interviewed. Using lifetime occupational histories, crude odds ratios were calculated for ever having worked in each occupation and industry listed. There was an excess risk for cancer of the lower urinary tract among men who had ever been employed in the petroleum extracting and refining industries (six cases; relative risk, 6.0; 95% CI, 0.7–49.8), which was not significant. [The Working Group noted that no data were given by duration of employment.]

A death certificate-based case-control study in 19 southern Louisiana parishes included 347 residents who had died between 1960 and 1975 and whose underlying cause of death was attributed to bladder cancer (Gottlieb & Pickle, 1981). An equal number of controls was selected from persons who had died from causes other than cancer, matched on age, sex, race and parish of residence. Usual industry and occupation listed on the death certificates of study subjects were compared, and a logistic regression model was used to calculate maximum likelihood estimates of the odds ratios for particular variables, adjusting for potential confounding factors. The odds ratio for bladder cancer among white men (176 case-control pairs) whose usual industry of employment was listed as petroleum refining was 4.5 (six cases). Cases who had lived near petroleum refineries also had slightly elevated odds ratios for bladder cancer (whites: 31 cases, odds ratio, 1.1; blacks: three cases, odds ratio, 1.4; based on 238 case-control pairs of whites and 109 of blacks).

In a hospital-based case-control study in La Plata, Argentina, the relationship of bladder cancer to occupational history was examined (Iscovich *et al.*, 1987). An incident series of 117 cases of carcinoma confirmed histologically between March 1983 and December 1985, from ten hospitals, was compared with 117 hospital controls and 117 neighbourhood controls, both groups matched with cases for sex and age. As part of a standardized, interviewer-based questionnaire, a detailed occupational history was obtained for the three occupations of longest duration and the most recent one; job titles were coded according to the ILO classification (International Labour Office, 1970). After pooling the two controls groups and controlling for age and level of cigarette smoking, the only significant increases in occupation-associated risk for bladder cancer were found for lorry or railway drivers (20 cases; odds ratio, 4.3) and for petroleum refinery workers (seven cases; [crude odds ratio calculated by the Working Group, 3.7; 95% CI, 1.1–11.6]); adjusted for age and tobacco use, 6.2). [The Working Group noted that the method of selecting neighbourhood controls, while described unclearly, could have entailed selection bias.]

(ii) *Lung*

Deaths from cancer of the trachea, bronchus and lung among men in two Canadian cities (London and Sarnia) between 1969 and 1973 (348 cases) were ascertained from vital statistics records, and usual industry and occupation were recorded from death certificates

(Wigle, 1977). An equal number of controls who had died from other causes were matched on city, calendar period of death and age. Fifty-seven study subjects were residents of Sarnia, where 28% of the male work force was employed in petroleum refining or the chemical industry; while 291 were from London, where 1% of the men were so employed. Five cases and 12 controls were employed in petroleum refining [odds ratio calculated by the Working Group, 0.42; 95% CI, 0.2–1.0]. [The Working Group noted that no information was available on smoking habits.]

Usual occupation and type of industry listed on the death certificates of residents of 19 southern Louisiana, USA, parishes were obtained for all lung cancer deaths (3327) that occurred between 1960 and 1975 and for an identical number of adults who had died from causes other than cancer, matched on sex, race, age and parish of usual residence (Gottlieb et al., 1979). A logistic model was used to calculate odds ratios (adjusted for age, marital status, year of death, birthplace and parish of residence) by sex and race to estimate the risk for lung cancer of specific occupational and industrial categories. Among men who had been employed in petroleum refining, the race-adjusted odds ratio for lung cancer was 1.3 (95% CI, 0.93–1.9). The sex-adjusted odds ratio for lung cancer among whites who had been employed in petroleum refining was 1.3 (95% CI, 0.88–1.8) and that among blacks was 2.2 (95% CI, 0.59–7.9). Odds ratios for lung cancer among subjects whose usual residence had been in a town in which there was a petroleum refinery were elevated in each sex-race group (white men: 306 cases; odds ratio, 1.2 (95% CI, 0.97–1.4); black men: 28 cases; odds ratio, 1.9 (0.99–3.6); white women: 58 cases; odds ratio, 1.3 (0.86–2.0); black women: ten cases; odds ratio, 1.7 (0.60–4.6)). However, none of the results was significant. Further analyses of specific occupations within the petroleum industry indicated a significantly elevated odds ratio for lung cancer among men who had been employed in skilled maintenance trades or operator jobs in petroleum refining and who had died at age 60 or older (25 cases; odds ratio, 2.4; 95% CI, 1.0–5.9; Gottlieb, 1980). When the study group was restricted to subjects whose length of residence at the location listed on the death certificate could be verified from public records, subjects who had lived within a mile of a petroleum industry work site for at least ten years had an elevated lung cancer risk (work site with <100 employees: 11 cases; odds ratio, 1.5; work sites with ⩾100 employees: 32 cases; odds ratio, 1.7). Among subjects who had lived near a petroleum industry work site and whose usual occupation had been in the petroleum industry, there was a significantly elevated risk for lung cancer (36 cases; odds ratio, 2.3), controlling for year of death, age, race, years of residence and industry size (Gottlieb et al., 1982). [No information on smoking habits or on exposure to asbestos was available.]

(iii) *Other sites*

A preliminary study of risk factors for pancreatic cancer in the same Louisiana parishes included 876 case-control pairs identified from death certificates for the years 1960–75, using the same methods as for the studies on bladder and lung cancer (Pickle & Gottlieb, 1980). There was a two-fold excess risk for pancreatic cancer among white men whose usual industry of employment had been petroleum refining (15 cases; odds ratio, 2.1; 95% CI, 0.86–5.2), but this was not significant. Pancreatic cancer risk was elevated among white men

(40 cases; odds ratio, 1.2), white women (36 cases; odds ratio, 1.2) and black women (three cases, odds ratio, 1.4) whose usual residence had been near a petroleum refinery, but not among black men (three cases; odds ratio, 1.0).

Usual industry and occupation on the death certificates of 718 white men aged 30 and over who had died from malignancies or unspecified tumours of the brain were compared with those of 738 white men who had died of other causes, excluding epilepsy and stroke, and were frequency matched for age and study area (Thomas et al., 1986). All study subjects were residents of three geographical areas of the USA with a heavy concentration of petroleum and chemical industries (southern New Jersey, Philadelphia area and Gulf Coast of Louisiana), who had died between 1979 and 1981, and for whom a death certificate was found (99.7%). Risk for brain tumours in each usual occupation and industry listed was estimated by calculating a maximum likelihood estimate of the odds ratio, adjusting for age, marital status and occupation status (blue-collar, white-collar). The odds ratio for petroleum refining was 1.2 (95% CI, 0.6–2.6).

In a further analysis, lifetime occupational histories were obtained through interviews with next-of-kin (Thomas et al., 1987); 483 cases and 386 controls agreed to be interviewed. The analysis was performed on 300 white men who had had confirmed astrocytic tumour of the brain (astrocytoma, glioblastoma multiforme or mixed glioma with astrocytic cells). Astrocytic tumour risk associated with ever having been employed in specific industries was estimated by maximum likelihood techniques. Among men who had ever been employed in petroleum refining, the odds ratio for astrocytic tumours was 1.5 (18 cases; 95% CI, 0.7–3.2). The elevated risk among men ever employed in petroleum refining was limited to those who had worked in production and maintenance jobs (15 cases; odds ratio, 1.7; 95% CI, 0.7–4.2); however, among those whose duration of employment was known, risk decreased with increasing duration of employment in the industry (<5 years: five cases, odds ratio, 6.7; 5–9 years: two cases, odds ratio, 1.3; ⩾20 years: four cases, odds ratio, 0.8). [The Working Group calculated that this trend was statistically significant.]

A death certificate-based case-control study was conducted in the counties of Cleveland, Humberside and Cheshire and the Wirral district of Merseyside in the UK to examine the relationship between occupation and risk for five cancers — of the oesophagus, pancreas, kidney and brain and melanoma (Magnani et al., 1987). Cases had been male residents of the study areas who had died from one of the five cancers between the ages of 18 and 54 during the periods 1959–63 and 1965–79 (data for 1964 were not available). One set of controls who had died from other causes was matched to each case on county of residence and another set on 'local authority area' of residence; both sets were matched on sex and age at death. Occupation and industry listed on the death certificates were used to classify subjects into occupational and exposure categories. There were 244 cases of oesophageal cancer with 935 controls, 343 of pancreatic cancer with 1315 controls, 99 of melanoma with 361 controls, 147 of kidney cancer with 556 controls, and 432 of brain cancer with 1603 controls. Significantly elevated odds ratios were not reported for oesophageal, pancreatic or kidney cancer in association with petroleum refining occupations; there were significantly elevated odds ratios for melanoma (odds ratio, 8.0; 95% CI, 1.5–43.7) and brain cancer (odds ratio, 3.5; 1.5–8.1) associated with occupational exposure to coal and petroleum products. Both results were due to clusters of workers employed in petroleum refining. The four melanoma cases so employed had the following occupations reported on their death certificates: process worker/blender, engineer, security officer and clerk of works. The odds ratio for brain cancer was significantly elevated among men employed in petroleum refining (odds ratio, 2.9; 95% CI, 1.2–7.0), and four of the seven cases had worked as process operators.

Several studies on parental occupation involving exposure to hydrocarbons and cancer risks in children are reviewed in the monograph on gasoline. One of the studies, described more fully in that monograph, looked specifically at petrochemical occupations and industries and included 499 Texas children who had died from intracranial and spinal cord tumours and 998 controls (Johnson *et al.*, 1987). On the basis of information on paternal occupation extracted from the birth certificate, an odds ratio of 2.0 (95% CI, 0.6–6.2) for children of petroleum refinery workers was observed.

(c) Correlation studies

A survey by county of the average annual age-adjusted lung cancer mortality rates for the years 1950–69 among white men in the USA indicated higher than expected lung cancer rates (1.32 per 100 000), when compared with total US rates, in counties where at least 1% of the population was employed in the petroleum industry (Blot & Fraumeni, 1976). A second survey examined cancer mortality rates in 39 US counties where at least 100 persons were employed in the petroleum industry and the estimated number of workers comprised at least 1% of the county population (Blot *et al.*, 1977). White male residents of the petroleum industry counties had significantly higher average age-adjusted mortality rates for cancers of the lung (rate ratio, 1.15), nasal cavity and sinuses (rate ratio, 1.48), stomach (rate ratio, 1.09), rectum (rate ratio, 1.07), testis (rate ratio, 1.10) and skin (rate ratio, 1.10) than those of control counties with similar demographic characteristics.

Average annual age-adjusted cancer incidence rates for the period 1971–77 among Kaiser Health Foundation plan members living near petroleum and chemical plants in the San Francisco Bay area of the USA were compared with those among other San Francisco Bay area residents who did not live near the plants (Hearey *et al.*, 1980). Site-specific rates for cancer were not elevated for members living near the petroleum and chemical plants.

Average annual age-adjusted cancer incidence rates for the period 1969–77 in Contra Costa County, CA, USA, were examined to determine whether there was any correlation with levels of air emissions from petroleum and chemical plants (Kaldor *et al.*, 1984). The county was divided into four exposure areas, from low to high, based on air levels of sulfur dioxide, hydrocarbons and nitrogen oxides. Among men, significantly increasing incidence rates by level of exposure were found for cancers of the buccal cavity and pharynx, of the stomach, trachea, bronchus and lung, of the prostate and of the kidney. For all cancer sites combined, rates increased by exposure level, and the trend was significant. Among women, significantly increasing trends were noted only for cancers of the buccal cavity and pharynx.

Average annual age-adjusted mortality rates for multiple myeloma by state economic area in the USA were calculated for the period 1950-75 for each sex and race (Blattner *et al.*, 1981). A multiple regression model was used to examine the relationship between the magnitude of the rates for multiple myeloma and various social, demographic and employment characteristics of the state economic areas. Rates for multiple myeloma among white men were elevated in areas where more than 1% of the population was employed in the petroleum industry, and the regression coefficient was significantly different from 0.

(*d*) *Case reports*

An employee of a petroleum refinery near Chicago, IL, USA, treated for an epithelioma [squamous-cell carcinoma] of the skin of the arm, was the subject of an early case report (Davis, 1914). The employee had worked for more than 20 years in a refinery department where crude paraffin was pressed to remove the petroleum oil distillate. The crude wax residue remaining in the presses was removed by a manual scraping process, and workers' bare arms were exposed to the oil-containing wax. Investigation at the plant indicated that most of the workers in the department had developed skin lesions in the form of 'wax boils', pigmented spots, wart-like growths and epithelioma.

A review of ten cases of cancer of the scrotum among wax pressmen at the Esso Baton Rouge, LA, USA, petroleum refinery was conducted by Lione and Denholm (1959). All of the men had been exposed to crude wax containing 20–40% petroleum oil distillate for a minimum of 15 years, the longest exposure period being 38 years. During the process of separating wax from crude distillate, the workers' clothing became contaminated with the crude wax, particularly in the lower abdominal and genital areas. Pathological diagnoses indicated that all ten of the cases were squamous-cell carcinomas. [The Working Group noted that these cases were included in the study by Hendricks *et al.* (1959), p. 91.]

Cases of leukaemia that occurred during the period 1962–71 among employees of eight Esso affiliates in Europe were studied to determine whether leukaemia had occurred more often than expected in association with exposure to benzene in petroleum refining (Thorpe, 1974). Eighteen cases were reported during the study period among employees of only four of the affiliates; the other four companies reported no case of leukaemia. Eight of the cases were considered to have been exposed to benzene in their jobs; these were two tank truck drivers, two refinery mechanics, two refinery operators, one marketing repair mechanic and one marketing superintendent. Expected mortality from leukaemia was estimated by applying the mortality data of the World Health Organization for 1966 to the estimates of person-years at risk for the eight companies; the ratio of observed to expected mortality from leukaemia among the benzene-exposed workers was 1.2, which was not significant.

4. Summary of Data Reported and Evaluation

4.1 Exposure data

Approximately 3000 million tonnes of petroleum fuels, solvents, lubricants, bitumens and other products are produced annually from crude oil. World-wide, the petroleum refining industry employs about 500 000 persons in more than 700 plants. Process operators and maintenance workers may be exposed to a large number of substances which occur in crude oil, process streams, intermediates, catalysts, additives and final products. Aliphatic and aromatic hydrocarbons and hydrogen sulfide have commonly been measured in the air of working environments. Less commonly, polycyclic aromatic compounds have been detected at specific process units. In general, the concentrations of benzene in modern refineries have been reported to be less than 3 mg/m^3, with higher levels in some operations. Exposure *via* the skin to high-boiling materials may also occur.

The major process streams are listed in Table 2, p. 44; the numbers given in square brackets below are those assigned to the streams.

4.2 Experimental data

Several refinery streams used in the manufacture of (or sold directly as) mineral lubricating oils and processing oils were evaluated in Volume 33 of the *IARC Monographs*. The Working Group that prepared that monograph concluded that there was *sufficient evidence* for the carcinogenicity in experimental animals of untreated vacuum distillates [19, 20], of hydrotreated vacuum distillates [based on 19 and 20] and of the high-boiling fraction of catalytically cracked oils [26, 27]. A more recent working group which met to re-evaluate all agents considered in volumes 1–42 of the *IARC Monographs*, resulting in Supplement 7, concluded that there was *sufficient evidence* for the carcinogenicity of untreated and mildly treated mineral oils in experimental animals. The following summary covers experiments on refinery streams that were not considered previously or which have been published since Supplement 7 was prepared. In most of these experiments, no distinction was made in the published reports between benign and malignant skin tumours.

Uncracked distillates and residues[1]

In a series of experiments of similar design, several atmospheric and vacuum distillates were tested by repeated skin application to mice. One sample of a light straight-run naphtha [3], one sample of light paraffinic vacuum distillate [19A], one sample of heavy paraffinic vacuum distillate [20A] and four samples of heavy naphthenic vacuum distillates [20B] produced a marked increase in the incidence of skin tumours. Two samples of straight-run kerosene [5] and one sample of hydrotreated kerosene [5A] also produced skin tumours.

Two samples of hydrotreated heavy naphthenic distillate [20D] and one sample of a chemically neutralized/hydrotreated heavy naphthenic distillate [20C/20D] tested in mice by skin application produced a marked increase in the incidence of skin tumours.

One sample of vacuum residue [21] was tested by skin application in mice; no significant skin tumour response was observed.

Cracked distillates and residues

One sample of light catalytically cracked naphtha [22], three light catalytically cracked

---

[1]Subsequent to the meeting, the Secretariat became aware of one study in which skin tumours were reported in mice after application to the skin of petroleum naphtha (boiling range, 53–213°C) [near 4] (Clark *et al.*, 1988) and of another study in which it was reported that skin tumours developed in mice after skin application of a virgin heating oil blending base (boiling range, 142–307°C) [probably 5] (Biles *et al.*, 1988).

distillates [24] and one intermediate catalytically cracked distillate [25] were tested in mice by skin application and induced skin tumours.

Several high-boiling distillates [26] and residues [27] of catalytically cracked oils and several thermally cracked residues [31] were tested in experiments in mice by skin application, producing high incidences of benign and malignant skin tumours.

Thermally-cracked residues [31] originating from two different sources were tested by skin application in rabbits, producing some skin tumours, but the study was considered inadequate for evaluation. In one study in mice, skin application of water-quench pyrolysis fuel oil or oil-quench pyrolysis fuel oil (steam-cracked residues [34]) produced carcinomas and papillomas of the skin.

Effluents

Two studies on petroleum refinery effluents were inadequate for evaluation.

4.3 Human data

Taking into consideration the overlap in cohort studies conducted in the USA, ten separate, company-specific cohorts were studied. Two industry-wide study cohorts from the USA comprised various combinations of these cohorts. The cohorts mentioned hereafter refer to the ten separate US cohorts, two from Canada and one from the UK.

Information on specific jobs or exposures was available in only a few of the epidemiological studies of petroleum refinery workers. Some caution should be applied in interpreting the relative risks for cancer in cohort studies of petroleum refinery workers. As for most cohorts of actively employed persons, the overall risk for cancer in all of the cohort studies reviewed here was lower than that in the general population. Yet, it is the cancer experience of the general population that has been conventionally used, in published papers, in evaluating the rates of specific cancers in refinery workers. Significant deficits were reported for cancers at some sites in certain studies; such findings are mentioned in this summary only when a consistent pattern emerged. Caution should also be applied in interpreting the findings from those case-control studies conducted within the general population setting. Most of the studies reported had positive findings, and are likely to be an incomplete selection of case-control studies in which occupational exposures have been investigated.

One case report and one case series describe clusters of skin cancer cases (squamous-cell carcinoma) among wax pressmen who had been exposed to crude paraffin wax saturated with aromatic oils. Significant excess mortality from skin cancer was reported among three refinery cohorts, one of which included the wax pressmen from the case series. In a second cohort, the overall excess was due to an elevated risk for malignant melanoma. In the third, excess skin cancer risk was experienced primarily by maintenance workers. Skin cancer mortality was elevated in three additional cohorts, but the increase was not significant. A case-control study showed a significantly elevated risk for malignant melanoma among men employed in the coal and petroleum products industry, with a cluster of cases employed in petroleum refineries.

Mortality from leukaemia was significantly elevated in two refinery cohorts; in one of these, mortality increased with duration employed and also with time since first employment. Nonsignificant excess mortality from leukaemia was reported among two additional cohorts; in one of these, the excess was significant for boiler makers and pipe fitters. Elevated mortality from unspecified lymphatic leukaemia, unspecified myeloid leukaemia and acute monocytic leukaemia, but not other cell types, was reported in a subset of workers in the British cohort whose exposures included benzene. A significantly elevated incidence of lymphocytic leukaemia was reported in a large cohort study which included many of the refineries in the USA. Excess mortality from 'cancer of other lymphatic tissues' (multiple myeloma, polycythaemia vera and non-Hodgkin's lymphoma, excluding lymphosarcoma and reticulum-cell sarcoma), which was not significant, was reported in five refinery cohorts. One report indicated significant excess mortality from leukaemia and 'cancer of other lymphatic tissues' combined.

Mortality from malignant neoplasms of the brain was elevated in six of the refinery cohorts, but this was significant in only one of the studies and only for workers with short duration of employment. The elevated mortality was seen in operators and in maintenance and laboratory workers. A case-control study of astrocytic brain tumours showed a decreasing trend in risk with duration employed among men who had ever worked in petroleum refining during their lifetime. Another case-control study showed a significantly elevated risk for malignant neoplasms of the brain among men employed in petroleum refining.

Stomach cancer mortality was elevated among six refinery cohorts, significantly so in only one, among labourers, riggers and fire and safety workers; it was associated with lubricating oil production in one refinery and with solvent dewaxing in another. Mortality increased with increasing duration of employment in one of the studies.

Kidney cancer mortality was elevated, but not significantly so, among three petroleum refinery cohorts, particularly among operators, labourers and maintenance workers. Kidney and bladder cancer mortality combined was elevated in one refinery cohort. Five case-control studies of bladder cancer showed excess risk associated with employment in petroleum refining; the results were significant in two of these.

Pancreatic cancer mortality was reported to be elevated in four petroleum refining cohorts, and was associated with employment in the petroleum refining industry in one case-control study; however, none of these results was significant.

Excess mortality from cancer of the prostate, which increased with duration of employment, was reported in two refinery cohorts, and an overall excess was reported in two others. The only result that attained significance was found for men employed for 20 years or more in one of the refineries.

Lung cancer mortality was elevated in two refinery cohorts but not significantly so. There was a significant excess of lung cancer among workers with daily exposure to petroleum and its products in one of these cohorts. In five cohort studies, significant deficits in mortality from lung cancer were seen. In a case-control study, refinery maintenance workers and operators had a significantly elevated risk for lung cancer.

Mortality from malignant neoplasms of bone was elevated in two cohorts; the excess was significant in one of them, and specifically in association with employment in lubricating oil manufacture.

4.4 Other relevant data

It was reported in one study that wives of maintenance (crafts) workers employed in the waste-water treatment area of a petroleum refinery experienced an excess risk of fetal loss. In one study, an increased prevalence of chromosomal aberrations and of sister chromatid exchange was found in a group of workers in the sewage-treatment unit of a petroleum refinery, but no such effect was observed among a group of workers in a catalytic cracking unit.

Light straight-run [3], full-range alkylate [13] and thermally cracked naphtha [28, 29] produced severe renal toxicity in male but not in female rats.

Previous working groups have reported that vacuum distillates from petroleum refining [19, 20] and hydrotreated oils induced mutation in bacteria (IARC, 1984, 1987).

Extracts of light paraffinic distillate [19A], heavy paraffinic distillate [20A], heavy naphthenic distillate [20B], straight-run kerosene [5], hydrotreated heavy naphthenic distillate [20D] and chemically neutralized/hydrotreated heavy naphthenic distillate [20C/20D] induced mutation in bacteria. Extracts of hydrotreated kerosene [5A], light straight-run naphtha [3] and vacuum residue [21] did not induce mutation in bacteria.

Extracts of an intermediate catalytically cracked distillate [25] and of a mixture of a heavy catalytically cracked distillate [26] and a catalytically cracked clarified oil [27] induced mutation in bacteria. (See Appendix 1.)

4.5 Evaluation[1]

There is *limited evidence* that working in petroleum refineries entails a carcinogenic risk. This limited evidence applies to skin cancer and leukaemia; for all other cancer sites on which information was available, the evidence is inadequate.

There is *sufficient evidence* for the carcinogenicity in experimental animals of light and heavy vacuum distillates, of light and heavy catalytically cracked distillates and of cracked residues derived from the refining of crude oil.

There is *limited evidence* for the carcinogenicity in experimental animals of light straight-run naphtha, of straight-run kerosene, of hydrotreated kerosene and of light catalytically cracked naphtha.

In formulating the overall evaluation, the Working Group also took note of the following supporting evidence reported in Supplement 7: benzene and untreated and mildly

---

[1]For definitions of the italicized terms, see Preamble, pp. 25–28.

treated mineral oils are carcinogenic to humans (Group 1). There is *sufficient evidence* for the carcinogenicity in experimental animals of several polycyclic aromatic hydrocarbons[1].

Overall evaluation

Occupational exposures in petroleum refining *are probably carcinogenic to humans (Group 2A)*.

5. References

Alderson, M.R. & Rattan, N.S. (1980) Mortality of workers in an isopropyl alcohol plant and two MEK dewaxing plants. *Br. J. ind. Med.*, 37, 85–89

Alderson, M.R. & Rushton, L. (1982) Mortality patterns in eight UK oil refineries. *Ann. N.Y. Acad. Sci.*, 381, 139–145

American Petroleum Institute (1985) *Job Code Classification System*, Part II, *Production Operations and Marketing/Transportation Operations*, Washington DC

American Petroleum Institute (1987) *Basic Petroleum Data Book, Petroleum Industry Statistics*, Vol. VII, No. 3, Washington DC

Anon. (1985) Observations of reproductive functions among workers in an oil refinery — Louisiana. *Morb. Mortal. wkly Rep.*, 34, 350–351

Austin, H., Cole, P. & McCraw, D.S. (1986) A case-control study of leukemia at an oil refinery. *J. occup. Med.*, 28, 1169–1173

Baird, V.C. (1967) Effects of atmospheric contamination on cancer mortality in petroleum refinery employees. *J. occup. Med.*, 9, 415–420

Biles, R.W., McKee, R.H., Lewis, S.C., Scala, R.A. & DePass, L.R. (1988) Dermal carcinogenic activity of petroleum-derived middle distillate fuels. *Toxicology*, 53, 301-314

Bingham, E. & Barkley, W. (1979) Bioassay of complex mixtures derived from fossil fuels. *Environ. Health Perspect.*, 30, 157–163

Blackburn, G.R., Deitch, R.A., Schreiner, C.A., Mehlman, M.A. & Mackerer, C.R. (1984) Estimation of the dermal carcinogenic activity of petroleum fractions using a modified Ames assay. *Cell Biol. Toxicol.*, 1, 67–80

Blackburn, G.R., Deitch, R.A., Schreiner, C.A. & Mackerer, C.R. (1986) Predicting carcinogenicity of petroleum distillation fractions using a modified *Salmonella* mutagenicity assay. *Cell Biol. Toxicol.*, 2, 63–84

Blattner, W.A., Blair, A. & Mason, T.J. (1981) Multiple myeloma in the United States, 1950–1975. *Cancer*, 48, 2547–2554

Blot, W.J. & Fraumeni, J.F., Jr (1976) Geographic patterns of lung cancer: industrial correlations. *Am. J. Epidemiol.*, 103, 539–550

Blot, W.J., Brinton, L.A., Fraumeni, J.F., Jr & Stone, B.J. (1977) Cancer mortality in US counties with petroleum industries. *Science*, 198, 51–53

Brandt, H.C.A. & Molyneux, M.K.B. (1985) Sampling and analysis of bitumen fumes. Part 2. Field exposure measurements. *Ann. occup. Hyg.*, 29, 47–58

British Petroleum Co. (1977) *Our Industry Petroleum*, London, p. 586

---

[1]Other agents previously evaluated in the *IARC Monographs* that may occur in petroleum refining are listed in Table 1 of the 'General Remarks', p. 32.

British Petroleum Co. (1986) *BP Statistical Review of World Energy, June 1986*, London

British Petroleum Co. (1988) *BP Statistical Review of World Energy, June 1988*, London

Brown, M.G. (1985) Fluoride exposure from hydrofluoric acid in a motor gasoline alkylation unit. *Am. ind. Hyg. Assoc. J.*, 46, 662–669

Bruevich, T.S. (1971) On occupational skin pathology developing in workers of oil refining plants (Russ.). *Vestn. Dermatol. Venereol.*, 45, 43–47

Burgess, W.A. (1981) *Recognition of Health Hazards in Industry. A Review of Materials and Processes*, New York, John Wiley & Sons, pp. 211–216

Butala, J.H., Strother, D.E., Thilagar, A.K. & Brecher, S. (1985) Cell transformation testing of unfractionated petroleum liquids (Abstract). *Environ. Mutagenesis*, 7 (*Suppl. 3*), 37

Carrano, A.V., Harrison, L.B., Mayall, B.H., Minkler, J.L. & Cohon, F. (1980) Sister chromatid exchange studies in petroleum refinery workers (Abstract No. Cc–3). *Environ. Mutagenesis*, 2, 263

Chiles, J.R. (1987) Spindletop. *Am. Heritage Invention Technol.*, 3, 34–43

Cicolella, A. & Vincent, R. (1987) *Occupational Exposure to Benzene Vapours. Summary of a Map Campaign in Several Companies* (Fr.) (*Working Document No. 297.001/RV*), Vandoeuvre, France, Institut National de Recherche et de Sécurité, pp. 34–47

Clark, C.R., Walter, M.K., Ferguson, P.W. & Katchen, M. (1988) Comparative dermal carcinogenesis of shale and petroleum-derived distillates. *Toxicol. ind. Health*, 4, 11–22

Clayton Environmental Consultants, Inc. (1982) *Medical Management of Chemical Exposures in the Petroleum Industry*, Washington DC, American Petroleum Institute

Commission of the European Communities (1981) *Constructing EINECS: Basic Documents. European Core Inventory*, Vol. 1, Brussels

CONCAWE (1985) *Health Aspects of Petroleum Fuels. Potential Hazards and Precautions for Individual Classes of Fuels* (*Report No. 85/51*), The Hague

CONCAWE (1986) *Review of European Oil Industry. Benzene Exposure Data* (*Report No. 3/86*), The Hague

CONCAWE (1987) *A Survey of Exposures to Gasoline Vapour* (*Report No. 4/87*), The Hague

Cruzan, G., Low, L.K., Cox, G.E., Meeks, J.R., Mackerer, C.R., Craig, P.H., Singer, E.J. & Mehlman, M.A. (1986) Systemic toxicity from subchronic dermal exposure, chemical characterization, and dermal penetration of catalytically cracked clarified slurry oil. *Toxicol. ind. Health*, 2, 429–444

Darby, G.H., Dukich, A., Hargens, C.W., Hill, H.G., Hsiao, S.-H., Liss-Suter, D., Mason, R. & Miller, L.M. (1978) *Information Profiles on Potential Occupational Hazards*, Rockville, MD, National Institute for Occupational Safety and Health, pp. 127–141

Davis, B.F. (1914) Paraffin cancer. Coal and petroleum products as causes of chronic irritation and cancer. *J. Am. med. Assoc.*, 62, 1716–1720

Decouflé, P., Blattner, W.A. & Blair, A. (1983) Mortality among chemical workers exposed to benzene and other agents. *Environ. Res.*, 30, 16–25

Divine, B.J. & Barron, V. (1986) Texaco mortality study. II. Patterns of mortality among white males by specific job groups. *Am. J. ind. Med.*, 10, 371–381

Divine, B.J., Barron, V. & Kaplan, S.D. (1985) Texaco mortality study. I. Mortality among refinery, petrochemical, and research workers. *J. occup. Med.*, 27, 445–447

Dynamac Corp. (1985) *Industrial Hygiene Assessment of Petroleum Refinery Turnaround Activities*, Washington DC, American Petroleum Institute

Energy Information Administration (1986) *Annual Energy Review 1986*, Washington DC, p. 60

Futagaki, S.K. (1983) *Petroleum Refinery Workers Exposure to PAHs at Fluid Catalytic Cracker, Coker, and Asphalt Processing Units (NIOSH Publ. No. 83*–111), Cincinnati, OH, National Institute for Occupational Safety and Health

Gafafer, W.M. & Sitgreaves, R. (1940) Disabling morbidity, and mortality from cancer among the male employees of an oil refining company with reference to age, site, and duration, 1933–38, inclusive. *Publ. Health Rep.*, 55, 1517–1526

Getmanets, I.Y. (1967) Comparative evaluation of the carcinogenic properties of cracking residues of high- and low-paraffin petroleum (Russ.). *Gig. Tr. prof. Zabol.*, 11, 53–55

Gottlieb, M.S. (1980) Lung cancer and the petroleum industry in Louisiana. *J. occup. Med.*, 22, 384–388

Gottlieb, M.S. & Pickle, L.W. (1981) Bladder cancer mortality in Louisiana. *J. Louisiana State med. Soc.*, 133, 6–9

Gottlieb, M.S., Pickle, L.W., Blot, W.J. & Fraumeni, J.F., Jr (1979) Lung cancer in Louisiana: death certificate analysis. *J. natl Cancer Inst.*, 63, 1131–1137

Gottlieb, M.S., Shear, C.L. & Seale, D.B. (1982) Lung cancer mortality and residential proximity to industry. *Environ. Health Perspect.*, 45, 157–164

Halder, C.A., Warne, T.M. & Hatoum, N.S. (1984) *Renal toxicity of gasoline and related petroleum naphthas in male rats*. In: Mehlman, M.A., Hemstreet, G.P., III, Thorpe, J.J. & Weaver, N.K., eds, *Advances in Modern Environmental Toxicology*, Vol. VII, *Renal Effects of Petroleum Hydrocarbons*, Princeton, NJ, Princeton Scientific Publishers, pp. 73–88

Hanis, N.M., Stavraky, K.M. & Fowler, J.L. (1979) Cancer mortality in oil refinery workers. *J. occup. Med.*, 21, 167–174

Hanis, N.M., Holmes, T.M., Shallenberger, L.G. & Jones, K.E. (1982) Epidemiologic study of refinery and chemical plant workers. *J. occup. Med.*, 24, 203–212

Hanis, N.M., Shallenberger, L.G., Donaleski, D.L. & Sales, E.A. (1985a) A retrospective mortality study of workers in three major US refineries and chemical plants. Part I: Comparisons with US population. *J. occup. Med.*, 27, 283–292

Hanis, N.M., Shallenberger, L.G., Donaleski, D.L. & Sales, E.A. (1985b) A retrospective mortality study of workers in three major US refineries and chemical plants. Part II: Internal comparisons by geographic site, occupation, and smoking history. *J. occup. Med.*, 27, 361–369

Hearey, C.D., Ury, H., Siegelaub, A., Ho, M.K.P., Salomon, H. & Cella, R.L. (1980) Lack of association between cancer incidence and residence near petrochemical industry in the San Francisco Bay area. *J. natl Cancer Inst.*, 64, 1295–1299

Hendricks, N.V., Berry, C.M., Lione, J.G. & Thorpe, J.J. (1959) Cancer of the scrotum in wax pressmen. I. Epidemiology. *Arch. ind. Health occup. Med.*, 19, 524–529

Hobson, H.L. (1982) *Petroleum refinery processing*. In: Cralley, L.V. & Cralley, L.J., eds, *Industrial Hygiene Aspects of Plant Operations*, Vol. 1, *Process Flows*, New York, MacMillan, pp. 373–395

Holmberg, B. & Lundberg, P. (1985) Benzene: standards, occurrence, and exposure. *Am. J. ind. Med.*, 7, 375–383

Howe, G.R., Burch, J.D., Miller, A.B., Cook, G.M., Estève, J., Morrison, B., Gordon, P., Chambers, L.W., Fodor, G. & Winsor, G.M. (1980) Tobacco use, occupation, coffee, various nutrients, and bladder cancer. *J. natl Cancer Inst.*, *64*, 701–713

Hueper, W.C. & Ruchhoft, C.C. (1954) Carcinogenic studies on adsorbates of industrially polluted raw and finished water supplies. *Arch. ind. Hyg. occup. Med.*, *9*, 488–495

IARC (1976) *IARC Monographs on the Evaluation of Carcinogenic Risk of Chemicals to Man*, Vol. 11, *Cadmium, Nickel, Some Epoxides, Miscellaneous Industrial Chemicals and General Considerations on Volatile Anaesthetics*, Lyon, pp. 75–112

IARC (1978) *IARC Monographs on the Evaluation of the Carcinogenic Risk of Chemicals to Man*, Vol. 16, *Some Aromatic Amines and Related Nitro Compounds — Hair Dyes, Colouring Agents and Miscellaneous Industrial Chemicals*, Lyon, pp. 111–142

IARC (1980) *IARC Monographs on the Evaluation of the Carcinogenic Risk of Chemicals to Humans*, Vol. 23, *Some Metals and Metallic Compounds*, Lyon, pp. 205–323

IARC (1982) *IARC Monographs on the Evaluation of the Carcinogenic Risk of Chemicals to Humans*, Vol. 29, *Some Industrial Chemicals and Dyestuffs*, Lyon, pp. 93–148, 391–398

IARC (1984) *IARC Monographs on the Evaluation of the Carcinogenic Risk of Chemicals to Humans*, Vol. 33, *Polynuclear Aromatic Compounds, Part 2, Carbon Blacks, Mineral Oils and Some Nitroarenes*, Lyon, pp. 87–168

IARC (1985) *IARC Monographs on the Evaluation of the Carcinogenic Risk of Chemicals to Humans*, Vol. 35, *Polynuclear Aromatic Compounds, Part 4, Bitumens, Coal-tars and Derived Products, Shale-oils and Soots*, Lyon, pp. 39–81, 243–247

IARC (1986) *Information Bulletin on the Survey of Chemicals Being Tested for Carcinogenicity*, No. 12, Lyon, pp. 285–289

IARC (1987a) *IARC Monographs on the Evaluation of the Carcinogenic Risk of Chemicals to Humans*, Vol. 42, *Silica and Some Silicates*, Lyon, pp. 39–143

IARC (1987b) *IARC Monographs on the Evaluation of Carcinogenic Risks to Humans*, Suppl. 7, *Overall Evaluations of Carcinogenicity: An Updating of* IARC Monographs *Volumes 1 to 42*, Lyon

International Labour Office (1970) *Uniform International Classification of Occupations*, rev. ed. 1968, Geneva

International Labour Office (1986) *Petroleum Committee, 10th Session, General Report*, Report I, Geneva, p. 146

Iscovich, J., Castelletto, R., Estève, J., Muñoz, N., Colanzi, R., Coronel, A., Deamezola, I., Tassi, V. & Arslan, A. (1987) Tobacco smoking, occupational exposure and bladder cancer in Argentina. *Int. J. Cancer*, *40*, 734–740

Jahnig, C.E. (1982) *Petroleum (refinery processes, survey)*. In: Grayson, M., ed., *Kirk-Othmer Encyclopedia of Chemical Technology*, 3rd ed., Vol. 17, New York, John Wiley & Sons, pp. 183–256

Johnson, C.C., Annegers, J.F., Frankowski, R.F., Spitz, M.R. & Buffler, P.A. (1987) Childhood nervous system tumors. An evaluation of the association with paternal occupational exposure to hydrocarbons. *Am. J. Epidemiol.*, *126*, 605–613

Kaldor, J., Harris, J.A., Glazer, E., Glaser, S., Neutra, R., Mayberry, R., Nelson, V., Robinson, L. & Reed, D. (1984) Statistical association between cancer incidence and major-cause mortality, and estimated residential exposure to air emissions from petroleum and chemical plants. *Environ. Health Perspect.*, *54*, 319–332

Kane, M.L., Ladov, E.N., Holdsworth, C.E. & Weaver, N.K. (1984) Toxicological characteristics of refinery streams used to manufacture lubricating oils. *Am. J. ind. Med.*, *5*, 183–200

Kaplan, S.D. (1986) Update of a mortality study of workers in petroleum refineries. *J. occup. Med.*, *28*, 514–516

Karimov, M.A., Artamonova, L.A. & Yermolenko, A.S. (1984) Carcinogenic effect of heavy catalytic gas oil (Russ.). *Vopr. Onkol.*, *30*, 40–45

Karimov, M.A., Yermolenko, A.S. & Artamonova, L.A. (1986) Preneoplastic and neoplastic lesions in the mouse esophagus and cardia following skin painting with heavy catalytic gas oil (Russ.). *Vopr. Onkol.*, *32*, 56–61

Lewis, S.C. (1983) Crude petroleum and selected fractions. Skin cancer bioassays. *Prog. exp. Tumor Res.*, *26*, 68–84

Lione, J.G. & Denholm, J.S. (1959) Cancer of the scrotum in wax pressmen. II. Clinical observations. *Arch. ind. Health occup. Med.*, *19*, 530–539

Lower, W.R., Drobney, V.K., Aholt, B.J. & Politte, R. (1983) Mutagenicity of the environments in the vicinity of an oil refinery and a petrochemical complex. *Teratog. Carcinog. Mutagenesis*, *3*, 65–73

Magnani, C., Coggon, D., Osmond, C. & Acheson, E.D. (1987) Occupation and five cancers: a case-control study using death certificates. *Br. J. ind. Med.*, *44*, 769–776

Malker, H.S.R., McLaughlin, J.K., Malker, B.K., Stone, B.J., Weiner, J.A., Ericsson, J.L.E. & Blot, W.J. (1986) Biliary tract cancer and occupation in Sweden. *Br. J. ind. Med.*, *43*, 257–262

McCraw, D.S., Joyner, R.E. & Cole, P. (1985) Excess leukemia in a refinery population. *J. occup. Med.*, *27*, 220–222

Metcalfe, C.D. & Sonstegard, R.A. (1985) Oil refinery effluents: evidence of cocarcinogenic activity in the trout embryo microinjection assay. *J. natl Cancer Inst.*, *75*, 1091–1097

Metcalfe, C.D., Sonstegard, R.A. & Quilliam, M.A. (1985) Genotoxic activity of particulate material in petroleum refinery effluents. *Bull. environ. Contam. Toxicol.*, *35*, 240–248

Morgan, R.W., Kheifets, L., Obrinsky, D.L., Whorton, M.D. & Foliart, D.E. (1984) Fetal loss and work in a waste water treatment plant. *Am. J. publ. Health*, *74*, 499–501

Najem, G.R., Louria, D.B., Seebode, J.J., Thind, I.S., Prusakowski, J.M., Ambrose, R.B. & Fernicola, A.R. (1982) Life time occupation, smoking, caffeine, saccharin, hair dyes and bladder carcinogenesis. *Int. J. Epidemiol.*, *11*, 212–217

National Institute for Occupational Safety and Health (1976) *Criteria for a Recommended Standard. Occupational Exposure to Ethylene Dichloride (1,2-Dichloroethane)* (*NIOSH Publ. No. 76-139*), Washington DC, US Government Printing Office, p. 84

National Institute for Occupational Safety and Health (1977) *Criteria for a Recommended Standard. Occupational Exposure to Ethylene Dibromide* (*NIOSH Publ. No. 77-221*), Washington DC, US Government Printing Office, pp. 121–125

Nau, C.A., Neal, J. & Thornton, M. (1966) C_9–C_{12} fractions obtained from petroleum distillates. An evaluation of their potential toxicity. *Arch. environ. Health*, *12*, 382–393

Nelson, N.A., Barker, D.M., Van Peenen, P.F.D. & Blanchard, A.G. (1983) Determining exposure categories for a refinery retrospective cohort mortality study. *Am. ind. Hyg. Assoc. J.*, *46*, 653–657

Nelson, N.A., Van Peenen, P.F.D. & Blanchard, A.G. (1987) Mortality in a recent oil refinery cohort. *J. occup. Med.*, *29*, 610–612

Nelson, W.L. (1960) *Guide to Refinery Operating Costs*, Tulsa, OK, Petroleum Publishing Co., pp. 3-4

Norell, S., Ahlbom, A., Olin, R., Erwald, R., Jacobson, G., Lindberg-Navier, I. & Wiechel, K.-L. (1986) Occupational factors and pancreatic cancer. *Br. J. ind. Med.*, 43, 775-778

Page, R.C. (1951) Symposium on a cancer control program for high-boiling catalytically cracked oils. Teamwork in control of occupational diseases. An introductory statement. *Arch. ind. Hyg. occup. Med.*, 4, 297-298

Petroleum Association for Conservation of the Canadian Environment (1979) *A Review of the Environmental and Occupational Health Hazards of Benzene in Canada* (*PACE Rep. No. 79-11*), Ottawa

Pickle, L.W. & Gottlieb, M.S. (1980) Pancreatic cancer mortality in Louisiana. *Am. J. publ. Health*, 70, 256-259

Rappaport, S.M., Selvin, S. & Waters, M.A. (1987) Exposures to hydrocarbon components of gasoline in the petroleum industry. *Appl. ind. Hyg.*, 2, 148-154

Rosenberg, M.J., Wyrobek, A.J., Ratcliffe, J., Gordon, L.A., Watchmaker, G., Fox, S.H., Moore, D.H., II & Hornung, R.W. (1985) Sperm as an indicator of reproductive risk among petroleum refinery workers. *Br. J. ind. Med.*, 42, 123-127

Royal Dutch/Shell Group of Companies (1983) *The Petroleum Handbook*, 6th ed., Amsterdam, Elsevier

Runion, H.E. & Scott, L.M. (1985) Benzene exposure in the United States 1978-1983: an overview. *Am. J. ind. Med.*, 7, 385-393

Rushton, L. & Alderson, M.R. (1980) The influence of occupation on health — some results from a study in the UK oil industry. *Carcinogenesis*, 1, 739-743

Rushton, L. & Alderson, M.R. (1981a) An epidemiological survey of eight oil refineries in Britain. *Br. J. ind. Med.*, 38, 225-234

Rushton, L. & Alderson, M.R. (1981b) A case-control study to investigate the association between exposure to benzene and deaths from leukaemia in oil refinery workers. *Br. J. Cancer*, 43, 77-84

Ruszczak, Z., Bienias, L. & Prószyńska-Kuczyńska, W. (1981a) Studies of skin in workers of selected departments of the refining and the petrochemical establishment in Flock (Pol.). *Przegl. Lek.*, 38, 637-639

Ruszczak, Z., Bienias, L. & Prószyńska-Kuczyńska, W. (1981b) Skin diseases in petrochemical industry workers (Pol.) *Przegl. Derm.*, 68, 435-439

Saffiotti, U. & Shubik, P. (1963) Studies on promoting action in skin carcinogenesis. *Natl Cancer Inst. Monogr.*, 10, 489-507

Schottenfeld, D., Warshauer, M.E., Zauber, A.G., Meikle, J.G. & Hart, B.R. (1981) *A prospective study of morbidity and mortality in petroleum industry employees in the United States — a preliminary report*. In: Peto, R. & Schneiderman, M., eds, *Quantification of Occupational Cancer* (*Banbury Report 9*), Cold Spring Harbor, NY, CSH Press, pp. 247-265

Shamsadinskaya, N.M., Kasimova, K.G., Pugacheva, G.M. & Guseynova, M.B. (1976) Menstrual and child bearing functions and gynecological morbidity in female workers of the Shavmyan region petroleum processing plants (Russ.). *Azerbajdzandskij med. Zu.*, 6, 56-59

Shapiro, D.D. & Getmanets, I.Y. (1962) Blastomogenic properties of petroleum of different sources (Russ.). *Gig. Sanit.*, 27, 38-42

Shubik, P. & Saffiotti, U. (1955) The carcinogenic and promoting action of low boiling catalytically cracked oils. *Acta unio int. contra cancrum*, *11*, 707–711

Silverman, D.T., Hoover, R.N., Albert, S. & Graff, K.M. (1983) Occupation and cancer of the lower urinary tract in Detroit. *J. natl Cancer Inst.*, *70*, 237–245

Smith, W.E., Sunderland, D.A. & Sugiura, K. (1951) Experimental analysis of the carcinogenic activity of certain petroleum products. *Arch. ind. Hyg. occup. Med.*, *4*, 299–314

Spear, R.C., Selvin, S., Schulman, J. & Francis, M. (1987) Benzene exposure in the petroleum refining industry. *Appl. ind. Hyg.*, *2*, 155–163

Suess, M.J., Grefen, K. & Reinisch, D.W., eds (1985) *Ambient Air Pollutants from Industrial Sources*, Amsterdam, Elsevier

Sukhanova, V.A. & Melnikova, V.V. (1974) Menstrual function in female workers at oil-refining plants suffering from chronic poisoning with petroleum products (Russ.) *Gig. Tr. prof. Zabol.*, *4*, 39–41

Thériault, G. & Goulet, L. (1979) A mortality study of oil refinery workers. *J. occup. Med.*, *21*, 367–370

Thériault, G. & Provencher, S. (1987) Mortality study of oil refinery workers: five-year follow-up. *J. occup. Med.*, *29*, 357–360

Thomas, T.L., Decouflé, P. & Moure-Eraso, R. (1980) Mortality among workers employed in petroleum refining and petrochemical plants. *J. occup. Med.*, *22*, 97–103

Thomas, T.L., Waxweiler, R.J., Crandall, M.S., White, D.W., Moure-Eraso, R., Itaya, S. & Fraumeni, J.F., Jr (1982a) Brain cancer among OCAW members in three Texas oil refineries. *Ann. N.Y. Acad. Sci.*, *381*, 120–129

Thomas, T.L., Waxweiler, R.J., Moure-Eraso, R., Itaya, S. & Fraumeni, J.F., Jr (1982b) Mortality patterns among workers in three Texas oil refineries. *J. occup. Med.*, *24*, 135–141

Thomas, T.L., Waxweiler, R.J., Crandall, M.S., White, D.W., Moure-Eraso, R. & Fraumeni, J.F., Jr (1984) Cancer mortality patterns by work category in three Texas oil refineries. *Am. J. ind. Med.*, *6*, 3–16

Thomas, T.L., Fontham, E.T.H., Norman, S.A., Stemhagen, A. & Hoover, R.N. (1986) Occupational risk factors for brain tumors: a case-referent death-certificate analysis. *Scand. J. Work Environ. Health*, *12*, 121–127

Thomas, T.L., Stewart, P.A., Stemhagen, A., Correa, P., Norman, S.A., Bleecker, M.L. & Hoover, R.N. (1987) Risk of astrocytic brain tumors associated with occupational chemical exposures. A case-referent study. *Scand. J. Work Environ. Health*, *13*, 417–423

Thorpe, J.J. (1974) Epidemiologic survey of leukemia in persons potentially exposed to benzene. *J. occup. Med.*, *16*, 375–382

Tsai, S.P., Wen, C.P., Weiss, N.S., Wong, O., McClellan, W.A. & Gibson, R.L. (1983) Retrospective mortality and medical surveillance studies of workers in benzene areas of refineries. *J. occup. Med.*, *25*, 685–692

US Environmental Protection Agency (1978) *Toxic Substances Control Act (TSCA) PL94-469. Candidate List of Chemical Substances*, Addendum 1, *Generic Terms Covering Petroleum Refinery Process Streams*, Washington DC, Office of Toxic Substances

US Environmental Protection Agency (1979) *Toxic Substances Control Act. Chemical Substance Inventory*, Washington DC, Office of Toxic Substances

Viau, C., Bernard, A., Lauwerys, R., Buchet, J.P., Quaeghebeur, L., Cornu, M.E., Phillips, S.C., Mutti, A., Lucertini, S. & Franchini, I. (1987) A cross-sectional survey of kidney function in refinery employees. *Am. J. ind. Med.*, *11*, 177–187

Wade, L. (1963) Observations on skin cancer among refinery workers. *Arch. environ. Health*, *6*, 730–735

Weaver, N.K., Gibson, R.L. & Smith, C.W. (1983) *Occupational exposure to benzene in the petroleum and petrochemical industries*. In: Mehlman, M.A., ed., *Advances in Modern Environmental Toxicology*, Vol. IV, *Carcinogenicity and Toxicity of Benzene*, Princeton, NJ, Princeton Scientific Publishers, pp. 63–75

Weil, C.S. & Condra, N.I. (1977) Experimental carcinogenesis of pyrolysis fuel oil. *Am. ind. Hyg. Assoc. J.*, *38*, 730–733

Wen, C.P., Tsai, S.P. & Gibson, R.L. (1982) A report on brain tumors from a retrospective cohort study of refinery workers. *Ann. N.Y. Acad. Sci.*, *381*, 130–138

Wen, C.P., Tsai, S.P., McClellan, W.A. & Gibson, R.L. (1983) Long-term mortality study of oil refinery workers. I. Mortality of hourly and salaried workers. *Am. J. Epidemiol.*, *118*, 526–542

Wen, C.P., Tsai, S.P., Moffitt, K.B., Bondy, M. & Gibson, R.L. (1984a) *Epidemiologic studies of the role of gasoline (hydrocarbon) exposure in kidney cancer risk*. In: Mehlman, M.A., Hemstreet, G.P., III, Thorpe, J.J. & Weaver, N.K., eds, *Advances in Modern Environmental Toxicology*, Vol. VII, *Renal Effects of Petroleum Hydrocarbons*, Princeton, NJ, Princeton Scientific Publishers, pp. 245–257

Wen, C.P., Tsai, S.P., Gibson, R.L. & McClellan, W.A. (1984b) Long-term mortality of oil refinery workers. II. Comparison of the experience of active, terminated and retired workers. *J. occup. Med.*, *26*, 118–127

Wen, C.P., Tsai, S.P., Weiss, N.S., Gibson, R.L., Wong, O. & McClellan, W.A. (1985) Long-term mortality study of oil refinery workers. IV. Exposure to the lubricating-dewaxing process. *J. natl Cancer Inst.*, *74*, 11–18

Wen, C.P., Tsai, S.P., Weiss, N.S. & Gibson, R.L. (1986) Long-term mortality study of oil refinery workers. V. Comparison of workers hired before, during, and after World War II (1940–1945) with a discussion on the impact of study designs on cohort results. *Am. J. ind. Med.*; *9*, 171–180

Wigle, D.T. (1977) The distribution of lung cancer in two Canadian cities. *Can. J. publ. Health*, *68*, 463–468

Witschi, H.P., Smith, L.H., Frome, E.L., Pequet-Goad, M.E., Griest, W.H., Ho, C.-H. & Guérin, M.R. (1987) Skin tumorigenic potential of crude and refined coal liquids and analogous petroleum products. *Fundam. appl. Toxicol.*, *9*, 297–303

Wong, O. & Raabe, G.K. (1989) Critical review of cancer epidemiology in petroleum industry employees, with a quantitative meta-analysis by cancer site. *Am. J. ind. Med*, *15*

Wong, O., Morgan, R.W., Bailey, W.J., Swencicki, R.E., Claxton, K. & Kheifets, L. (1986) An epidemiological study of petroleum refinery employees. *Br. J. ind. Med*, *43*, 6–17

Zhou, X., Li, L., Cui, M., Yu, R., Li, L. & Yan, Z. (1986) Cytogenetic monitoring of petrochemical workers. *Mutat. Res.*, *175*, 237–242

Žuškin, D.J. & Žuškin, E. (1964) Occupational dermatoses in oil refining (Slav.). *Arh. Hig. Rada*, *15*, 15–25

CRUDE OIL

1. Chemical and Physical Data

1.1 Synonyms and trade names

Chem. Abstr. Services Reg. No.: 8002-05-9
Chem. Abstr. Name: Petroleum
IUPAC Systematic Name: −
Synonyms: Naphtha; petrol; rock oil; Seneca oil

1.2 Description

Crude oil is a product of the remains of prehistoric plants and animals, buried in the primaeval mud of swamps, lakes and oceans. Over the centuries, layers of mud and organic debris were subjected to enormous pressures and high temperatures, and a petroleum-saturated rock was formed.

Four elements must be present for oil to accumulate in commercially useful quantities: source rock, reservoir rock, trap and seal. These elements allow the crude oil to remain underground and available in large quantities. A source rock is usually sedimentary rock rich in organic matter. The crude oil created by the decayed matter migrates from the source rock to a reservoir rock. The reservoir rock contains many tiny pores that store the oil. A trap, either stratigraphic layers of impermeable rock or structural traps, prevents the oil from migrating from the reservoir rock. An impermeable layer, or seal, prevents the oil from rising through or around the trap to the surface (American Petroleum Institute, 1984).

Crude oil has been defined as a 'highly complex mixture of paraffinic, cycloparaffinic (naphthenic) and aromatic hydrocarbons, containing low percentages of sulfur and trace amounts of nitrogen and oxygen compounds'(Hawley, 1981). Crude oils are often classified on the basis of chemical composition, according to the proportion of hydrocarbon constituents. Paraffinic crude oils are rich in straight-chain and branched paraffin hydrocarbons, whereas naphthenic crude oils contain mainly naphthenic and aromatic hydrocarbons. The composition and classification of many crude oils are obtained by ring analysis and by determination of the other constituents (Sachanen, 1950). Crude oil constituents are further described in section 1.3.

Crude oils may also be classified by geological source, as arising from productive sands, sandstones and limestones. The fractional and chemical compositions of crude oil from the same producing sand are usually very similar, even if they are drawn from fairly distant pools. However, some oilfields that are close together may produce quite different crude oils from the same stratum or from different oil-bearing sands. For instance, in East Texas, USA, Woodbine sand produces almost identical crude oils in different fields (specific gravity, 0.825–0.835; sulfur content, 0.25–0.40%); and crude oils from other Woodbine oilfields close to the East Texas field differ only slightly from the East Texas crude oil. In contrast, crude oils produced from the New and Old Grozny fields in the USSR are quite different, despite being only ten miles (16 km) from each other; New Grozny crude oil is highly paraffinic, whereas Old Grozny crude oil is highly naphthenic or asphaltic (Sachanen, 1950).

A similar phenomenon is found among different oil-bearing sands of the same pool. The Old Grozny field yields at least three different types of crude oil from its 16 producing sands, while Pennsylvania fields commonly produce similar types of crude oil in a range of different producing sands and the New Grozny field produces almost identical crude oils from 24 producing sands (Sachanen, 1950).

There is no clear-cut relationship between the chemical composition of crude oils and their geological age or origin. A commonly accepted generalization for US crude oils is that those that are geologically old are paraffin- and mixed-based, while those that are geologically new are naphthenic or asphaltic. Oilfields in other countries, however, are different: in Poland, crude oils that are geologically new are asphaltic, naphthenic and paraffinic. In practice, crude oils are often identified by the oilfield alone (Sachanen, 1950).

Crude oils are also referred to as light, medium (intermediate) or heavy, depending on their density. A light crude oil generally has an API (American Petroleum Institute) gravity (see section 1.3) greater than 40 (specific gravity, <0.82), a medium crude oil between 15 and 40 (specific gravity, 0.82–0.97) and a heavy crude oil less than 15 (specific gravity, >0.97).

Crude oils are designated in industry according to their suitability for use in various products. Thus, a crude oil may be referred to as a 'gasoline crude', a 'wax crude', a 'lube crude', an 'asphalt crude', and so forth.

1.3 Chemical composition and physical properties

Crude oils are complex mixtures of a vast number of individual chemical compounds. Each crude oil is a unique mixture, not matched exactly in composition or properties by any other sample of crude oil. Two typical crude oils, for example, have been characterized by the American Petroleum Institute as shown in Figure 1. Although the mid-points of their respective boiling ranges are similar, they differ considerably in other physical properties, hydrocarbon composition and distribution and sulfur content.

The bulk of the compounds present in crude oils are hydrocarbons (Speight, 1980). Crude oils generally contain the classes of hydrocarbons and other compounds described below (Cuddington & Lowther, 1977).

Fig. 1. Characteristics of two samples of crude oil

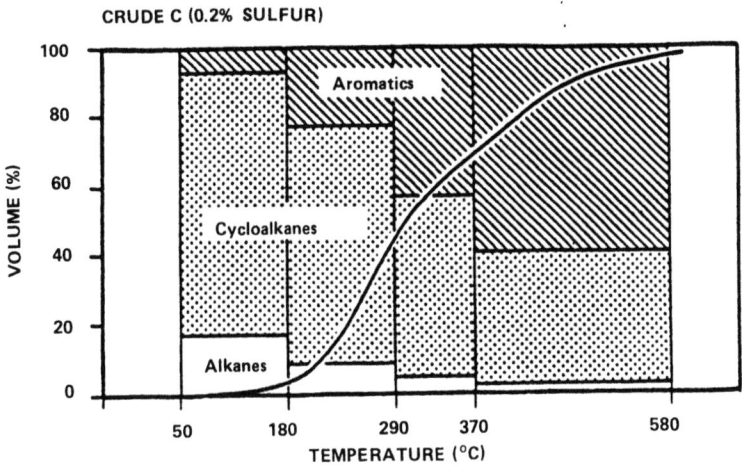

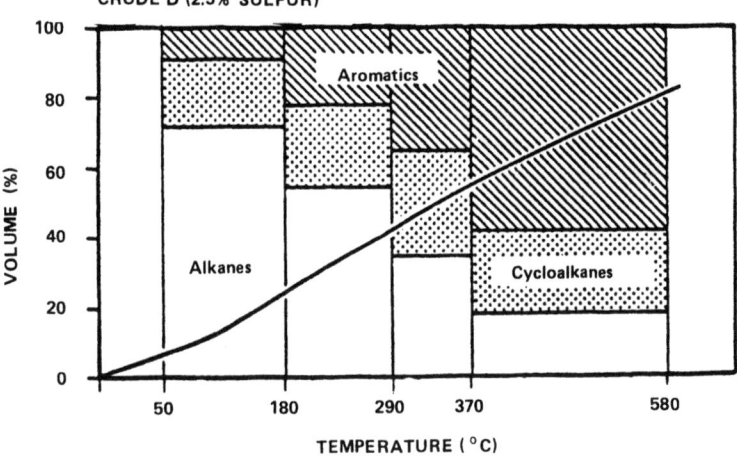

(a) *Hydrocarbon compounds*

(i) *Alkanes (paraffins)*

Alkanes are straight-chain normal alkanes and branched iso-alkanes with the general formula C_nH_{2n+2}. The major paraffinic components of most crude oils are in the range C_1 to C_{35} (Speight, 1980), although smaller quantities of alkanes up to C_{60} or higher may be present. Crude oils vary widely in alkane content (Dickey, 1981). The ratio of *n*-alkanes to isoalkanes is shown in Table 1 for one crude oil sample (Ponca). The ratio ranges from a minimum of 1.7 for heptanes to a maximum of 6.9 for octanes (Speight, 1980). A Pennsylvania crude oil sample had *n*-alkane:isoalkane ratios of 1.3, 1.7 and 1.5 for pentanes,

Table 1. Alkanes isolated from a crude oil sample[a]

Compound	Vol. %	n-Alkane:isoalkane
C_6		2.2
n-Hexane	1.8	
2-Methylpentane	0.4	
3-Methylpentane	0.3	
2,2-Dimethylbutane	0.04	
2,3-Dimethylbutane	0.08	
C_7		1.7
n-Heptane	2.3	
3-Methylhexane	0.5	
3-Ethylpentane	0.05	
2-Methylhexane	0.7	
2,3-Dimethylpentane	0.1	
C_8		6.9
n-Octane	1.9	
2,2-Dimethylhexane	0.01	
2,3-Dimethylhexane	0.06	
2,4-Dimethylhexane	0.06	
2,5-Dimethylhexane	0.06	
3,3-Dimethylhexane	0.03	
2-Methyl-3-ethylpentane	0.04	
2,2,3-Trimethylpentane	0.004	
2,3,3-Trimethylpentane	0.006	
2,3,4-Trimethylpentane	0.005	
C_9		2.6
n-Nonane	1.8	
2-Methyloctane	0.4	
3-Methyloctane	0.1	
4-Methyloctane	0.1	
2,3-Dimethylheptane	0.05	
2,6-Dimethylheptane	0.05	
Higher alkanes		
n-Decane	1.8	
n-Undecane	1.7	
n-Dodecane	1.7	

[a]From Speight (1980); a Ponca crude oil

hexanes and heptanes, respectively (Tiratsoo, 1951). Alkenes are not generally found in crude oils (Speight, 1980).

(ii) *Cycloalkanes (naphthenes)*

Cycloalkanes (or cycloparaffins), also called naphthenes in the petroleum industry, are saturated hydrocarbons containing structures with carbon atoms linked in a ring. The cycloalkane composition in crude oil worldwide typically varies from 30% to 60% (see also

Table 3). The predominant monocycloalkanes in crude oil are in the cyclopentane series, having five carbon atoms in the ring, and in the cyclohexanes, having a six-membered ring. The most predominant monocycloalkanes and their composition ranges in crude oil are shown in Table 2 (Bestougeff, 1967). In the higher boiling fractions, such as lubricating oils, cycloalkanes with two or more rings are common, and structures containing up to ten rings have been reported. These polycyclic structures are usually composed of fused five- and six-membered rings (Table 2; Mair, 1964).

Table 2. Predominant cycloalkanes isolated from crude oil[a]

Cycloalkane	Carbon atom number	% in crude oil		
		Min	Max	%
Monocycloalkanes[b]				
Methylcyclopentane	C_6	0.11	2.35	
Cyclohexane	C_6	0.08	1.4	
Methylcyclohexane	C_7	0.25	2.8	
trans-1,2-Dimethylcyclopentane	C_7	0.05	1.2	
cis-1,3-Dimethylcyclopentane	C_7	0.04	1.0	
cis-1,3-Dimethylcyclohexane	C_8	–	0.9	
cis-1,2-Dimethylcyclohexane	C_8	–	0.6	
1,1,3-Trimethylcyclohexane	C_9	–	0.7	
Polycycloalkanes[c]				
Methylbicyclo[2.2.1]heptane	C_8			0.001
cis-Bicyclo[3.3.0]octane	C_8			0.06
Bicyclo[3.2.1]octane	C_8			0.008
trans-Decahydronaphthalene	C_{10}			0.2
Tricyclo[3.3.1.1^{3,7}]decane	C_{10}			0.0004
cis-Decahydronaphthalene	C_{10}			0.01

[a]Reference crude oil from American Petroleum Institute
[b]From Bestougeff (1967)
[c]From Mair (1964)

(iii) *Aromatic hydrocarbons*

The most common aromatic compounds in crude oils are benzene (see IARC, 1982, 1987a), benzene derivatives (e.g., alkylbenzenes) and fused benzene ring compounds. The concentration of benzene in crude oil has been reported to range between 0.01% and 1% (Bestougeff, 1967). Table 3 shows the overall composition of three crude oil samples, including the major classes of aromatic hydrocarbons, and Table 4 gives the levels of seven specific polycyclic aromatics in two of these samples (National Research Council, 1985).

Table 3. Composition and physical characteristics of three crude oils[a]

Characteristic or component	Crude oil		
	Prudhoe Bay	South Louisiana	Kuwait
API gravity (20°C; °API)	27.8	34.5	31.4
Sulfur (wt %)	0.94	0.25	2.44
Nitrogen (wt %)	0.23	0.69	0.14
Nickel (ppm; mg/kg)	10	2.2	7.7
Vanadium (ppm; mg/kg)	20	1.9	28.0
Naphtha fraction[b] (wt %)	23.2	18.6	22.7
Alkanes	12.5	8.8	16.2
Cycloalkanes	7.4	7.7	4.1
Aromatic hydrocarbons	3.2	2.1	2.4
Benzenes	0.3[c]	0.2	0.1
Toluene	0.6	0.4	0.4
C_8 aromatics	0.5	0.7	0.8
C_9 aromatics	0.06	0.5	0.6
C_{10} aromatics	–	0.2	0.3
C_{11} aromatics	–	0.1	0.1
Indans	–	–	0.1
High-boiling fraction[d] (wt %)	76.8	81.4	77.3
Saturates	14.4[e]	56.3	34.0
n-Alkanes	5.8[f]	5.2	4.7
C_{11}	0.12	0.06	0.12
C_{12}	0.25	0.24	0.28
C_{13}	0.42	0.41	0.38
C_{14}	0.50	0.56	0.44
C_{15}	0.44	0.54	0.43
C_{16}	0.50	0.58	0.45
C_{17}	0.51	0.59	0.41
C_{18}	0.47	0.40	0.35
C_{19}	0.43	0.38	0.33
C_{20}	0.37	0.28	0.25
C_{21}	0.32	0.20	0.20
C_{22}	0.24	0.15	0.17
C_{23}	0.21	0.16	0.15
C_{24}	0.20	0.13	0.12
C_{25}	0.17	0.12	0.10
C_{26}	0.15	0.09	0.09
C_{27}	0.10	0.06	0.06
C_{28}	0.09	0.05	0.06
C_{29}	0.08	0.05	0.05
C_{30}	0.08	0.04	0.07
C_{31}	0.08	0.04	0.06
C_{32} plus	0.07	0	0.06

Table 3 (contd)

Characteristic or component	Crude oil		
	Prudhoe Bay	South Louisiana	Kuwait
Isoalkanes	–	14.0	13.2
1-ring cycloalkanes	9.9	12.4	6.2
2-ring cycloalkanes	7.7	9.4	4.5
3-ring cycloalkanes	5.5	6.8	3.3
4-ring cycloalkanes	5.4	4.8	1.8
5-ring cycloalkanes	–	3.2	0.4
6-ring cycloalkanes	–	1.1	–
Aromatic hydrocarbons (wt %)	25.0	16.5	21.9
Benzenes	7.0	3.9	4.8
Indans and tetralins	–	2.4	2.2
Dinaphthenobenzenes	–	2.9	2.0
Naphthalenes	9.9	1.3	0.7
Acenapthenes	–	1.4	0.9
Phenanthrenes	3.1	0.9	0.3
Acenaphthalenes	–	2.8	1.5
Pyrenes	1.5	–	–
Chrysenes	–	–	0.2
Benzothiophenes	1.7	0.5	5.4
Dibenzothiophenes	1.3	0.4	3.3
Indanothiophenes	–	–	0.6
Polar material[g] (wt %)	2.9	8.4	17.9
Insolubles[h]	1.2	0.2	3.5

[a]These analyses represent values for one typical crude oil from each of the three geographical regions; variations in composition can be expected for oils produced from different formations or fields within each region. From National Research Council (1985)

[b]Fraction boiling from 20 to 205°C

[c]Reported for fraction boiling from 20 to 150°C

[d]Fraction boiling above 205°C

[e]Reported for fraction boiling above 220°C

[f]Prudhoe Bay crude oil weathered two weeks to duplicate fractional distillation equivalent to approximately 205°C n-alkane percentages from gas chromatography over the range C_{11}–C_{32} plus

[g]Clay-gel separation according to ASTM method D-2007 using pentane on unweathered sample

[h]Pentane-insoluble materials according to ASTM method D-893

–, not measured

Table 4. Concentrations of individual polynuclear aromatic hydrocarbons in crude oil (10^{-6} g/g oil)[a]

Compound	South Louisiana crude oil	Kuwaiti crude oil
Pyrene	4.3	4.5
Fluoranthene	6.2	2.9
Benz[a]anthracene	3.1	2.3
Chrysene	23	6.9
Triphenylene	13	2.8
Benzo[a]pyrene	1.2	2.8
Benzo[e]pyrene	3.3	0.5

[a]From National Research Council (1985)

(b) *Nonhydrocarbon compounds*

(i) *Sulfur compounds*

Crude oils vary widely in sulfur content, which can range from <0.1% to 10% by weight. The following types of sulfur compounds have been identified in crude oils: thiols (mercaptans), sulfides, disulfides and thiophenes (Costantinides & Arich, 1967).

In the lower distillation range up to about 150°C, the most abundant sulfur compounds are thiols. In the 150–250°C distillation range, the most abundant compounds are thiocyclo-, thiobicyclo- and thiotricycloalkanes and thiophenes. These sulfur compounds are replaced, in turn, by benzothiophenes and more complex ring structures in the higher distillation ranges (Costantinides & Arich, 1967).

(ii) *Nitrogen compounds*

The nitrogen content of crude oils ranges from trace amounts to 0.9% by weight. The bulk of the nitrogen in fractions that boil below about 200°C is basic nitrogen. The basic nitrogen compounds often found in crude oils include pyridines and quinolines, e.g., 3-methylpyridine and quinoline, while nonbasic nitrogen compounds include pyrroles, indoles and carbazoles, e.g., carbazole, and amides (Costantinides & Arich, 1967).

(iii) *Oxygen compounds*

The oxygen content of crude oils ranges from 0.06% to 0.4% by weight, the majority of components being alkane and cycloalkane (naphthenic) acids. Other minor components include ketones and phenols (Costantinides & Arich, 1967). The oxygen content of crude oils increases with boiling range, so that more oxygen-containing compounds are found in distillates that boil above 400°C.

(iv) *Metal-containing compounds*

Traces of many metallic compounds can be found in crude oils. Nickel (see IARC, 1976, 1987b) and vanadium compounds have been identified in crude oils at levels ranging from a few parts per million to 200 ppm (mg/kg) nickel and up to 1200 ppm (mg/kg) vanadium. These metals occur primarily as complexes (porphyrins; Costantinides & Arich, 1967) which are stable and can be distilled at temperatures above 500°C.

Table 5 is a compilation of some other trace elements reported in crude oil and their typical concentrations either in crude oil or in crude oil ash (Magee et al., 1973; Valković, 1978). Most of these elements occur naturally in crude oil as a result of their presence in the rock formation or in salt-water deposits from which the crude oil was drawn, although some

Table 5. Elements in crude oil[a]

Element	Concentration (ppm)
Calcium	5000–50 000[b]
Aluminium	2000–20 000[b]
Magnesium	200–10 000[b]
Titanium	100–5000[b]
Strontium	100–1000[b]
Barium	20–500[b]
Potassium	4.9
Sodium	2.9–20.3
Chlorine	1.5–39.3
Iron	1–125
Molybdenum	<1–10
Tin	<1–2.2
Zinc	0.67–62.9
Lead	0.17–0.31
Fluorine	0.14–1.1
Copper	0.13–6.3
Bromine	0.072–1.33
Manganese	0.05–11.4
Selenium	0.03–1.4
Antimony	0.03–0.15
Mercury	0.02–30
Rubidium	0.015 (average)
Gallium	0.01–0.30
Rhenium	<0.005–2.5
Gold	0.004 (average)
Cobalt	0.003–13.5
Arsenic	0.002–0.66
Europium	0.001 (average)
Caesium	0.0004
Cadmium	0.0003–0.027
Scandium	0.0003–0.008
Chromium	0.00023–0.640
Uranium	0.00004–0.014

[a]From Magee et al. (1973); Valković (1978)
[b]Ash

may also be introduced during the process of drilling, pumping, preparing and transporting crude oil to a refinery.

(v) *Miscellaneous contaminants*

Crude oil, as it emerges from the well-head, is typically a heterogeneous mixture of solids, liquids and gases, including, in addition to the constituents described above, sand and other sediments, water and water vapour, salts and acid gases such as hydrogen sulfide and carbon dioxide. These contaminants are at least partially separated from the crude oil in surface treatment at the well-head (see p. 132) to prepare it for transportation to the refinery (Baker *et al.*, 1986a).

Crude oils are not analysed routinely for their content of various classes of hydrocarbons and nonhydrocarbons; rather, they are usually characterized by their physical properties (specific gravity or density, viscosity) and their sulfur content. Crude oils are also characterized in pilot-scale distillations by the volume or weight percentage in various boiling-point ranges ('straight-run fractions').

One of the most important physical properties of crude oil is its specific gravity —the ratio of the density of oil to the density of water, both taken at the same temperature and pressure. From the specific gravity, the ratio of aromatic (high density) to saturated (low density) hydrocarbons in crude oil samples may be estimated. An alternative expression for specific gravity, developed for petroleum applications, is:

$$\text{Degrees API (°API)} = \frac{141.5}{\text{specific gravity at 16°C}} - 131.5.$$

The specific gravities of petroleum usually range from about 0.8 (45.3°API) for the lighter crude oils to over 1.0 (10°API) for the heavier asphaltic crude oil (Dickey, 1981).

Crude oil is also characterized by its viscosity. Viscosity is expressed in Saybolt universal seconds (SUS) at 38°C. This value is determined by the time it takes for 60 cm^3 of crude oil to flow by gravity through an orifice in a calibrated viscometer (Dickey, 1981). Viscosity may also be expressed in centipoises.

Sulfur content is the third important property of crude oil because of its effect on the refining process (in poisoning catalysts) and the malodorous and toxic properties of hydrogen sulfide and other sulfur compounds. Table 6 gives the API gravity, sulfur content and viscosity of several crude oils.

Table 7 summarizes the composition of crude oils throughout the world, based on analysis by the US Department of Energy of 800 crude oil samples from 691 major oilfields in the USA (Coleman *et al.*, 1978) and on analysis by the US Bureau of Mines of the Department of the Interior of 169 samples of crude oil from 122 fields in 27 countries outside the USA (Ferrero & Nichols, 1972).

Table 6. Characteristics of some typical crude oils[a]

Name, area	Specific gravity (°API)	Sulfur content (%)	Viscosity (SUS at 38°C)
Smackover, AR, USA	20.5	2.30	270
Kern River, CA, USA	10.7	1.23	6000+
Kettleman, CA, USA	37.5	0.32	
London, IL, USA	38.8	0.26	45
Rodessa, LA, USA	42.8	0.28	
Oklahoma City, OK, USA	37.3	0.11	
Bradford, PA, USA	42.4	0.09	40
East TX, USA	38.4	0.33	40
Leduc, Alberta, Canada	40.4	0.29	37.8
Boscan, Venezuela	9.5	5.25	
Poza Rica, Mexico	30.7	1.67	67.9
La Rosa, Venezuela	25.3	1.76	
Kirkuk, Iraq	36.6	1.93	42
Abqaiq, Saudi Arabia	36.5	1.36	
Seria, Brunei, Malaysia	36.0	0.05	

[a]From Dickey (1981)

Table 7. Summary of worldwide crude oil compositions and characteristics[a]

Geographical region	Volume % in crude oil		General characteristics (wt %)	
	Light gasoline and naphtha	Kerosene and gas oil	Sulfur	Carbon residue[b]
Africa				
Maximum	48.9	43.0	2.06	10.8
Minimum	2.4	19.5	0.05	0.1
Average	24.2	28.9	0.50	2.5
(n = 47 [35])				
Asia (Far East)				
Maximum	37.1	41.1	0.28	8.6
Minimum	4.5	18.0	0.10	0.3
Average	16.9	26.0	0.15	3.3
(n = 7 [6])				
Asia (Middle East)				
Maximum	35.6	28.8	3.91	6.9
Minimum	12.1	8.8	0.62	1.3
Average	26.9	23.7	2.08	4.0
(n = 44 [34])				

Table 7 (contd)

Geographical region	Volume % in crude oil		General characteristics (wt %)	
	Light gasoline and naphtha	Kerosene and gas oil	Sulfur	Carbon residue[b]
Australia				
Maximum	50.6	56.3	0.44	3.9
Minimum	12.8	24.6	0.02	0.2
Average	37.2	33.9	0.10	0.7
($n = 9$ [8])				
Caribbean				
Maximum	30.9	30.7	3.26	6.3
Minimum	0.6	20.6	0.88	2.6
Average	16.3	25.2	1.92	4.1
($n = 8$ [3])				
Europe				
Maximum	26.0	46.5	4.34	9.7
Minimum	2.9	14.2	0.14	0.3
Average	14.7	23.6	1.16	4.4
($n = 8$ [8])				
North America (USA)				
Maximum	84.5	68.6	5.1	14.0
Minimum	0.4	9.7	0.01	0.0
Average	27.7	28.3	0.7	2.6
($n = 800$ [691])				
North America (Canada)				
Maximum	36.1	28.3	3.38	11.0
Minimum	6.3	20.2	0.11	1.2
Average	26.7	24.1	1.1	3.6
($n = 10$ [7])				
South America				
Maximum	43.5	40.1	5.54	8.4
Minimum	1.9	14.3	0.09	0.02
Average	18.9	23.9	1.34	4.4
($n = 36$ [26])				

[a]From Ferrero & Nichols (1972) and Coleman *et al.* (1978). Averages are simple numerical (unweighted) averages of the data for the various oilfields in the region, where n is the number of samples and [] the number of oilfields used to calculate the average and establish the range.

[b]% of carbon residue, after thermic treatment, determined by the method of Conradson

2. Production, Use, Occurrence and Analysis

2.1 Production and use

(a) Production

Crude oil production is the process of raising well fluids to the surface and preparing them for further processing at the refinery. Since 1972, about 60 million barrels of crude oil have been produced each day worldwide, mostly in areas of sparse population or of limited industrial development (Anderson, 1984; American Petroleum Institute, 1987a; British Petroleum Company, 1988). Crude oil production begins with preparation of a well, followed by the application of a variety of natural and artificial lift mechanisms to bring the oil to the surface. There it is treated superficially to prepare it for transport to the refinery by tanker or barge, by pipeline, or by truck or rail (Baker *et al.*, 1986a).

Worldwide, about 500 000 workers are employed in oil exploration and production (International Labour Office, 1986).

(i) Preparing the well

The production operation begins after the well has been drilled and has been evaluated as being economically favourable for production. Pipe or casing is inserted into the well bore in a concentric series to prevent contamination by fresh water, loss of circulation, sloughing or charging of shallow sands with abnormal pressures (American Petroleum Institute, 1983). The first such casing placed into a well is the conductor pipe, which may be pile driven or cemented into place and may extend to a depth of 150–1500 m.

The conductor pipe and all other casings are attached at the surface to the casing head (American Petroleum Institute, 1983). Surface casing is inserted through the conductor pipe and deeper into the well to prevent underground formations of fresh water from becoming contaminated with well fluids and to provide a mechanism for controlling the flow of fluid from the well.

(ii) Pumping the crude

Once the well has been completed, oil begins to flow up the well as a result of the inherent reservoir energy, which is manifested by an oil displacement process involving water, gas or a combination of both. Reservoir drive mechanisms — the processes by which the reservoir energy displaces the crude oil — include dissolved-gas drive, gas-cap drive, water drive and combination drive (Baker *et al.*, 1986a; Gray, 1986). Natural drive mechanisms may, at some point in the economic life of the well, lose their inherent energy and the well will require a mechanical force to draw the oil from the reservoir. The common methods of artificial lift are surface pumping, submersible pumping and gas lift (Baker *et al.*, 1986a; Gray, 1986).

The natural and artificial lift mechanisms provide a means of raising reservoir fluids capable of flowing into the well bore. However, fractures, channels and perforations through which the fluids flow often become blocked and diminish the production capacity of a well. These passages may be cleared and new ones created by using reservoir stimulation techniques such as acidizing and hydraulic fracturing (Baker *et al.*, 1986a).

Acidizing is the process of treating the formation — limestone or dolomite — with hydrochloric, acetic or hydrofluoric acid. Additives such as corrosion inhibitors, surface active agents, sequestering agents and antisludge agents are mixed with the acids to prevent acid attack on tubing and casing, to help disperse the acid in the formation, to prevent precipitation of ferric iron during acidizing and to prevent formation of insoluble sludge (Giuliano, 1981; Baker *et al.*, 1986a).

Hydraulic fracturing is used extensively and successfully on formations composed of sandstone. A fluid, such as water charged with nitrogen, is pumped under high pressure at high rates into the well to create deep penetrating fractures in the reservoir. Charging the water with nitrogen facilitates the flow of water back out of the well (Giuliano, 1981; Baker *et al.*, 1986a).

(iii) *Surface treatment*

When the crude oil has been brought to the surface, the final production step is to reduce it to the form in which it will be sent to the refinery for processing. Contaminants such as sediment and water are removed, and volatile components are separated and treated by the use of separators (Giuliano, 1981; Baker *et al.*, 1986a; Gray, 1986).

Natural gases must be treated to remove water vapour and acid gases such as carbon dioxide and hydrogen sulfide. Water vapour may be removed by bubbling the gas through a solid or liquid desiccant; the acid gases may also be removed from a natural gas stream by adsorption or absorption with an appropriate liquid or solid desiccant. This process of removing acid gases from a natural gas stream is commonly referred to as sweetening (Baker *et al.*, 1986a).

(iv) *Transportation and storage*

The primary means of transporting crude oil are tankers and pipelines; trucks and railways fulfil much smaller yet significant roles. Barges are used to transport oil on inland waterways and to off-load large tankers.

Modern tankers carry over two-thirds of all crude oil produced to modern industrial societies (Baker *et al.*, 1986b). Oil can be loaded onto tankers either from onshore facilities after transport from inland fields or from offshore platforms. The single-point (or single-buoy) mooring system is a common method for loading tankers. Oil is pumped from an offshore or onshore facility through a pipeline on the ocean bed to a marine riser which is suspended at the surface by a large mooring buoy. The oil is passed from the pipeline into a flexible hose connected to the riser, through the riser to a floating base and from there to the ship (Giuliano, 1981).

An individual oil field may contain several hundred wells. Flow lines connect individual wells in an oil field to field storage tanks and transport oil to a central location for treatment, testing and measurement. Following treatment, oil is transported from a central tank battery by intermediate 'gathering' lines which, like the flow lines, generally range from 5 to 30 cm in diameter (Giuliano, 1981; Baker *et al.*, 1986b).

Pumps at a pump station move the oil into and through a pipeline. A gathering station in or close to an oil field receives oil from producers' tanks via a pipeline gathering system and moves it on to a trunk-line station located on the main 'trunk' line. Trunk lines are large-diameter (up to 120 cm) pipelines that carry oil over long distances to refineries, central storage or ports. Booster pump stations are placed along the trunk line as necessary to compensate for loss of pressure as the oil is moved through the line (Giuliano, 1981; Baker et al., 1986b).

Tank farms may be located along pipelines, where oil can be temporarily side-tracked from transit for holding, sorting, measuring or rerouting. A tank farm may function as a receiving station for oil that is to be moved into the pipeline transportation system. Pipelines from a tank farm converge at a station manifold which can split, merge or reroute the flow of oil as needed (Baker et al., 1986b). Highly viscous crude oil can be heated and transported via an insulated pipeline, along which reheating stations may be employed (Watkins, 1977).

Deposits accumulate on the inside wall of a pipe during the course of operations. Some crude oils deposit substantial coatings of wax on cooling; salts and other foreign materials may also build up. To clean the pipeline and remove deposits, 'pigs' equipped with scrapers and brushes are run through it periodically, entering and leaving via locks or pig traps, so that the line can continue to operate under pressure (Anderson, 1984).

Crude oil is also transported by truck, especially from new fields where pipeline gathering lines have not been built. However, motor carrier transport represents only a small fraction of US domestic transportation of crude oil, accounting for less than 0.3% of that total in 1982. An even smaller percentage (0.05% in 1982) of domestic crude oil transportation is by rail. Rail tank cars are used to move crude oil from ocean tankers or waterways to small inland refineries (Baker et al., 1986b).

(v) *Production volumes*

World crude oil production from 1947 to 1986 is shown in Table 8 by geographical region. Over the past 40 years, production has increased more than seven fold, from 3000 million barrels to 22 000 million barrels per year. Table 9 gives production data for the 20 countries that produced the most crude oil in 1976 and 1986.

In 1986, proven worldwide reserves of crude oil were estimated to be 700 000 million barrels (Table 10).

(b) *Use*

The direct use of raw crude oil was reported as far back as 3000 BC. Crude oil seeping to the earth's surface was collected and used in ancient times by the Chinese, Babylonians, Assyrians and other early civilizations. With only rudimentary methods of discovery and extraction, these early peoples often located crude oil by observing natural gas escaping from the earth's crust with the petroleum liquid. They used this natural resource for its four principal components — oil, grease, asphalt and wax. The source of the crude oil and its composition determined the petroleum products for which it was useful. Among the early uses of the unrefined natural product were fuel for oil lamps, heating fuel, bitumens mixed with fibre, sand, etc. for buildings, roads and dams, medicinal oils (e.g., Seneca oil), paints,

Table 8. World crude oil production, 1947–86 (millions of barrels per year)[a]

Geographical region	1947	1956	1966	1976	1987
Canada and USA	1 865	2 789	3 348	3 465	4 312
Latina America	574	1 128	1 670	1 625	2 409
Western Europe	13	73	144	312	1 531
Middle East	306	1 261	3 408	8 116	4 787
Africa	9	13	1 030	2 135	1 907
Asia and Australasia	25	146	256	923	1 230
Centrally planned economies[b]	231	715	2 165	4 616	5 796
Total world	3 023	6 125	12 021	21 192	21 972

[a]From American Petroleum Institute (1987a), not including natural gas liquids; British Petroleum Company (1988), for 1987 data only, which include natural gas liquids which typically comprise ~7% of total world crude oil production (6.86–7.47%, 1981–86)

[b]Albania, Bulgaria, China, Cuba, Czechoslovakia, Democratic Kampuchea, the Democratic People's Republic of Korea, the German Democratic Republic, Hungary, the Lao People's Democratic Republic, Mongolia, Poland, Romania, the USSR, Viet Nam and Yugoslavia

Table 9. World crude oil production (thousands of barrels per year): 20 leading regions[a]

1976		1986	
Region	Production	Region	Production
1. USSR	3 839 800	1. USSR	4 584 000
2. USA	3 553 300	2. USA	3 741 300
3. Saudia Arabia	3 111 600	3. Saudia Arabia	1 879 800
4. Iran (Islamic Republic of)	2 160 800	4. Mexico	1 003 800
5. Iraq	881 500	5. United Kingdom	972 700
6. Venezuela	866 900	6. China	960 000
7. Nigeria	753 700	7. Iran (Islamic Republic of)	695 300
8. Kuwait	717 200	8. Venezuela	673 400
9. Libyan Arab Jamahiriya	704 500	9. Canada	671 600
10. China	611 400	10. Iraq	637 000
11. Canada	585 800	11. Nigeria	534 700
12. United Arab Emirates (Abu Dhabi)	582 200	12. Indonesia	511 000
13. Indonesia	549 300	13. Kuwait	456 300
14. Algeria	392 400	14. United Arab Emirates (Abu Dhabi)	397 900
15. Mexico	319 400	15. Algeria	386 900
16. Qatar	180 700	16. Libyan Arab Jamihiriya	381 400
17. Neutral zone[b]	169 700	17. Norway	332 200
18. Argentina	142 400	18. Egypt	304 800
19. Oman	133 200	19. Brazil	217 200
20. Egypt	118 600	20. Oman	204 400

[a]From British Petroleum Company (1986, 1988); includes natural gas liquids
[b]Of the Middle East

Table 10. Proven reserves at end 1987[a]

Region	Proven reserves	
	Thousand million barrels	Share of total (%)
North America	41.1	4.6
Latin America	114.3	12.9
Western Europe	22.4	2.5
Middle East	564.8	63.0
Africa	55.2	6.1
Asia and Australasia	19.5	2.1
Centrally planned economies[b]	79.2	8.8
Total world	896.5	

[a]Estimated quantities of crude oil demonstrated with reasonable certainty by geological and engineering data to be recoverable from known reservoirs under existing economic and operating conditions. From British Petroleum Company (1988)

[b]See footnote b to Table 8.

waterproofing wicker and mats, adhesives for inlay work, insecticides and rodenticides, and tool manufacture. Historical uses in Europe include lubricants for axles, lamp oil, preservatives for wood used in shipbuilding, and other applications in navigation (Cross, 1983).

During the twentieth century, crude oil has become one of the world's most important natural raw materials. Commercial quantities are extracted from all large land masses, except Antarctica and Greenland, as well as from the earth beneath major bodies of water. The petroleum or crude oil thus obtained is a major source of the world's energy and the main feedstock for the petrochemical industry (Considine, 1974).

According to the American Petroleum Institute (1984), the use of oil refinery products as feed stocks for the petrochemical industry has resulted in more than 3000 petrochemical intermediates and products. Hoffman (1982) has published a useful table of 'Petroleum Products, Their Uses and Compositions'.

Because crude oil varies markedly in composition and properties and, therefore, lacks consistency and reproducibility, it is no longer used directly in consumer applications, even as fuel. Today, virtually all recovered crude oil is sent to a refinery for processing into products or intermediates.

A significant and growing amount of the world's elemental sulfur is also recovered as a by-product of sour crude oil. Refineries process more sour crude oils under stricter pollution controls, with the result that the production of recovered sulfur has increased in recent years (West, 1983). The *Oil and Gas Journal Data Book* (Anon., 1987) lists three countries as producers of sulfur derived from crude oil, reporting production levels in tonnes per day at 1 January 1986 of 120 in Brazil, 51 in Hungary and 121.4 in the USA.

Demand for refined petroleum products by geographical region during the past two decades is shown in Table 11. Consumption of petroleum products by group (gasoline, middle distillates, fuel oil, others) is given in Table 4 of the monograph on occupational exposures in petroleum refining.

Table 11. Estimated world demand for refined petroleum products by region (millions of barrels per year)[a]

Region	1966	1976	1986
Canada and USA	4 850	7 029	6 210
Latin America	824	1 375	1 655
Western Europe	3 051	4 922	4 508
Middle East	300	620	785
Africa	213	393	617
Asia	1 248	2 921	3 176
Centrally planned economies[b]	1 765	3 916	4 920
Total world	12 251	21 176	21 871

[a]From American Petroleum Institute (1987a) for 1966 and 1976; adapted from British Petroleum Company (1988) for 1986

[b]See footnote b to Table 8.

(c) *Regulatory status and guidelines*

Occupational exposure limits have been established or recommended for various petroleum fractions, as well as for many of the individual substances found in crude oil. However, for crude oil itself, no exposure limit has been set.

Several national laws and multinational agreements have been established to prevent pollution of the seas and other environments by oil (Reitze, 1972; Myhre, 1980; Duck, 1983).

2.2 Occurrence

(a) *Natural occurrence*

Crude oil is a naturally occurring complex mixture which is found in subsurface deposits in most regions of the world.

(b) *Occupational exposure*

Since crude oil is a complex liquid, there is potential occupational exposure to a variety of substances: various hydrocarbons and other organic compounds, dissolved gases and metal compounds. Exposure is possible in all operations involving the product, including drilling, pumping and treating steps; transport by pipeline, ships or rail cars; storage and refinery processing (Suess *et al.*, 1985).

The primary route of exposure is through skin contact. However, some sour crude oils contain high concentrations of hydrogen sulfide, and control of exposures, particularly during sampling and maintenance operations, is critical. Some known carcinogens, such as benzene, certain polycyclic aromatic compounds and nickel and arsenic compounds, are commonly found in crude oils. Certain crude oil condensates can contain up to 15 vol % benzene.

Other airborne contaminants identified in operations involving crude oil are mercaptans and gaseous and volatile hydrocarbons. Explosive concentrations of airborne hydrocarbons and lethal levels of hydrogen sulfide can be found at the well head and in compartments and confined spaces (Duck, 1983). No data were available to quantify occupational exposure levels to crude oil components.

(c) Environmental exposure

A recent estimate of the total input of petroleum into the marine environment from all sources is 1.7–8.8 million tonnes per year, with a best estimate of 3.2 million tonnes per year. Table 12 presents the approximate annual input of petroleum hydrocarbons into the oceans from various man-made and natural sources (Koons, 1984).

The total amount of oil produced in Nigeria between 1980 and 1983 was approximately 350 million m^3 (370 million tonnes), averaging 88 million m^3 (93 million tonnes) per year and generating an average of 13 million m^3 of waste water per year. The average concentration of oil dissolved in the water ranged from 11.2 to 53.9 mg/l (total range, 0.9–96.7 mg/l; Ibiebele, 1986).

In a study of estuarine and seawater samples from three Australian bodies of water, it was found that a probable source of aromatic hydrocarbons in the dissolved and particulate phases from the estuarine samples was crude oil. Other probable sources included refined petroleum products, including lubricating oil and residual fuel oil, and distillates, including gasoline and diesel fuel (Smith & Maher, 1984).

In a study of petroleum residues in the waters of the Shatt al-Arab River in the northwest region of the Arabian Gulf, DouAbul (1984) found that average total hydrocarbon concentrations ranged from 2.7 to 86.7 μg/l Kuwaiti crude oil equivalents. The highest concentrations were found at sites that were near port areas. These results were within the range of values reported for comparable areas in other parts of the world (UK marine waters, 24.0–74.0 μg/l; Canadian marine waters, 1.0–90.0 μg/l; Corella river, 2.2–200 μg/l; Halifax harbour, 1.2–71.7 μg/l).

In a similar study of seasonal variations in oil residues in the waters of the Shatt al-Arab River in Iraq, DouAbul and Al-Saad (1985) found that concentrations varied between 1.7 to 35.4 μg/l Kuwaiti crude oil equivalents. The results suggested that petroleum hydrocarbons found in the river originated from diverse sources. Hydrocarbon concentrations were highest in winter (averaging 17.4 μg/l) and lowest in summer (averaging 3.1 μg/l).

Table 12. Petroleum hydrocarbons in the marine environment[a]

Source	Input rate (million tonnes/year)	
	Estimate	Probable range
Natural sources		
Marine seepage	0.2	0.02–2.0
Sediment erosion	0.5	0.005–0.5
Offshore production	0.05	0.04–0.06
Transportation		
Tanker operations	0.7	0.4–1.5
Dry docking	0.03	0.02–0.05
Marine terminals	0.02	0.01–0.03
Bilge and fuel oils	0.3	0.2–0.6
Tanker accidents	0.4	0.3–0.4
Non-tanker accidents	0.02	0.02–0.04
Atmospheric deposition	0.3	0.05–0.5
Waste-water, run-off and ocean dumping		
Municipal wastes	0.7	0.4–1.5
Refineries	0.1	0.06–0.6
Non-refining industrial wastes	0.2	0.1–0.3
Urban run-off	0.12	0.01–0.2
River run-off	0.04	0.01–0.5
Ocean dumping	0.02	0.005–0.02
Total	3.7	1.7–8.8

[a]From Koons (1984)

Table 13 lists some accidental releases of crude oil that have been reported in the recent past.

2.3 Analysis

Because of the extreme complexity of the composition of petroleum and petroleum products, no single analytical method can be used to measure all the components in an environmental sample. For example, methods suitable for sampling and analysis of the volatile paraffinic (alkanes) hydrocarbon components are not directly applicable to the high molecular weight aromatic and polar fractions or to metals. Moreover, because petroleum is a complex and labile mixture, the composition of a sample released into the environment begins to change almost immediately. Fractionation and separation of components begins to take place by evaporation (or condensation), dissolution (e.g., of more polar components into water) and adsorption/absorption (e.g., into soils, sediments or biological tissues). Chemical, photochemical and biochemical reactions occur, leading to further selective changes and the appearance of degradation products and metabolites.

Table 13. Major accidental releases of crude oil in the recent past

Place	Date	Type	Quantity	Reference
UK	1967	Wreck of *Torrey Canyon* tanker	91 000 tonnes	Anon. (1973)
Santa Barbara, CA, USA	January 1969– October 1969	Ocean platform leak	11 290–112 900 tonnes (78 000– 780 000 barrels)	Foster *et al.* (1971)
La Coruña, Spain	May 1976	Persian Gulf crude oil from grounding of *Urquiola* tanker	90 000–91 000 tonnes	Gundlach & Hayes (1977)
Brittany coast, France	March 1978	Light Arabian and Iranian oil from wreck of *Amoco Cadiz* tanker	200 000 tonnes	Berne & Bodennec (1984)
Arabian Gulf	February 1983	Two damaged Iranian oil wells	4000 barrels per day	Sadiq & Zaidi (1984)
Cape Town, South Africa	August 1983	Light crude oil from wreck of *Castillo de Bellver* tanker	145 000–172 000 tonnes	Moldan *et al.* (1985)
Claymont, DE, USA	September 1985	Wreck of *Grand Eagle* tanker	435 000 gallons [1 650 000 l]	Miller & Ott (1986)

The problem of identification and quantification of petroleum released into the environment is further complicated by the fact that many petroleum components are ubiquitous and may arise from other sources such as the incomplete combustion of fossil fuels or biogenesis.

For these reasons, a number of analytical techniques have been applied in environmental analyses of petroleum, ranging from low-resolution, relatively nonspecific techniques, such as extraction/gravimetry and infrared spectrometry, to high-resolution, specific techniques involving capillary gas chromatography, high-pressure liquid chromatography and mass spectrometry (National Research Council, 1985). The choice of a method in any particular case depends on several factors, including the objective of the study, the medium (air, water, soil, sediment), what is known about the sample(s) and practical considerations such as cost, time restrictions and availability of equipment.

A number of reviews have been published on the environmental analysis of crude oil (e.g., Egan *et al.*, 1979; National Research Council, 1985; US Environmental Protection Agency, 1986; American Petroleum Institute, 1987b).

3. Biological Data Relevant to the Evaluation of Carcinogenic Risk to Humans

3.1 Carcinogenicity studies in animals

Skin application[1]

Mouse: Groups of 25 male and 25 female outbred albino mice [stock unspecified], 10–12 weeks of age, received twice weekly skin applications of 0.2 ml of one of three crude oils: from Kuwait (paraffinic-asphaltic base), Lagunillas/Venezuela (naphthenic) and Oklahoma [unspecified] or laboratory distilled fractions of the oils (obtained by fractionation using vacuum and steam in an apparatus selected to preclude cracking) or residues for 52 weeks. A similar experiment, using the same samples and numbers of mice of different strains was carried out in another laboratory. Skin from the treated area of all mice that survived 12 weeks of treatment was prepared for histology. Surviving animals were killed at week 52 [survival rate and effective number of animals unspecified]. In 18 groups each of 50 mice in laboratory 1, the skin tumour yield per group varied between 0 and 5; that in laboratory 2 varied between 0 and 2 [tumour type unspecified]. With the crude oils and residues, only two tumours developed among mice treated with Kuwaiti crude oil and one among mice treated with its residue (Hieger & Woodhouse, 1952). [The Working Group noted the lack of information on untreated controls, lack of histological classification and the short duration of the study.]

A group of 30 mice [age, sex and strain unspecified] received thrice-weekly skin applications of crude oil (natural Saratov; 28% methane, 68% naphthenes (cycloalkanes), 4% aromatic hydrocarbons, 2.86% paraffins (alkanes), 0.34% sulfur [quantity unspecified]) for six months, followed by twice weekly applications for life. All mice died within 13 months; the first death occurred after 40 treatments (94 days) and the last after 142 treatments (393 days). Hyperkeratosis was observed at the site of treatment in 13 of 23 animals of which the skin was examined histologically, and three mice developed papillomas within 147, 149 and 154 days, respectively (Antonov & Lints, 1960). [The Working Group noted the small number of animals, the lack of controls and absence of experimental detail, and the short duration of the experiment.]

Three groups of 30 mice [sex, age and strain unspecified] received twice weekly skin applications [not otherwise specified] of crude oils [quantities unspecified] of different origins (Bitkovsk, Gozhansk and Kokhanovsk) containing different amounts of paraffins, sulfur and tar, for ten months. No squamous-cell tumour was observed, but an angiosarcoma of the skin developed in two mice treated with the Bitkovsk and Gozhansk crude oils (Shapiro & Getmanets, 1962). [The Working Group noted the absence of experimental detail and the short duration of treatment.]

---

[1]The Working Group was aware of studies by skin painting in progress in mice using three distillate fractions of a high-nitrogen crude oil (IARC, 1986).

Groups of ten male and ten female C3H/Bd$_f$ mice [age unspecified] received twice weekly applications on shaved skin of 3, 6, 12 or 25 mg crude oil (Wilmington, CA; benzo[a]pyrene content, 1 µg/g) in 70% cyclohexane: acetone (final volume, 50 µl) for 30 weeks and were observed for a further 20 weeks. A group of 50 mice received applications of vehicle only. No skin tumour was observed in either treated or control animals (Holland et al., 1979). [The Working Group noted the small number of animals and the short duration of treatment.]

Groups of 15 male and 15 female C3H/Bd$_f$ mice [age unspecified] received thrice weekly applications on shaved skin of 25 mg of a composite petroleum sample (Wilmington, CA, USA (20%); South Swan Hills, Alberta, Canada (20%); Prudhoe Bay, AK, USA (20%); Gach Sach, Iran (20%); Louisiana-Mississippi, USA, Sweet (10%); Arabian Light (10%); polycyclic aromatic hydrocarbon content, 2.6%; benzo[a]pyrene content, 1 µg/g) in 70% cyclohexane:30% acetone (final volume, 50 µl) for 22 weeks, followed by a 22-week observation period. A group of 25 males and 25 females received the vehicle only. None of the animals developed skin tumours (Holland et al., 1979). [The Working Group noted the small number of animals and short duration of treatment.]

Groups of 25 male and 25 female C3H/Bd$_f$ mice [age unspecified] received thrice weekly applications on shaved skin of 0, 0.08, 0.3, 0.4 or 2.0 mg of the same composite petroleum samples as described above for 24 months. A group of 25 males and 25 females served as vehicle controls. Among mice treated with the highest dose, four skin carcinomas developed (8%), with an average latency of 658 (± 22) days. No tumour was observed among mice treated with lower doses or with the solvent only (Holland et al., 1979). [The Working Group noted the low doses tested.]

Groups of 20 male C3H mice [age unspecified] were treated on the clipped dorsal skin with 50 µl of a crude oil sample of Texan origin (benzo[a]pyrene content, 0.002%) or 50 µl of an asphaltic type (benzo[a]pyrene content, 0.0005%) two to three times per week [duration not specified]. No skin tumour developed in the animals. Benzo[a]pyrene (0.005% and 0.2% in toluene) produced high numbers of skin papillomas (6/50 and 3/30) and carcinomas (1/50 and 27/30; Bingham & Barkley, 1979). [The Working Group noted the small number of animals and the lack of experimental details.]

Groups of 25 male and 25 female C3H/Bd$_f$ mice, ten weeks of age, received thrice weekly applications on shaved skin of 0.08, 0.3, 0.4 or 2.0 mg of a natural composite petroleum sample (Wilmington, CA, USA (10%); South Swan Hills, Alberta, Canada (20%); Prudhoe Bay, AK, USA (20%); Gach Sach, Iran (20%); Louisiana-Mississippi, USA, Sweet (10%); Arabian Light (20%)) in 70% acetone:30% cyclohexane (final volume, 50 µl) for 24 months. The numbers of animals that died in the respective groups were 15, 11, 14 and 10. No skin tumour developed in the mice. Further groups of 25 males and 25 females treated with 0.006, 0.03 or 0.15 mg benzo[a]pyrene per week developed skin tumours at the application site: low-dose, 43/50; mid-dose, 49/50; high-dose, 48/50. No skin tumour was observed among solvent-treated mice (Holland et al., 1981). [The Working Group noted the low doses of the petroleum mixture tested.]

Groups of 50 C3H mice [sex and age unspecified] received twice weekly skin applications of 50 mg crude oil from either Kuwait (paraffinic with high sulfur content) or southern

Louisiana, USA (naphthenic with low sulfur content), for 80 weeks and were observed for a further 40 weeks. Of the Kuwaiti oil-treated animals, 38% developed squamous-cell tumours [histological type not specified] with an average tumour latency of 64 weeks; of the Louisiana oil-treated mice, 20% had skin tumours with an average tumour latency of 69 weeks. In a similar experiment conducted separately, a group of 20 mice received skin applications of southern Louisiana crude oil; tumour incidence was also 20%, but average tumour latency was 86 weeks. In an experiment conducted in another laboratory, 40 C3H mice [sex and age unspecified] received thrice weekly applications of 5 mg southern Louisiana crude oil (as described above) in a 30:70% cyclohexane:acetone mixture on the skin for 78 weeks and were observed for an additional 22 weeks. Skin tumours [histologically unspecified] developed in 92% of animals with an average tumour latency of 67 weeks (Coomes & Hazer, 1984). [The Working Group noted the lack of appropriate controls and of histological characterization of the tumours.]

Groups of 50 male C3H/HeJ mice, eight weeks of age, received twice weekly applications of 50 mg of one of two undiluted samples of crude oils ('C', predominantly naphthenic; 'D', predominantly paraffinic with a high sulfur content) or distilled fractions of the oils with boiling ranges corresponding to various refinery streams (petroleum ether, D-1; naphthas or gasoline components, C-2 and D-2; kerosene, C-3 and D-3; gas oil, C-4 and D-4; heavy oils, C-5 and D-5; and residual, C-6 and D-6) on clipped interscapular skin for 18 months. One group of mice received no treatment on the clipped skin and another treated with toluene only on the clipped skin served as negative controls; a further group treated with 0.05 or 0.15% benzo[a]pyrene in toluene on clipped skin served as positive controls. Total polycyclic aromatic hydrocarbon and benzo[a]pyrene contents, when determined, and details of the experiments are summarized in Table 14 [effective number of animals unspecified]. Fractions D-1 and C-6 produced no tumour and fractions D-4 and D-6 produced one carcinoma and one papilloma, respectively. All other samples produced numerous tumours, the most potent being the C-5 and D-5 fractions (boiling range, 371–577°C). Both crude oils induced tumours; however, the paraffinic sample (D) produced more tumours with slightly shorter arithmetic average time to appearance of the first tumour in weeks than the naphthenic (C) sample (56% and 64 weeks *versus* 30% and 69 weeks; Lewis, 1983; Lewis *et al.*, 1984; Cragg *et al.*, 1985). [The Working Group noted that the authors were not the original investigators of the study.]

Rabbit: A group of 30 male rabbits (from different stocks) [age unspecified] received twice weekly applications of 0.3 ml of crude oils from Kuwait (paraffinic-asphaltic), Lagunillas/Venezuela (naphthenic) or Oklahoma, USA [unspecified], on six different areas (~3 cm²) of shaved skin for 52 weeks. Another group of 75 male rabbits received twice weekly applications of 0.3 ml of laboratory distilled fractions (obtained by fractionation using vacuum and steam in an apparatus selected to preclude cracking) or residues of the same crude oils on seven different areas of shaved skin for 52 weeks. A similar experiment using the same samples and equal numbers of animals of different stocks was carried out in another laboratory (2). Surviving animals were killed at 52 weeks. Treatment with Oklahoma crude oil resulted in the development of two skin tumours in laboratory 2. Twenty-one, 34 and six skin tumours were induced by the fractions in laboratory 1 and 13,

Table 14. Carcinogenic activity of crude oil samples and their fractions[a]

Crude sample	Distillation range[b] (°C)	Average latency (weeks)	% Mice with skin tumours	Ratio of malignant: benign	Total PAH[c] (ppm)	BaP[d] (ppm)
No treatment		–	0	–		
Toluene		97	2	0/1		
Naphthenic						
C	OP–>577	69	30	2.3		1.2
C–2	OP–177	85	21	0.3		10^{-4}
C–3	177–288	70	30	0.8		
C–4	288–371	85	34	1.6	48	0.1
C–5	371–577	50	81	2.9	137	6.5
C–6	>577	>110[e]	0	–		
Paraffinic						
D	OP–>577	64	56	2.2		2.8
D–1	OP–49	>110[e]	0	–		
D–2	49–177	85	25	4.5		10^{-4}
D–3	177–288	62	15	1.0		
D–4	288–371	40	3	1/0	1.7	<0.1
D–5	371–577	34	91	9.3	62	1.9
D–6	>577	70	2	0/1		
0.05% BaP		46	74	2.1		
0.15% BaP		29	97	6.2		

[a]From Cragg et al. (1985)
[b]OP, overpoint; similar to initial boiling-point
[c]Polycyclic aromatic hydrocarbons
[d]Benzo[a]pyrene
[e]From Levis (1983)

12 and 12 by the fractions and residues in laboratory 2 by the Kuwaiti, Lagunillas and Oklahoma oils, respectively. The heavy fraction of each crude oil was the most active (Hieger & Woodhouse, 1952). [The Working Group noted the lack of information on controls and the lack of histological classification.]

A group of eight rabbits [sex, strain and age unspecified] received thrice weekly applications of crude oil (natural Saratov; 28% methane, 68% naphthenes, 4% aromatic hydrocarbons, 2.86% paraffins, 0.34% sulfur) [quantity unspecified] on the entire internal surface of one ear for six months followed by twice weekly applications for life. The first death occurred at 25 months and the last at 31 months from the start of the experiment. Six rabbits that were studied microscopically had all developed papillomas at the application site; the first tumour appeared 14 months after the start of the experiment (Antonov & Lints, 1960). [The Working Group noted the small number of animals and the lack of controls and the uncertainty about the cause of death.]

Five groups of six rabbits [sex, strain and age unspecified] received thrice weekly skin applications [not otherwise specified] of crude oils [quantity unspecified] of different origin (Bitkovsk, Gozhansk, Kokhanovsk, Romashkinsk and Radchenkovsk) with different paraffin, sulfur and tar contents for 10–17 months. Papillomas developed in all groups [survival, effective number of animals and number of tumours unspecified] (Shapiro & Getmanets, 1962). [The Working Group noted the lack of experimental details.]

(a) *Experimental systems*

Absorption, distribution, excretion and metabolism

No data were available to the Working Group on the absorption, distribution, excretion and metabolism of crude oil in laboratory animals.

Toxicokinetic studies have been reported in non-laboratory mammals, birds and aquatic organisms (Engelhardt *et al.*, 1977; Lee, 1977; Lawler *et al.*, 1978a,b; Gay *et al.*, 1980; Engelhardt, 1981; Neff & Anderson, 1981; Oritsland *et al.*, 1981).

Toxic effects

Oral administration of Prudhoe Bay crude oil (5.0 ml/kg bw daily for two days) to male Charles River CD-1 mice resulted in increases in liver weight, hepatic proteins, RNA, glycogen, total lipids, cholesterol, triglycerides and phospholipids (Khan *et al.*, 1987a).

Epidermal ornithine decarboxylase was induced following application of Prudhoe Bay crude oil to the backs of female Charles River CD-1 mice; a maximal induction of over 60 fold was seen 6 h after application of 50 μl. Concurrently, epidermal putrescine levels were elevated 4.7 fold over those in controls. Intraperitoneal administration of the crude oil led to an increase (15–20 fold, maximal activity 12 h following administration of 4 ml/kg bw) in hepatic ornithine decarboxylase activity but to a 45% decrease in the renal enzyme activity. Hepatic putrescine levels were elevated 34 fold over those in controls (Rahimtula *et al.*, 1987).

Application of Kuwaiti crude oil (0–200 μg) to the skin of male Sprague-Dawley rats increased dermal benzo[*a*]pyrene 3-hydroxylase by 15 fold and diphenyloxazole hydroxylase by six fold (Rahimtula *et al.*, 1984).

Platelets isolated from male Sprague-Dawley rats 24 h after oral treatment with a Prudhoe Bay crude oil showed a substantial inhibition of aggregation induced by adenosine diphosphate, arachidonic acid or epinephrine (Chaudhury *et al.*, 1987a). Inhibition of aggregation was effected with as little as 0.1 ml crude oil/kg bw (Chaudhury *et al.*, 1987b). Aggregation was also inhibited by aliphatic, heterocyclic and aromatic fractions of the crude oil (Chaudhury *et al.*, 1987a).

Alteration in cellular calcium sequestration has been postulated to be a primary mechanism in initiating irreversible cell damage. Administration of 5 ml/kg bw Prudhoe Bay crude oil intraperitoneally or orally daily for two days to male Sprague-Dawley rats that were sacrificed 24 h later resulted in an abrupt drop in liver mitochondrial and microsomal adenosine triphosphate-dependent calcium uptake. *In-vitro* incubation of either mitochondria or microsomes with dimethyl sulfoxide (DMSO) extracts of the crude oil resulted in a concentration-dependent inhibition of calcium influx. The release of calcium from calcium-loaded mitochondria and microsomes was also observed in the presence of the crude oil extract. At concentrations which affect calcium sequestration, the crude oil extract produced swelling of mitochondria. Microsomal adenosine triphosphatase activity in the presence or absence of calcium was unaffected by the crude oil. The results indicate that increased permeability of the mitochondrial and microsomal membranes to calcium is a contributing factor in the inhibition of calcium uptake by Prudhoe Bay crude oil (Khan et al., 1986).

Administration of a single oral dose (5–10 ml/kg bw) of Prudhoe Bay crude oil to pregnant Sprague-Dawley rats resulted in induction in maternal hepatic microsomal cytochrome P450 levels and various monooxygenases in a dose-dependent manner after 24 h. Maximal induction of glutathione S-transferase, uridine 5′-diphospho (UDP) glucuronyltransferase and DT-diaphorase (NADH, NADPH quinone oxido reductase) activities were observed 72 h after administration of the crude oil (Khan et al., 1987b).

Many studies on the toxic effects of crude oil in non-laboratory mammals, birds, and aquatic organisms have been reported and reviewed (Rice et al., 1977; Engelhardt, 1984; Holmes, 1984; Engelhardt, 1985; Leighton et al., 1985; Payne et al., 1987).

Effects on reproduction and prenatal toxicity

The effects of petroleum and petroleum products on reproduction have been reviewed (Schreiner, 1984).

Prudhoe Bay crude oil was administered orally to pregnant Sprague-Dawley rats as a single dose (5 ml/kg bw) on various gestation days (3, 6, 11, 15 or 17), as a single variable dose (2–10 ml/kg bw) on gestation day 6, or as daily doses (1 or 2 ml/kg bw) on days 6–17 of pregnancy. Administration during the earlier stages of pregnancy (day 3, 6 or 11) significantly increased the number of resorptions and decreased fetal weight and length. No adverse effect was observed following administration on gestation day 15 or 17. Multiple exposure to crude oil also caused a significant reduction in maternal body weight (Khan et al., 1987c). [The Working Group noted that no information on gross external abnormalities was reported and that the embryotoxic effects might have been a consequence of maternal toxicity.]

Both placental and fetal hepatic enzyme systems were induced on gestation day 18 following treatment of pregnant Sprague-Dawley rats with a single 5 ml/kg bw dose of Prudhoe Bay crude oil on gestation days 11, 15 or 17. Liver microsomal P450 levels, benzo[a]pyrene hydroxylase and ethoxyresorufin O-deethylase activities were increased two, two to three and 10–12 fold, respectively in 18-day-old fetuses. Similar trends were noticed in the placenta. Activities of phase II enzymes such as glutathione S-transferase, UDP glucuronyltransferase and DT-diaphorase were also significantly elevated (Khan et al., 1987b).

Several studies have demonstrated pronounced effects of crude oil on the reproductive capacity of birds (decreased hatchability, deformed bills, incomplete ossification, incomplete feather formation, gross structural abnormalities, dead embryos) after application on the shell surface or after oral administration (Grau et al., 1977; Albers, 1978; Holmes et al.,

1978; Hoffman, 1978, 1979a,b; Lee *et al.*, 1986; Walters *et al.*, 1987). [The Working Group noted that the avian system is a sensitive model for embryotoxic effects; results should be interpreted with caution with respect to possible effects in mammalian systems.]

Genetic and related effects

A large number of studies have been reported on the mutagenicity of crude oil and its fractions to *Salmonella typhimurium* (Table 15). Crude oil did not induce mutagenicity in any of the studies reported, either in the presence or absence of an exogenous metabolic system. Some neutral/aromatic (including polycyclic aromatic) fractions of crude oil were mutagenic in the presence of an exogenous metabolic system.

Aromatic fractions (one to three rings and four rings and more) of Prudhoe Bay crude oil caused a significant increase in the frequency of sister chromatid exchange in cultured Chinese hamster ovary cells only in the presence of an exogenous metabolic system; no increase in the frequency of chromosomal aberrations was observed (Ellenton & Hallett, 1981). Wilmington crude oil did not increase the number of sister chromatid exchanges in human lymphocytes *in vitro* in the presence of an exogenous metabolic system (Lockard *et al.*, 1982).

Intraperitoneal administration of Wilmington crude oil (five doses of 1 or 2.1 g/kg bw) did not induce sperm abnormalities in $B6C3F_1$/Hap mice, and micronuclei were not induced in bone marrow of outbred Swiss male mice given 6.1 g/kg bw intraperitoneally; an increase in the number of sister chromatid exchanges in bone-marrow cells of male outbred Swiss mice was observed at 7.2 g/kg bw intraperitoneally, but not at 1.8 or 3.6 g/kg (Lockard *et al.*, 1982).

(*b*) *Humans*

Absorption, distribution, excretion and metabolism

No data were available to the Working Group.

Toxic effects

A labourer who had aspirated crude oil developed aspiration pneumonia and hepatic and renal toxicity, from which he recovered completely (Wojdat & Winnicki, 1964).

Adverse skin effects including dryness, pigmentation, hyperkeratosis, pigmented plane warts and eczematous reactions have been observed among petroleum field workers in contact with crude oil (Mierzecki, 1965; Dzhafarov, 1970; Gusein-Zade, 1982). In one study in the USSR, a higher prevalence of skin effects was noted among transport workers in crude oil production than among petroleum field workers (Gusein-Zade, 1982). Skin diseases (hyperkeratosis and follicular lesions) were 1.5–2.5 times more frequent in petroleum field workers than in control groups (Chernov *et al.*, 1970).

Effects on reproduction and prenatal toxicity

No data were available to the Working Group.

Genetic and related effects

No data were available to the Working Group.

Table 15. Mutagenicity of crude oils[a] and their fractions in *Salmonella typhimurium*

Crude oil source	Crude sample, fraction or specified extract	Test strain	Results reported -S9	Results reported +S9	Test method	Reference
Louisiana-Mississippi sweet crude	Neutral fraction	TA98	NT[b]	+	Plate	Epler et al. (1978)
Composite crude	Neutral fraction	TA98	NT	+		
Arabian crude		TA1535	−	−	Plate	Petrilli et al. (1980)
		TA1537	−	−		
		TA1538	−	−		
		TA98	−	−		
		TA100	−	−		
	Extract (mechanical shaking with DMSO)	TA1535	−	−	Plate	
		TA1537	−	−		
		TA1538	−	−		
		TA98	−	−		
		TA100	−	−		
Prudhoe Bay crude	Aliphatic fraction	TA1535	−	−	Plate	Ellenton & Hallett (1981)
		TA1537	−	−		
		TA1538	−	−		
		TA98	−	−		
		TA100	−	−		
	Aromatic fraction (1–3-ring PAH[c])	TA1535	−	−	Plate	
		TA1537	−	−		
		TA1538	−	−		
		TA98	−	−		
		TA100	−	+		
	Aromatic fraction (≥4-ring PAH)	TA1535	−	−		
		TA1537	−	−		
		TA1538	−	−		
		TA98	−	−		
		TA100	−	+		
Wilmington, CA, crude (5301)[d]	Polyaromatic sub-fraction of neutral fraction	TA98	NT	+	Plate	Guerin et al. (1981)
Recluse (5305)			NT	+		
Louisiana-Mississippi sweet crude (5101)			NT	+		
South Swan Hills, Alberta, Canada, crude (5106)			NT	+		
Gach Saran Iran crude (5104)			NT	−		
Prudhoe Bay, Alaska, crude (5105)			NT	−		
Arabian light crude (5102)			NT	−		
Composite (5107)			NT	−		
Prudhoe Bay crude	Acid-base solvent extraction	TA98	−	−	Plate	Pelroy et al. (1981)

Table 15 (contd)

Crude oil source	Crude sample, fraction or specified extract	Test strain	Results reported −S9	Results reported +S9	Test method	Reference
Wilmington crude		TA98	−	−	Plate	Lockard et al. (1982)
		TA100	−	−	Plate	
US Gulf Coast Crude C (naphthenic)	Crude sample and 5 distilled fractions (different boiling ranges)	TA1535 TA1537 TA1538 TA98	−[e]	−[e]	Spot and plate	MacGregor et al. (1982)
Crude D (paraffinic)	Crude sample and 6 distilled fractions (different boiling ranges)	TA100				
Petroleum crude CRM3	Dewaxed	TA98	NT	−	Plate	Ma et al. (1983)
	Suspended in Tween 80		NT	−		
	DMSO slurry		NT	−		
Prudhoe Bay crude		TA98	−	−	Plate	Sheppard et al. (1983)
	Acid fraction		+	+		
	Basic fraction		−	?		
	Neutral fraction		−	+		
Crude C (naphthenic)	Distilled	TA98	NT	+	Plate at high amounts of S9	Carver et al. (1984)
		TA100	NT	+		
	Aromatic fraction	TA98	NT	+		
		TA100	NT	+		
Kuwaiti crude		TA1535	−	−	Spot and plate	Vandermeulen et al. (1985)
		TA1538	−	−		
		TA98	−	−		
		TA100	−	−		
Saran Gach crude		TA1535	−	−	Spot and plate	
		TA1538	−	−		
		TA98	−	−		
		TA100	−	−		
Kuwaiti crude	Hexane	Not specified	−	−	Spot and plate	
	10% benzene-hexane		−	−		
	50% benzene-hexane		−	−		
	Acetone		+	+		

[a]Dimethyl sulfoxide (DMSO) extracts, unless otherwise specified
[b]NT, not tested
[c]Polycyclic aromatic hydrocarbon
[d]Repository number
[e]Data for each fraction tested in different strains not reported

3.3 Epidemiological studies and case reports of carcinogenicity to humans

(a) Cohort study

A large retrospective cohort mortality study of US petroleum producing and pipeline workers was reported by Divine and Barron (1987). To be included in the study, men had to have been employed for at least six months at a producing or pipeline location and to have worked at some time during the period 1946–80. Vital status was ascertained for 97.8% of the cohort, which comprised 11 098 white men; death certificates were obtained for all but 3.4% of the deceased. Complete occupational histories were available from company records. Standardized mortality ratios (SMRs) were calculated in comparison with rates for US white males, and mortality was studied by length of employment, latency, whether producing or pipeline workers, and selected job categories. The SMR for all causes of death was significantly low (1886 observed; SMR, 0.63; 95% confidence interval [CI], 0.61–0.66), as was that for all cancers (393 observed; SMR, 0.68; 95% CI, 0.61–0.75). There was a significant excess of thyroid cancer among men employed as pumper-gaugers in petroleum production, but this was based on four cases only. A significant deficit of lung cancer (109 observed; SMR, 0.61; 95% CI, 0.50–0.73) was found among producing and pipeline workers, and no death from testicular cancer was observed although 3.2 were expected.

(b) Case-control studies

(i) Lung cancer

In an attempt to explain an excess of lung cancer cases observed in a cluster of parishes in Louisiana, USA, Gottlieb et al. (1979) conducted a case-control study, the design of which is described in the monograph on occupational exposures in petroleum refining (p. 102). An elevated risk for lung cancer was observed among black men aged over 53 years who had been employed in petroleum exploration and production (odds ratio, 1.6; 95% CI, 1.0–2.6). By logistic analysis, the ratio associated with crude oil exploration and drilling was three fold among persons over the age of 62 in parishes with petroleum or paper industries. [The Working Group noted that, since information used in this study was extracted directly from death certificates and since no account was taken of cigarette smoking, caution should be applied in interpreting the results.]

Gottlieb (1980) reanalysed the risk of lung cancer in relation to work in the petroleum mining and refining industry in the men included in the previous study. A group of 200 men with lung cancer and 170 control men who had worked in petroleum mining (125 cases, 112 controls) and refining (75 cases, 58 controls) were identified. The odds ratio for lung cancer associated with employment in the petroleum industry (mining and refining combined) was estimated at 1.2 (95% CI, 1.1–1.4). For welders, operators, boiler makers and painters, and oil-field workers taken as a group (mining and refining combined), the odds ratio was 2.3 (95% CI, 1.4–3.9). [The Working Group noted that information on exposure was extracted directly from death certificates; that no information on cigarette smoking was available; that cases were older than controls, which, in itself, may explain the difference observed; and that mining and refining occupations were combined.]

(ii) *Testicular cancer*

Mills *et al.* (1984) studied 347 hospital patients with histologically confirmed germ-cell tumour of the testis in the USA and matched them by age, sex, race and residence with 347 hospital controls, most of whom had tumours other than cancer of the testis. The ascertainment period was from 1 January 1977 to 31 August 1980. Occupational histories were extracted from medical records; when the type of industry was not apparent in the record, this was ascertained from the employer. An excess risk for testicular cancer was observed among petroleum and natural gas extraction workers (odds ratio, 2.3; 95% CI, 1.0–5.1). [The Working Group noted that information was obtained only on current occupation.]

Sewell *et al.* (1986) conducted a population-based study in New Mexico, USA, in which cases were identified at the New Mexico Tumor Registry. In order to be included in the study, the cases had to have had histologically confirmed testicular cancer registered in 1966–84, to have been 15 years old or more at the time of diagnosis and to have died of the disease. Controls consisted of persons who had died from other cancers, matched by age, year of diagnosis, race and sex. A total of 81 cases and 311 controls was identified. The source of occupational data was either death certificates (99%) or information on file at the tumour registry (1%). No excess risk for testicular cancer was observed among petroleum and gas workers (odds ratio, 0.57; 95% CI, 0.16–2.0). The authors noted the limited power of the study, that an association might have been obscured by the restriction to fatal cases and that information on exposure was limited.

(iii) *Multiple sites*

In a large case-control study of cancer at many sites conducted in Montreal, Canada, which is described in detail in the monograph on gasoline, p. 185, an association was seen between exposure to crude oil and rectal cancer (five cases; adjusted odds ratio 3.7; 90% CI, 1.3–10.6) and squamous-cell lung cancer (seven cases; adjusted odds ratio, 3.5; 90% CI, 1.5–8.2) (Siemiatycki *et al.*, 1987). It was indicated, however, that these associations might only be apparent since they are based on very small numbers. The authors suggested that one of the main groups exposed to crude oil, namely seamen, would probably have had life styles very different from those of the rest of the study population.

4. Summary of Data Reported and Evaluation

4.1 Exposure data

Crude oil, which may be broadly characterized as paraffinic or naphthenic, is a complex mixture of alkanes, cycloalkanes and aromatic hydrocarbons containing low percentages of sulfur, nitrogen and oxygen compounds and trace quantities of many other elements. Worldwide, about 500 000 workers are employed in crude oil exploration and production. Occupational exposures during drilling, pumping and transportation of crude oil, including maintenance of equipment used for these processes, may involve inhalation of volatile compounds, including hydrocarbons and hydrogen sulfide. Skin contact with crude oils, which contain polycyclic aromatic compounds, may also occur during these operations. Accidental releases of crude oil into the aquatic environment are also potential sources of human exposure.

4.2 Experimental data[1]

Samples of crude oil from single sources and composite blends were tested for carcinogenicity by skin application in ten experiments in mice. Four samples of crude oil from single sources produced benign and malignant or unspecified skin tumours in two experiments. In one experiment, a composite sample produced a low incidence of skin carcinomas; in a similar experiment using the same treatment regimen but a blend of slightly different composition, no skin tumour was observed. The conduct and/or reporting of the results of six other experiments in mice were inadequate for evaluation.

Skin application to mice of fractions of two crude oil samples distilled under laboratory conditions and corresponding to various refinery streams produced skin tumours.

One sample of crude oil produced skin papillomas in rabbits in one experiment. Two other experiments were inadequate for evaluation.

4.3 Human data

In a retrospective cohort mortality study of a large group of male employees in petroleum producing and pipeline operations, mortality from all types of cancer was low, except from thyroid cancer. There was a significant deficit of lung cancer and no death from testicular cancer.

In a population-based case-control study, an elevated risk for lung cancer was observed among older men who had been employed in petroleum exploration and production. Reanalysis of the risk for lung cancer among men who had worked in the petroleum mining and refining industry showed an elevated risk for lung cancer among welders, operators, boiler makers, painters and oil-field workers taken as a group; no data were available on smoking habits.

In one of two case-control studies, an excess risk for testicular cancer was observed among petroleum and natural gas extraction workers. No such excess was found in the other study.

In a case-control study of cancer at many sites, an association was observed between exposure to crude oil and rectal and squamous-cell lung cancer. However, the association was based on small numbers and may have been confounded by life style factors.

---

[1]Subsequent to the meeting, the Secretariat became aware of a study in which skin tumours were reported in mice after application to the skin of East Wilmington crude oil (Clark *et al.*, 1988).

4.4 Other relevant data

Crude oil induces dermal xenobiotic metabolizing enzymes and ornithine decarboxylase after skin application in mice.

In single studies of mice treated *in vivo*, crude oil induced an increase in the number of sister chromatid exchanges at the highest dose tested but did not induce micronuclei in bone-marrow cells or sperm abnormalities. Crude oil did not increase the number of sister chromatid exchanges in cultured human lymphocytes. Aromatic fractions of crude oil induced sister chromatid exchange, but not chromosomal aberrations, in cultured mammalian cells. Crude oil extracts did not induce mutation in bacteria; when fractionated, neutral fractions of crude oil, which contain aromatic or polycyclic aromatic compounds, generally had mutagenic activity in bacteria. (See Appendix 1.)

4.5 Evaluation[1]

There is *inadequate evidence* for the carcinogenicity in humans of crude oil.

There is *limited evidence* for the carcinogenicity in experimental animals of crude oil.

Overall evaluation

Crude oil *is not classifiable as to its carcinogenicity to humans (Group 3)*.

5. References

Albers, P.H. (1978) The effects of petroleum on different stages of incubation in bird eggs. *Bull. environ. Contam. Toxicol., 19*, 624-630

American Petroleum Institute (1983) *Introduction to Oil and Gas Production*, Book 1, 4th ed., Dallas, TX

American Petroleum Institute (1984) *Facts About Oil*, Washington DC, pp. 8-9

American Petroleum Institute (1987a) *Basic Petroleum Data Book: Petroleum Industry Statistics*, Vol. VII, No. 3, Washington DC

American Petroleum Institute (1987b) *Manual of Sampling and Analytical Methods for Petroleum Hydrocarbons in Groundwater and Soil (API Publ. No. 4449)*, Washington DC

Anderson, R.O. (1984) *Fundamentals of the Petroleum Industry*, Norman, OK, University of Oklahoma Press

Anon. (1973) Oil spils: how serious a problem? *J. Water Pollut. Control, 45*, 583-585

Anon. (1987) *Oil and Gas Journal Data Book*, Tulsa, OK, PennWell Publishing

Antonov, A.M. & Lints, A.M. (1960) The blastomogenic action of natural Saratov oil. *Probl. Oncol., 6*, 1629-1634

Baker, A.M., Baker, R., Cyrus, C., Gerding, M., House, R., Morris, J., Pietrobono, J.T., Stelzner, I. & Stemerick, M. (1986a) *Production*. In: Gerding, M., ed., *Fundamentals of Petroleum*, 3rd ed., Austin, TX, Petroleum Extension Service, pp. 176-245

Baker, A.M., Baker, R., Cyrus, C., Gerding, M., House, R., Morris, J., Pietrobono, J.T., Stelzner, I. & Stemerick, M. (1986b) *Transportation*. In: Gerding, M., ed., *Fundamentals of Petroleum*, 3rd ed., Austin, TX, Petroleum Extension Service, pp. 247-320

---

[1]For definitions of the italicized terms, see Preamble, pp. 25-28.

Berne, S. & Bodennec, G. (1984) Evaluation of hydrocarbons after the Tanio oil spill — a comparison with the Amoco Cadiz accident. *Ambio*, *13*, 109–114

Bestougeff, M.A. (1967) *Petroleum hydrocarbons*. In: Nagy, B. & Colombo, U., eds, *Fundamental Aspects of Petroleum Geochemistry*, Amsterdam, Elsevier, pp. 77–108

Bingham, E. & Barkley, W. (1979) Bioassay of complex mixtures derived from fossil fuels. *Environ. Health Perspect.*, *30*, 157–163

British Petroleum Company (1986) *BP Statistical Review of World Energy, June 1986*, London

British Petroleum Company (1988) *BP Statistical Review of World Energy, June 1988*, London

Carver, J.H., MacGregor, J.A. & King, R.W. (1984) Mutagenicity and chemical characterization of two petroleum distillates. *J. appl. Toxicol.*, *4*, 163–169

Chaudhury, S., Macko, S. & Rahimtula, A.D. (1987a) Inhibition of rat platelet aggregation by a Prudhoe Bay crude oil and its aliphatic, aromatic, and heterocyclic fractions. *Toxicol. appl. Pharmacol.*, *90*, 347–356

Chaudhury, S., Martin, M., Payne, J.F. & Rahimtula, A. (1987b) Alterations in platelet aggregation and microsomal benzo-α-pyrene hydroxylase activities after exposure of rats to a Prudhoe Bay crude oil. *J. Biochem. Toxicol.*, *2*, 93–104

Chernov, B.S., Karimov, M.A. & Rakhimova, G.K. (1970) Dermatoses in workers in oil-fields (Russ.). *Vestn. Dermatol. Venereol.*, *44*, 65–68

Clark, C.R., Walter, M.K., Ferguson, P.W. & Katchen, M. (1988) Comparative dermal carcinogenesis of shale and petroleum-derived distillates. *Toxicol. ind. Health*, *4*, 11–22

Coleman, H.J., Shelton, E.M., Nichols, D.T. & Thompson, C.J. (1978) *Analyses of 800 Crude Oils from United States Oilfields (BETC/RI-78/14)*, Bartlesville, OK, Bartlesville Energy Technology Center

Considine, D.M., ed. (1974) *Chemical and Process Technology Encyclopedia*, New York, McGraw-Hill, pp. 848–861

Coomes R.M. & Hazer, K.A. (1984) *Statistical analyses of crude oil and shale oil carcinogenic test data*. In: MacFarland, H.N., Holdsworth, C.E., MacGregor, J.A., Call, R.W. & Lane, M.L., eds, *Advances in Modern Environmental Toxicology*, Vol. VI, *Applied Toxicology of Petroleum Hydrocarbons*, Princeton, NJ, Princeton Scientific Publishers, pp. 167–186

Costantinides, G. & Arich, G. (1967) *Non-hydrocarbon compounds in petroleum*. In: Nagy, B. & Colombo, U., eds, *Fundamental Aspects of Petroleum Geochemistry*, Amsterdam, Elsevier, pp. 109–175

Cragg, S.T., Conaway, C.C. & MacGregor, J.A. (1985) Lack of concordance of the *Salmonella*/microsome assay with the mouse dermal carcinogenesis bioassay for complex petroleum hydrocarbon mixtures. *Fundam. appl. Toxicol.*, *5*, 382–390

Cross, W. (1983) *Petroleum*, Chicago, IL, Regensteiner

Cuddington, K.S. & Lowther, N.F. (1977) *The character of crude oil*. In: *Our Industry Petroleum*, London, British Petroleum Company, pp. 208–221

Dickey, P.A. (1981) *Petroleum Development Geology*, 2nd ed., Tulsa, OK, PennWell Publishing, pp. 194–226

Divine, B.J. & Barron, V. (1987) Texaco mortality study: III. A cohort study of producing and pipeline workers. *Am. J. ind. Med.*, *11*, 189–202

DouAbul, A.A.Z. (1984) Petroleum residues in the waters of the Shatt al-Arab River and the northwest region of the Arabian Gulf. *Environ. int.*, *10*, 265–267

DouAbul, A.A.Z. & Al-Saad, H.T. (1985) Seasonal variations of oil residues in water of Shatt al-Arab River, Iraq. *Water Air Soil Pollut., 24*, 237–246

Duck, B.W. (1983) *Petroleum, extraction and transport by sea of*. In: Parmeggiani, L., ed., *Encyclopaedia of Occupational Health and Safety*, 3rd (rev.) ed., Vol. 2, Geneva, International Labour Office, pp. 1652–1656

Dzhafarov, F.A. (1970) Results of dermatological examination of oilmen occupationally exposed to the effect of crude oil (Russ.). *Gig. Tr. prof. Zabol., 14*, 37–41

Egan, H., Castegnaro, M., Bogovski, P., Kunte, H. & Walker, E.A., eds (1979) *Environmental Carcinogens — Selected Methods of Analysis*, Vol. 3, *Analysis of Polycyclic Aromatic Hydrocarbons in Environmental Samples (IARC Scientific Publications No. 29)*, Lyon, International Agency for Research on Cancer

Ellenton, J.A. & Hallett, D.J. (1981) Mutagenicity and chemical analysis of aliphatic and aromatic fractions of Prudhoe Bay crude oil and fuel oil No. 2. *J. Toxicol. environ. Health, 8*, 959–972

Engelhardt, F.R. (1981) *Oil pollution in polar bears: exposure and clinical effects*. In: *Proceedings of the Fourth Arctic Marine Oilspill Program Technical Seminar, Edmonton, Alberta*, Ottawa, Environmental Protection Service, pp. 139–179

Engelhardt, F.R. (1984) *Environmental effects of petroleum on mammals*. In: Hodgson, E., ed., *Reviews in Environmental Toxicology*, Vol. I, Amsterdam, Elsevier, pp. 319–337

Engelhardt, F.R. (1985) *Effects of petroleum on marine mammals*. In: Engelhardt, F.R., ed., *Petroleum Effects in the Arctic Environment*, London, Elsevier, pp. 217–243

Engelhardt, F.R., Geraci, J.R. & Smith, T.G. (1977) Uptake and clearance of petroleum hydrocarbons in the ringed seal, *Phoca hispida*. *J. Fish. Res. Board Can., 34*, 1143–1147

Epler, J.L., Young, J.A., Hardigree, A.A., Rao, T.K., Guerin, M.R., Rubin, I.B., Ho, C.-H. & Clark, B.R. (1978) Analytical and biological analyses of test materials from the synthetic fuel technologies. I. Mutagenicity of crude oils determined by the *Salmonella typhimurium*/microsomal activation system. *Mutat. Res., 57*, 265–276

Ferrero, E.P. & Nichols, D.T. (1972) *Analyses of 169 Crude Oils from 122 Foreign Oilfields (Information Circular 8542)*, Washington DC, US Department of the Interior

Foster, M., Charters, A.C. & Neushul, M. (1971) The Santa Barbara oil spill. Part 1: Initial quantities and distribution of pollutant crude oil. *Environ. Pollut., 2*, 97–113

Gay, M.L., Belisle, A.A. & Patton, J.F. (1980) Quantification of petroleum-type hydrocarbons in avian tissue. *J. Chromatogr., 187*, 153–160

Giuliano, F.A., ed. (1981) *Introduction to Oil and Gas Technology*, 2nd ed., Boston, MA, International Human Resources Development Corp.

Gottlieb, M.S. (1980) Lung cancer and the petroleum industry in Louisiana. *J. occup. Med., 22*, 384–388

Gottlieb, M.S., Pickle, L.W., Blot, W.J. & Fraumeni, J.F., Jr (1979) Lung cancer in Louisiana: death certificate analysis. *J. natl Cancer Inst., 63*, 1131–1137

Grau, C.R., Roudybush, T., Dobbs, J. & Wathen, J. (1977) Altered yolk structure and reduced hatchability of eggs from birds fed single doses of petroleum oils. *Science, 195*, 779–781

Gray, F. (1986) *Petroleum Production for the Nontechnical Person*, Tulsa, OK, PennWell Publishing

Guerin, M.R., Rubin, I.B., Rao, T.K., Clark, B.R. & Epler, J.L. (1981) Distribution of mutagenic activity in petroleum and petroleum substitutes. *Fuel, 60*, 282–288

Gundlach, E.R. & Hayes, M.O. (1977) The Urquiola oil spill, La Coruna, Spain: case history and discussion of methods of control and clean-up. *Mar. Pollut. Bull.*, *8*, 132–136

Gusein-Zade, K.M. (1982) Characteristics of dermatoses morbidity in workers of Apsheron oil fields in relation to physico-chemical properties of the oil produced (Russ). *Vestn. Dermatol. Venereol.*, *9*, 63–66

Hawley, G.G. (1981) *The Condensed Chemical Dictionary*, 10th ed., New York, Van Nostrand Reinhold, p. 792

Hieger, I. & Woodhouse, D.L. (1952) The value of the rabbit for carcinogenicity tests on petroleum fractions. *Br. J. Cancer*, *6*, 293–299

Hoffman, D.J. (1978) Embryotoxic effects of crude oil in mallard ducks and chicks. *Toxicol. appl. Pharmacol.*, *46*, 183–190

Hoffman, D.J. (1979a) Embryotoxic and teratogenic effects of petroleum hydrocarbons in mallards (*Anas platyrhynchos*). *J. Toxicol. environ. Health*, *5*, 835–844

Hoffman, D.J. (1979b) Embryotoxic and teratogenic effects of crude oil on mallard embryos on day one of development. *Bull. environ. Contam. Toxicol.*, *22*, 632–637

Hoffman, H.L. (1982) *Petroleum (products)*. In: Grayson, M., ed., *Kirk-Othmer Encyclopedia of Chemical Technology*, 3rd ed., Vol. 17, New York, John Wiley & Sons, pp. 257–271

Holland, J.M., Rahn, R.O., Smith, L.H., Clark, B.R., Chang, S.S. & Stephens, T.J. (1979) Skin carcinogenicity of synthetic and natural petroleums. *J. occup. Med.*, *21*, 614–618

Holland, J.M., Wolf, D.A. & Clark, B.R. (1981) Relative potency estimation for synthetic petroleum skin carcinogens. *Environ. Health Perspect.*, *38*, 149–155

Holmes, W.N. (1984) *Petroleum pollutants in the marine environment and their possible effects on seabirds*. In: Hodgson, E., ed., *Reviews in Environmental Toxicology*, Vol. I, Amsterdam, Elsevier, pp. 251–317

Holmes, W.N., Cavanaugh, K.P. & Cronshaw, J. (1978) The effects of ingested petroleum on oviposition and some aspects of reproduction in experimental colonies of mallard ducks (*Anas platyrhynchos*). *J. Reprod. Fertil.*, *54*, 335–347

IARC (1976) *IARC Monographs on the Evaluation of Carcinogenic Risk of Chemicals to Man*, Vol. 11, *Cadmium, Nickel, Some Epoxides, Miscellaneous Industrial Chemicals, and General Considerations on Volatile Anaesthetics*, Lyon, pp. 75–112

IARC (1982) *IARC Monographs on the Evaluation of the Carcinogenic Risk of Chemicals to Humans*, Vol. 29, *Some Industrial Chemicals and Dyestuffs*, Lyon, pp. 93–148, 391–398

IARC (1986) *Information Bulletin on the Survey of Chemicals Being Tested for Carcinogenicity*, No. 12, Lyon, p. 287

IARC (1987a) *IARC Monographs on the Evaluation of Carcinogenic Risks to Humans*, Suppl. 7, *Overall Evaluations of Carcinogenicity: An Updating of* IARC Monographs *Volumes 1 to 42*, Lyon, pp. 120–122

IARC (1987b) *IARC Monographs on the Evaluation of Carcinogenic Risks to Humans*, Suppl. 7, *Overall Evaluations of Carcinogenicity: An Updating of* IARC Monographs *Volumes 1 to 42*, Lyon, pp. 264–269

Ibiebele, D.D. (1986) Point-source inputs of petroleum wastewater into the Niger Delta, Nigeria. *Sci. total Environ.*, *52*, 2330238

International Labour Office (1986) *Petroleum Committee, 10th Session, Report I, General Report*, Geneva, p. 146

Khan, S., Payne, J.F. & Rahimtula, A.D. (1986) Mechanisms of petroleum hydrocarbon toxicity: destruction of liver microsomal and mitochondrial calcium pump activities by Prudhoe Bay crude oil. *J. Biochem. Toxicol.*, *1*, 31–43

Khan, S., Irfan, M. & Rahimtula, A.D. (1987a) The hepatotoxic potential of a Prudhoe Bay crude oil: effect on mouse liver weight and composition. *Toxicology*, *46*, 95–105

Khan, S., Martin, M., Rahimtula, A.D. & Payne, J.F. (1987b) Effect of a Prudhoe Bay crude oil on hepatic and placental drug metabolism in rats. *Can. J. Physiol. Pharmacol.*, *65*, 2400–2408

Khan, S., Martin, M., Payne, J.F. & Rahimtula, A.D. (1987c) Embryotoxic evaluation of a Prudhoe Bay crude oil in rats. *Toxicol. Lett.*, *38*, 109–114

Koons, C.B. (1984) Input of petroleum to the marine environment. *Mar. Technol. Soc. J.*, *18*, 4–10

Lawler, G.C., Loong, W.-A. & Laseter, J.L. (1978a) Accumulation of saturated hydrocarbons in tissues of petroleum-exposed mallard ducks (*Anas platyrhynchos*). *Environ. Sci. Technol.*, *12*, 47–51

Lawler, G.C., Loong, W.-A. & Laseter, J.L. (1978b) Accumulation of aromatic hydrocarbons in tissues of petroleum-exposed mallard ducks (*Anas platyrhynchos*). *Environ. Sci. Technol.*, *12*, 51–54

Lee, R.F. (1977) *Accumulation and turnover of petroleum hydrocarbons in marine organisms*. In: Wolfe, D.A., ed., *Fate and Effect of Petroleum in Marine Organisms and Ecosystems*, Oxford, Pergamon Press, pp. 60–70

Lee, Y.-Z., O'Brien, P.J., Payne, J.F. & Rahimtula, A.D. (1986) Toxicity of petroleum crude oils and their effect on xenobiotic metabolizing enzyme activities in the chicken embryo *in ovo*. *Environ. Res.*, *39*, 153–163

Leighton, F.A., Lee, Y.-Z., Rahimtula, A.D., O'Brien, P.J. & Peakall, D.B. (1985) Biochemical and functional disturbances in red blood cells of herring gulls ingesting Prudhoe Bay crude oil. *Toxicol. appl. Pharmacol.*, *81*, 25–31

Lewis, S.C. (1983) Crude petroleum and selected fractions. Skin cancer bioassays. *Progr. exp. Tumor Res.*, *26*, 68–84

Lewis, S.C., King, R.W., Cragg, S.T. & Hillman, D.W. (1984) *Skin carcinogenic potential of petroleum hydrocarbons: crude oil, distillate fractions and chemical class subfractions*. In: MacFarland, H.N., Holdsworth, C.E., MacGregor, J.A., Call, R.W. & Lane, M.L., eds, *Advances in Modern Environmental Toxicology*, Vol. VI, *Applied Toxicology of Petroleum Hydrocarbons*, Princeton, NJ, Princeton Scientific Publishers, pp. 139–150

Lockard, J.M., Prater, J.W., Viau, C.J., Enoch, H.G. & Sabharwal, P.S. (1982) Comparative study of the genotoxic properties of eastern and western US shale oils, crude petroleum and coal-derived oil. *Mutat. Res.*, *102*, 221–235

Ma, C.Y., Ho, C.-H., Quincy, R.B., Guerin, M.R., Rao, T.K., Allen, B.E. & Epler, J.L. (1983) Preparation of oils for bacterial mutagenicity testing. *Mutat. Res.*, *118*, 15–24

MacGregor, J.A., Conaway, C.C. & Cragg, S.T. (1982) *Predictivity of the* Salmonella/microsome *assay for carcinogenic and noncarcinogenic complex petroleum hydrocarbon mixtures*. In: MacFarland, H.N., Holdsworth, C.E., MacGregor, J.A., Call, R.W. & Kane, M.L., eds, *Proceedings of the Symposium on the Toxicology of Petroleum Hydrocarbons*, Washington DC, American Petroleum Institute

Magee, E.M., Hall, H.J. & Varga, G.M., Jr (1973) *Potential Pollutants in Fossil Fuels (EPA-R2-72-249/PB 225-039)*, Linden, NJ, Esso Research and Engineering

Mair, B.J. (1964) Here's a complete up-to-date list of the hydrocarbons isolated from petroleum. *Oil Gas J.*, 62, 130–134

Mierzecki, H. (1965) Chemical sensitization in the petroleum industry (Ger.). *Berufsdermatosen*, 13, 350–359

Miller, A.J. & Ott, G.L. (1986) Major oil spill on the Delaware River, September 1985. *US Geol. Surv. Water-Supply Pap.*, 2300, 47–48

Mills, P.K., Newell, G.R. & Johnson, D.E. (1984) Testicular cancer associated with employment in agriculture and oil and natural gas extraction. *Lancet*, i, 207–210

Moldan, A.G.S., Jackson, L.F., McGibbon, S. & van der Westhuizen, J. (1985) Some aspects of the Castillo de Bellver oil spill. *Mar. Pollut. Bull.*, 16, 97–102

Myhre, W. (1980) *Review of Federal and State Oil Pollution Laws*, Washington DC, Preston, Thorgrimson, Ellis & Holman

National Research Council (1985) *Oil in the Sea. Inputs, Fates and Effects*, Washington DC, National Academy Press

Neff, J.M. & Anderson, J.W. (1981) *Response of Marine Animals to Petroleum and Specific Petroleum Hydrocarbons*, London, Applied Science Publishers, pp. 93–142

Oritsland, N.A., Engelhardt, F.R., Juck, F.A., Hurst, R.J. & Watts, P.D. (1981) *Effect of Crude Oil on Polar Bears (Environmental Studies No. 24)*, Ottawa, Northern Environmental Protection Branch, Indian and Northern Affairs

Payne, J.F., Fancey, L.L., Rahimtula, A.D. & Porter, E.L. (1987) Review and perspective on the use of mixed-function oxygenase enzymes in biological monitoring. *Comp. Pharmacol. Physiol.*, 86C, 233–245

Pelroy, R.A., Sklarew, D.S. & Downey, S.P. (1981) Comparison of the mutagenicities of fossil fuels. *Mutat. Res.*, 90, 233–245

Petrilli, F.L., De Renzi, G.P. & De Flora, S. (1980) Interaction between polycyclic aromatic hydrocarbons, crude oil and oil dispersants in the *Salmonella* mutagenesis assay. *Carcinogenesis*, 1, 51–56

Rahimtula, A.D., O'Brien, P.J. & Payne, J.F. (1984) *Induction of xenobiotic metabolism in rats on exposure to hydrocarbon-based oils*. In: MacFarland, H.N., Holdsworth, C.E., MacGregor, J.A., Call, R.W. & Lane, M.L., eds, *Advances in Modern Environmental Toxicology*, Vol. VI, *Applied Toxicology of Petroleum Hydrocarbons*, Princeton, NJ, Princeton Scientific Publishers, pp. 71–79

Rahimtula, A.D., Lee, Y.-Z. & Silva, J. (1987) Induction of epidermal and hepatic ornithine decarboxylase by a Prudhoe Bay crude oil. *Fundam. appl. Toxicol.*, 8, 408–414

Reitze, A.W., Jr (1972) *Environmental Law*, 2nd ed., Washington DC, North American International

Rice, S.D., Short, J.W. & Karinen, J.F. (1977) *Comparative oil toxicity and comparative animal sensitivity*. In: Wolfe, D.A., ed., *Fate and Effect of Petroleum in Marine Organisms and Ecosystems*, Oxford, Pergamon Press, pp. 78–94

Sachanen, A.N. (1950) *Hydrocarbons in petroleum*. In: Brooks, B.T. & Dunstan, A.E., eds, *The Science of Petroleum*, Vol. V, Part I, *Crude Oils. Chemical and Physical Properties*, London, Oxford University Press, pp. 72–77

Sadiq, M. & Zaidi, T.H. (1984) Vanadium and nickel content of Nowruz spill tar flakes on the Saudi Arabian coastline and their probable environmental impact. *Bull. environ. Contam. Toxicol.*, 32, 635–639

Schreiner, C.A. (1984) *Petroleum and petroleum products: a brief review of studies to evaluate reproductive effects*. In: Christian, M.S., Galbraith, W.M., Voytek, P. & Mehlman, M.A., eds, *Advances in Modern Environmental Toxicology*, Vol. III, *Assessment of Reproductive and Teratogenic Hazards*, Princeton, NJ, Princeton Scientific Publishers, pp. 29–45

Sewell, C.M., Castle, S.P., Hull, H.F. & Wiggins, C. (1986) Testicular cancer and employment in agriculture and oil and natural gas extraction. *Lancet*, i, 553

Shapiro, D.D. & Getmanets, I.Y. (1962) Blastomogenic properties of petroleum of different sources (Russ.). *Gig. Sanit.*, 27, 38–42

Sheppard, E.P., Wells, R.A. & Georghiou, P.E. (1983) The mutagenicity of a Prudhoe Bay crude oil and its residues from an experimental in situ burn. *Environ. Res.*, 30, 427–441

Siemiatycki, J., Dewar, R., Nadon, L., Gérin, M., Richardson, L. & Wacholder, S. (1987) Associations between several sites of cancer and twelve petroleum-derived liquids. Results from a case-referent study in Montreal. *Scand. J. Work Environ. Health*, 13, 493–504

Smith, J.D. & Maher, W.A. (1984) Aromatic hydrocarbons in waters of Port Phillip bay and the Yarra river estuary. *Aust. J. mar. Freshwater Res.*, 35, 119–128

Speight, J.G. (1980) *The Chemistry and Technology of Petroleum*, New York, Marcel Dekker, pp. 49–78

Suess, M.J., Grefen, K., Reinisch, D.W., eds (1985) *Ambient Air Pollutants from Industrial Sources*, Amsterdam, Elsevier, pp. 279–282

Tiratsoo, E.N. (1951) *Petroleum Geology*, London, Methuen, pp. 1–22

US Environmental Protection Agency (1986) *Test Methods for Evaluating Solid Waste. Physical/Chemical Methods* (*Publ. SW-846*), 3rd ed., Washington DC

Valković, V. (1978) *Trace Elements in Petroleum*, Part 2, *Trace Element Levels in Crude Oils and Products*, Tulsa, OK, Petroleum Publishing, pp. 62-101

Vandermeulen, J.H., Foda, A. & Stuttard, C. (1985) Toxicity vs mutagenicity of some crude oils, distillates and their water soluble fractions. *Water Res.*, 19, 1283–1289

Walters, P., Khan, S., O'Brien, P.J., Payne, J.F. & Rahimtula, A.D. (1987) Effectiveness of a Prudhoe Bay crude oil and its aliphatic, aromatic and heterocyclic fractions in inducing mortality and aryl hydrocarbon hydroxylase in chick embryo in ovo. *Arch. Toxicol.*, 60, 454–459

Watkins, R.E. (1977) *Transport of crude oil, gas and products by pipeline*. In: *Our Industry Petroleum*, London, British Petroleum Company, pp. 179–196

West, J.R. (1983) *Sulphur recovery*. In: Grayson, M., ed., *Kirk-Othmer Encyclopedia of Chemical Technology*, 3rd ed., Vol. 22, New York, John Wiley & Sons, pp. 267–297

Wojdat, W. & Winnicki, S. (1964) A case of bronchial aspiration pneumonia due to crude oil (Pol.). *Bull. Inst. mar. Med. Gdansk*, 15, 83–85

GASOLINE

1. Chemical and Physical Data

1.1 Synonyms and trade names

Automotive gasoline

    Chem. Abstr. Services Reg. No.: not assigned (8006-61-9 for natural gasoline)
    Chem. Abstr. Name: not assigned
    IUPAC Systematic Name: −
    Synonyms: Benzin; benzine; casinghead (natural gasoline); essence; ethyl; gasohol (with up to 10% ethanol in blend); mogas; motor gasoline; naphtha; petrol; premium leaded; premium low-lead; premium unleaded; regular leaded; regular unleaded; super premium leaded; super premium unleaded

Aviation gasoline

    Chem. Abstr. Services Reg. No.: not assigned
    Chem. Abstr. Name: not assigned
    IUPAC Systematic Name: −
    Synonyms: Avgas; Avgas (Grade) 80; Avgas (Grade) 100; Grade 100LL; Avgas (Grade) 115

1.2 Description

'Gasoline' is a generic term used to describe volatile, inflammable petroleum fuels used primarily in internal combustion engines to power passenger cars and other types of vehicle, such as buses, trucks, motorbikes and aircraft. It is a complex mixture of volatile hydrocarbon compounds with a nominal boiling-point range of 50–200°C (USA) or 25–220°C (Europe) for automotive gasoline and 25–170°C for aviation gasoline (CONCAWE, 1985). Hydrocarbons are predominantly in the C_4-C_{12} range (Ladefoged & Prior, 1984; Ward, 1984; CONCAWE, 1986, 1987).

Automotive gasolines are blended from several refinery process streams, including any of the various naphtha streams from direct distillation of crude oil at atmospheric pressure (light straight-run naphtha [3]) by catalytic [22] and thermal [28] cracking processes, by catalytic reforming [15] processes and from alkylation [13] and isomerization [14] of the lighter distillate streams[1]. They may also contain one or more additional components. The actual composition of gasolines varies widely, depending on the crude oils used, the refinery processes available, the overall balance of product demand, and the product specifications.

Gasoline is marketed as several products, and, within each product line, in various grades. Definitions have been developed for gasolines (American Petroleum Institute, 1981).

(a) Automotive gasoline

Automotive gasoline is a complex mixture of relatively volatile hydrocarbons, with or without additives, obtained by blending appropriate refinery streams to form a fuel suitable for use in spark ignition engines. Gasoline also includes all refinery products within the gasoline range (American Society for Testing and Materials (ASTM) Specification D 439) that are to be marketed as automotive gasoline without further processing in any refinery operation other than mechanical blending. In Europe and, to a lesser extent, in the USA, oxygenated compounds are also part of automotive gasoline components. Their nature and amounts are regulated. Gasoline includes leaded and unleaded grades, both of which are manufactured from blends of straight-run, cracked, reformed and other naphtha streams. A typical composition of unleaded gasoline is qualitatively similar to premium leaded grade but without lead antiknock additives (Hoffman, 1982). The two common grades of gasoline, premium and regular, differ chiefly in their octane number: regular, 91–93; premium, 96–99 (Ladefoged & Prior, 1984; Langdon, 1986).

(i) *Finished leaded automotive gasoline*

This automotive gasoline is produced by the addition of any lead (see IARC, 1980, 1987a) additive or which contains more than 0.013 g lead/l or more than 0.0013 g phosphorus/l. The differences among US grades are based primarily on the octane rating; these include super premium, premium and regular. Lead compounds are deliberately added to increase octane number and to suppress pre-ignition. In European countries, the amount of lead additive is limited to 0.15 g lead/l (Council of the European Communities, 1987), except in France, Ireland, Italy, Portugal and Spain, where the limit is 0.4 g/l (CONCAWE, 1988). The current grades are premium and regular. Phosphorus additives were used in the past but are now no longer added to gasolines.

(ii) *Finished unleaded automotive gasoline*

This US automotive gasoline contains no more than 0.013 g lead/l and no more than 0.0013 g phosphorus/l (American Petroleum Institute, 1981); lead and phosphorus additives are prohibited by regulation. The same grades as for leaded gasoline are produced. This definition of unleaded automotive gasoline also applies in Europe, except that only premium and regular grades are available. Furthermore, in central Europe and Scandinavia, facilities are installed in service stations which allow blending of leaded and unleaded premium gasoline in a 50:50 ratio, to produce 'intermediate' or 'low lead' grade. Such blends typically contain 0.075 g lead/l and include oxygenated compounds.

---

[1]See p. 41 of the monograph on occupational exposures in petroleum refining for characteristics of principal refinery process streams.

(iii) *Gasohol*

Gasohol is a mixture of gasoline with up to 10% volume anhydrous ethanol (Royal Dutch/Shell Group of Companies, 1983).

(b) *Aviation gasoline*

This category covers all special grades of gasoline for use in aviation reciprocating engines, as given in ASTM Specification D 910 and Military Specification MIL-G-5572, and includes all refinery products within the gasoline range that are to be marketed straight, or in blends, as aviation gasoline without further processing in any refinery operation other than mechanical blending (American Petroleum Institute, 1981).

1.3 Chemical composition and physical properties of technical products

(a) *Automotive gasoline*

Automotive gasoline is a volatile, inflammable, liquid hydrocarbon mixture used almost exclusively to fuel internal combustion engines. It has a typical density of about 0.7–0.8 g/cm³ (CRCS, 1985) and has a Reid vapour pressure (which is about 10% less than the true vapour pressure at 37.8°C) ranging between 8 and 15 psi [0.4–0.9 atm] (CONCAWE, 1985), depending on the season and geographical location.

The chemical composition of gasoline is highly variable because a product with the desired automotive fuel properties can be formulated in a number of ways. The composition by hydrocarbon type of typical automotive gasolines is given in Table 1. The hydrocarbon components are predominantly in the range C_5–C_{10} with an overall carbon number range of C_4–C_{12}. In Europe, the amount of each component process stream used would normally be

Table 1. Composition by hydrocarbon type of typical automotive gasolines[a]

Composition	Range
Alkanes	4–8 wt %
Alkenes	2–5 wt %
Isoalkanes	25–40 wt %
Cycloalkanes	3–7 wt %
Cycloalkenes	1–4 wt %
Total aromatics	20–50 wt %
Benzene	0.5–2.5 wt %
Paraffins (naphthenes)	30–90 vol. %
Olefins	0–30 vol. %
Aromatics	10–50 vol. %

[a]Adapted from CONCAWE (1985, 1987)

expected to fall within the range indicated in Table 2. A laboratory-blended reference sample of US unleaded gasoline has been reported to contain 44.5% heavy catalytically cracked naphtha [23], 22% light alkylate naphtha [13], 21.3% light reformed naphtha [16], 7.6% light catalytically cracked naphtha [22], 3.8% added butane and 0.8% added benzene (MacFarland et al., 1984; CRCS, 1985). According to CONCAWE, the aromatic fraction of gasoline contains benzene at a normal range of 0–7 vol % and typically at 2–3 vol %.

Table 2. Major component streams in automotive and aviation gasolines[a]

TSCA inventory name and identification number[b]	Refinery process stream (nomenclature used in Europe)	Automotive gasoline (vol. %)	Aviation gasoline (vol. %)
n-Butane [12]	Butanes	0–10	0–2
Light straight-run naphtha [3]	Light straight-run gasoline	0–30	0
Full-range reformed naphtha [15]	Catalytic reformate	30–80	0–40
Catalytically cracked naphthas [22, 23]	Catalytically cracked gasoline	0–60	0
Isomerization naphtha [14]	C_5/C_6 Isomerate	0–30	0–15
Full-range alkylate naphtha [13]	Alkylate	0–5	50–70
Thermally cracked naphthas [28, 29]	Thermally cracked gasoline	0–5	0
Light steam-cracked naphtha [33]	Steam-cracked (pyrolysis) gasoline[c]	0–50	0

[a]From CONCAWE (1985)

[b]See Table 2 and Figure 1 in the monograph on occupational exposures in petroleum refining

[c]Not widely used

A list of specific hydrocarbons detected in US 'midcontinent' gasolines at concentrations of 1 wt % or more is given in Table 3. ASTM specifications for automotive gasolines are provided in Table 4. No European standard is available for leaded automotive gasoline, but in most countries national specifications apply.

Gasoline also contains other additives, used to raise the octane number of leaded gasolines, to keep carburettors clean, to prevent oxidation of gasoline, to prevent corrosion in distribution systems and to differentiate grades of gasoline (Huddle, 1983). A list of typical additives used in automotive gasoline is given in Table 5. A number of contaminants must be removed to provide good quality gasoline, including water, particulate matter, nitrogen compounds, mercaptans and hydrogen sulfide (Huddle, 1983).

(b) Aviation gasoline

Many of the gasoline requirements of the automotive engine are shared by gasoline-powered aviation engines. However, aeroplane engines have several additional requirements because many involve direct fuel injection into the cylinders and some also have superchargers.

Table 3. Detectable hydrocarbons found in US finished gasolines at a concentration of 1% or more[a]

Chemical	Weight %	
	Estimated range	Weighted average[b]
Toluene	5–22	10
2-Methylpentane + 4-Methyl-*cis*-2-pentene + 3-Methyl-*cis*-2-pentene[c]	4–14	9
n-Butane	3–12	7
iso-Pentane	5–10	7
n-Pentane	1–9	5
Xylene (three isomers)	1–10	3
2,2,4-Trimethylpentane	<1–8	3
n-Hexane	<1–6	2
n-Heptane	<1–5	2
2,3,3-Trimethylpentane	<1–5	2
2,3,4-Trimethylpentane	<1–5	2
3-Methylpentane	<1–5	2
Methylcyclohexane + 1-*cis*-2-Dimethylcyclopentane + 3-Methylhexane[c]	<1–5	1
Benzene	<1–4	2
2,2,3-Trimethylpentane	<1–4	2
Methyl tertiary butyl ether	<1–4	1
Methylcyclopentane	<1–3	2
2,4-Dimethylpentane	<1–3	1
Cyclohexane	<1–3	1
1,2,4-Trimethylbenzene	<1–3	1
2-Methyl-2-butene	<1–2	2
2,3-Dimethylbutane	<1–2	1
trans-2-Pentene	<1–2	1
Methylcyclohexane	<1–2	1
3-Ethyltoluene	<1–2	1
2,3-Dimethylpentane	<1–2	1
2,5-Dimethylpentane	<1–2	1
2-Methyl-1-butene	<1–2	1
Ethyl benzene	<1–2	1

[a] Provided by American Petroleum Institute

[b] The sum of the weighted averages does not equal 100% because numerous components were detected at less than 1%.

[c] These chemicals could not be distinguished by gas chromatography because of similar retention times.

Table 4. Detailed requirements for gasoline (ASTM D439-79)[a]

Volatility class	Distillation temperature (°C) at % evaporated at 101.3 kPa					Distillation residue (vol % max)	Vapour:liquid ratio at 10.3 kPa (V:L)		
	10 Vol % max	50 Vol % min	50 Vol % max	90 Vol % max	End-point max		Test temperature (°C)	V:L max	
A	70	77	121	190	225	2	60	20	
B	65	77	118	190	225	2	56	20	
C	60	77	116	185	225	2	51	20	
D	55	77	113	185	225	2	47	20	
E	50	77	110	185	225	2	41	20	

Volatility class	Reid vapour pressure, max (kPa)	Lead content (max g/l)		Copper strip corrosion max	Existent gum, max (mg/100 ml)	Sulfur max (mass %)		Oxidation stability min (minutes)
		Unleaded[b]	Leaded[c]			Unleaded	Leaded	
A	62	0.013	1.1	No. 1	5	0.10	0.15	240
B	69	0.013	1.1	No. 1	5	0.10	0.15	240
C	79	0.013	1.1	No. 1	5	0.10	0.15	240
D	93	0.013	1.1	No. 1	5	0.10	0.15	240
E	103	0.013	1.1	No. 1	5	0.10	0.15	240

[a]From Hoffman (1982); CRCS (1985); CONCAWE (1988)

[b]The intentional addition of lead or phosphorus compounds is not permitted. US Environmental Protection Agency regulations limit their maximum concentrations to 0.05 g lead per gallon (0.013 g/l) and 0.005 g phosphorus per gallon (0.0013 g/l; by Test Method D 3231), respectively (Huddle, 1983).

[c]The US Environmental Protection Agency in 1986 limited the concentration in leaded gasoline to no more than 0.1 g/gallon (0.026 g/l), averaged for quarterly production of leaded gasoline (CONCAWE, 1988); 1.1 g/l is the maximum amount of lead permitted in leaded gasoline.

Table 5. Typical additives used in automotive gasoline[a]

Purpose	Compound
Antiknock	Tetraethyllead
	Tetramethyllead
	2-Methyl cyclopentadienyl manganese tricarbonyl[b]
Lead scavengers	1,2-Dibromoethane
	1,2-Dichloroethane
Detergents	Amino hydroxy amide
	Amines
	Alkyl ammonium dialkyl phosphate[b]
	Imidazolines
	Succinimides
Antirust	Fatty acid amines
	Sulfonates
	Amine/alkyl phosphates[b]
	Alkyl carboxylates
Antioxidants	Hindered phenols[c]
	para-Phenylenediamine[c]
	Aminophenols
	2,6-Di-tert-butyl-para-cresol
	ortho-Alkylated phenols combined with phenylenediamine
Dyes	Red: alkyl derivatives of azobenzene-4-azo-2-naphthol
	Orange: benzene-azo-2-naphthol
	Yellow: para-diethyl aminoazobenzene
	Blue: 1,4-diisopropylaminoanthraquinone
Anti-icing	Alcohols
	Amides/amines
	Organophosphate ammonium salts[b]
	Glycols
Upper cylinder lubricants	Light mineral oils
	Cycloparaffins
Metal deactivators	N,N'-Disalicylidene-1,2-diaminopropane
Oxygenates[d]	Ethanol
	Methanol
	Methyl-tert-butyl ether (MTBE)
	tert-Butyl alcohol (TBA)
	tert-Amyl methyl ether

[a]From Lane (1980); Huddle (1983); CRCS (1985)

[b]Not used in Europe

[c]Prevalent in Europe

[d]Oxygenates used commonly in Europe are methanol in conjunction with TBA or MTBE. Typical oxygenate contents are 3% methanol + 2% TBA or 5% MTBE. The methanol content in automotive gasolines should not exceed 3%; the MTBE content should not exceed 10%, and total amount of oxygen should not exceed 2.5% (CONCAWE, 1988).

Three grades of fuel are specified for use in aeroplanes: Avgas (Grade) 80 (formerly referred to as 80–87), Avgas (Grade) 100 (formerly called 100–130) and Grade 100LL (a low-lead formulation of Grade 100). A higher octane formulation, Avgas (Grade) 115 (115–145), is no longer in common use (see, e.g., Ward, 1984).

The same types of blending materials as those used in automotive gasolines may be used in aviation gasolines (Table 2), but higher percentages of some stocks (especially alkylates) and additional tetraethyllead (see IARC, 1980, 1987a) are used to meet the higher octane number requirement. The heat of combustion (energy content) is important in aviation fuels — the more energy available per unit of fuel, the less fuel load required for a specific trip. Because aviation gasolines may be subjected to low temperatures in high-altitude flight, the freezing-point of the fuel cannot be above −58°C. Only three additives are permitted in aviation gasoline: dye, tetraethyllead and antioxidant. Each of the three grades of gasoline has a standard colour to ensure that the correct grade is used (Ward, 1984). ASTM specifications for aviation gasoline are provided in Table 6.

Table 6. Detailed requirements for aviation gasoline (ASTM D 910–79)[a]

Requirement	Grade 80	Grade 100	Grade 100LL
Knock value, min, octane number, lean rating[b]	80	100	100
Knock value, min, rich rating[c]	87	100	100
Minimum performance number	87	130	130
Colour	red	green	blue
Dye content:			
Permissible blue dye, max, mg/gallon [mg/l]	0.5 [0.13]	4.7 [1.2]	5.7 [1.5]
Permissible yellow dye, max, mg/gallon [mg/l]	none	5.9 [1.6]	none
Permissible red dye, max, mg/gallon [mg/l]	8.65 [2.3]	none	none
Tetraethyllead, max, ml/gallon [g/l]	0.5 [0.13]	4.0 [1.1]	2.0 [0.5]

Requirement	All grades
Distillation temperature, °C:	
10% evaporated, max	75
40% evaporated, max	75
50% evaporated, max	105
90% evaporated, max	135
Final boiling-point, max °C	170
Sum of 10% and 50% evaporated temperatures, min, °C	135
Distillation recovery, min %	97
Distillation residue, max %	1.5
Distillation loss, max %	1.5
Net heat of combustion, min, Btu/lb [kJ/kg]	18 720 [43 520]
Vapour pressure	
min (kPa) [atm]	38 [0.4][d]
max (kPa) [atm]	48 [0.5]
Copper strip corrosion, max	No. 1

Table 6 (contd)

Requirement	All grades
Potential gum (5-h ageing), max, mg/100 ml	6
Visible lead precipitate, max, mg/100 ml	3
Sulfur, weight max, %	0.05
Freezing-point, max °C	−58
Water reaction	volume change not to exceed ± 2 ml
Permissible antioxidants, max lb/1000 bbl (42 gallons) [g/l]	4.2 [12]

[a]From Hoffman (1982)
[b]For cruising conditions
[c]For takeoff conditions
[d]From CONCAWE (1988)

2. Production, Use, Occurrence and Analysis

2.1 Production and use

(a) Production

Both automotive gasolines and aviation gasolines are produced primarily by blending component streams from petroleum refinery processing units. Blending of various stocks is a large volume operation. Gasoline components, including alkylates and other high-octane components, are blended with octane-improving additives (such as methyl *tert*-butyl ether), carburettor detergents, antirust agents, anti-icing agents and other additives.

Production volumes of automotive gasoline and aviation gasoline for the period 1970-85 at five-year intervals are shown in Table 7. Production in 1985 is shown for major geographical areas of the world in Table 8 (International Energy Agency, 1987).

(b) Use

Prior to the early 1900s, gasoline was an undesirable by-product of the manufacture of kerosene. The supply exceeded the demand, so the cut from gasoline to kerosene was processed to produce the minimal amount of gasoline and a maximum of kerosene. Under these conditions, the yield of gasoline was about 10% of crude oil, which was still too great for market needs (Guthrie, 1960). In time, uses were developed for gasoline. Varnish and paint makers used it as a solvent, and special lamps burnt it to illuminate parks and streets (Purdy, 1958).

With the rapid development of the automobile in the early 1900s, gasoline demand began to exceed supply. Over the ensuing decades, many processes were developed to produce gasoline, and it became the primary product of most petroleum refineries and remains so today (Purdy, 1958; Guthrie, 1960). Consumption volumes for use as automotive and aviation gasolines are presented in Tables 7 and 8.

Table 7. Production and consumption (in thousands of tonnes) of gasoline in the USA and countries of the Organisation for Economic Cooperation and Development (OECD), 1970–85[a]

Area/product	Production/consumption	1970	1975	1980	1985
USA					
Automotive gasoline	Production	244 495	285 133	284 843	270 562
	Consumption	247 520	286 639	285 052	289 922
Aviation gasoline	Production	2 215	1 561	1 385	969
	Consumption	2 234	1 598	1 459	1 204
OECD					
Automotive gasoline	Production	359 399	429 979	457 053	445 934
	Consumption	362 964	434 325	455 151	459 438
Aviation gasoline	Production	2 919	2 020	2 000	1 453
	Consumption	3 015	2 178	1 934	1 583

[a]From International Energy Agency (1987)

Table 8. Production and consumption (in thousands of tonnes) of automotive gasoline and aviation gasoline by geographical area, 1985[a]

Region/organization	Automotive gasoline		Aviation gasoline	
	Production	Consumption	Production	Consumption
North America	295 241	313 980	1 096	1 329
USA	270 562	289 922	969	1 204
Canada	24 679	24 058	127	125
OECD[b] (Europe)	111 854	105 416	232	150
European Economic Community	99 569	91 081	232	121
Pacific[c]	38 839	40 042	125	104
OECD (All)	445 934	459 438	1 453	1 583

[a]From International Energy Agency (1987)
[b]Organisation for Economic Cooperation and Development
[c]Australia, Japan, New Zealand

(c) *Regulatory status and guidelines*

In Sweden, occupational exposure standards of 220 mg/m^3 (8-h time-weighted average (TWA)) and 300 mg/m^3 (15-min TWA) have been established for gasoline with an assumed aromatic content of 46% (CONCAWE, 1987).

In the USA, occupational exposure limits for gasoline have been recommended at 900 mg/m^3 (8-h TWA) and 1500 mg/m^3 (15-min TWA; American Conference of Governmental Industrial Hygienists, 1987). A compilation of national occupational exposure limits for gasoline components has been published (CONCAWE, 1987).

As of 1 January 1986, the US Environmental Protection Agency promulgated as a final rule a low-lead standard of 0.10 g lead per gallon (0.026 g/l) of leaded gasoline (CONCAWE, 1988). An EEC Directive requires Member States to ensure that unleaded gasoline (as defined in section 1.2) is available and evenly distributed throughout their territory from 1 October 1989 onwards (Council of the European Communities, 1987).

2.2 Occurrence

(a) *Occupational exposure*

Exposure to gasoline in the work environment has been associated with the following operations or jobs (CONCAWE, 1985, 1987): refinery operations leading to the production of gasoline; tank dipping, pipeline and pump repairs and filter cleaning in refineries, distribution terminals and depots; maintenance, inspection and cleaning of gasoline storage tanks; gasoline distribution via bulk transfer in refineries and terminals; service station attendants; engine and vehicle maintenance; and routine sampling and laboratory analysis of gasoline. Other operations or jobs involving gasoline exposure include: adjustment of gasoline pumps in service stations (Andersson *et al.*, 1984), and the use of gasoline as a metal cleaning solvent (Verwilghen *et al.*, 1975).

Quantitative exposure data typical of various activities are summarized in Table 9 for total hydrocarbons and benzene (see IARC, 1982, 1987b), the two most commonly reported measures of gasoline vapours.

Because of the lower volatility of hydrocarbons with a higher number of carbons, the hydrocarbon composition of gasoline vapours in most occupational situations is different from that of liquid gasoline. Thus, vapours from several European gasolines were found to contain an average of 90% by volume of C_3–C_5 nonaromatic hydrocarbons (compared to 26% by weight in the liquid) and about 2% of C_6–C_8 aromatics (compared to 31% by weight in the liquid; CONCAWE, 1987).

Highest overall 8-h TWA concentrations have been observed for drum filling and marine loading operations, while service station attendants have the lowest exposure levels. High short-term concentrations in air may occur during loading operations on tank trucks with no vapour recovery system; lower levels are observed over the full working day of loader-drivers (Phillips & Jones, 1978).

Table 9. Concentrations (time-weighted average measurements) of airborne gasoline constituents in various operations and occupations

Operation/occupation (region)	Exposure and sampling duration	Concentration (mg/m³)		Reference
		Total hydrocarbons arithmetic mean (range) [no. of samples]	Benzene mean (range) [no. of samples]	
Top loading of road tankers, no vapour recovery (western Europe)	<1 h	451 (6.4–3030) [142]	6.1 (ND[a]–60.5) [142]	CONCAWE (1987)
Top loading of road tankers, no vapour recovery (USA)	8 h	46.4 (9.9–109) [10]	0.9 (0.1–2.3) [43]	Halder et al. (1986)
Bottom loading of road tankers, no vapour recovery (western Europe)	<1 h	76 (8.2–234) [59]	1.4 (ND–5.5) [59]	CONCAWE (1987)
Bottom loading of road tankers, no vapour recovery (USA)	8 h	89.8 (21.9–184) [7]	1.1 (0.2–5.9) [38]	Halder et al. (1986)
Bottom loading of road tankers, vapour recovery (USA)	8 h	39.6 (9.4–195)[b] [8]	1.0 (0.2–8.9)[b] [56]	Halder et al. (1986)
Road tankers during driving (western Europe)	8 h		0.1 (ND–0.3) [20]	Arbetarskyddsstyrelsen (1981)
Marine loading, tanker and barge (USA)	8 h	246 (9.1–1580) [11]	2.3 (0.1–19.5) [11]	Halder et al. (1986)
Marine loading deck crews, barges (western Europe)	8 h	263 (1.5–1750) [11]	4.7 (ND–31.5) [11]	CONCAWE (1987)
Railcar top loading (western Europe)	8 h	84.7 (2.0–535) [32]	1.5 (ND–9.5) [32]	CONCAWE (1987)
Drum filling (western Europe)	8 h	858 (61–1748) [9]	27.2 (ND–116) [9]	CONCAWE (1987)
Service station attendants (western Europe)	8 h	29.3 (7.9–101) [13]	0.35 (ND–1.3) [13]	CONCAWE (1987)

Table 9 (contd)

Operation/occupation (region)	Exposure and sampling duration	Concentration (mg/m³) Total hydrocarbons arithmetic mean (range) [no. of samples]	Benzene mean (range) [no. of samples]	Reference
Service station attendants (USA)	8 h	10–67[c] (range of means) [84] from 7 locations	0.06–0.75[c] (range of means) [84] from 7 locations	McDermott & Vos (1979)
Service station attendants (USA)	6–7 h	4.6[d] (1.9–14.3) [8]		Kearney & Dunham (1986)
Service station mechanics (USA)	7 h	2.9[d] (1.1–22.3) [4]		Kearney & Dunham (1986)
Cleaning of gasoline storage tanks (western Europe)	<1 h		(64–1680)[e] [10]	Arbetarskyddsstyrelsen (1981)
Refinery operators, gasoline production (western Europe)	8 h	52.8 (0.7–1820) [62]	0.9 (ND–23.8) [62]	CONCAWE (1987)
Refinery operators, ancillary (western Europe)	8 h	66.0 (3.8–923) [27]	1.0 (ND–14.1) [27]	CONCAWE (1987)
Gasoline truck drivers (USA)	7–8 h	45.8 (19–72.5)[f] [49]	0.45 (0.25–0.65)[f] [47]	Rappaport et al. (1987)
Service station attendants (USA)	7–8 h	70 (53–86.8)[f] [49]	0.65 (0.48–0.81)[f] [49]	Rappaport et al. (1987)
Rail tanker top loaders (UK)	4 and 5 h		5.1 and 8.0[c] [39] (means for 2 loaders)	Sherwood (1972)
Rail tanker weigher (UK)	6 h		64[c] [23]	Sherwood (1972)

Table 9 (contd)

Operation/occupation (region)	Exposure and sampling duration	Concentration (mg/m³)		Reference
		Total hydrocarbons arithmetic mean (range) [no. of samples]	Benzene mean (range) [no. of samples]	
Loading, rail and road tankers (UK)	35 min–3 h		0.96–21[g] [70]	Parkinson (1971)
Service station attendants (UK)	3.5–14 h		0.96–7.7[c] (range of means) [121] from 9 stations	Parkinson (1971)

[a]ND, not detected
[b]Values for one of three terminals
[c]Converted from ppm
[d]Geometric mean
[e]No mean value given because of highly varying concentration
[f]Approximate 95% confidence interval
[g]Range of means covering 24 operators; converted from ppm

The general trend seen in Table 9 is confirmed in studies focusing on benzene exposure (Irving & Grumbles, 1979; Runion & Scott, 1985). Furthermore, moderate levels of benzene have been measured during the following operations: dismantling of pump filters by pump servicemen (20 mg/m^3) and carburettor and cylinder head demounting in automobile garages (<16 mg/m^3; Holmberg & Lundberg, 1985). Besides benzene, a variety of other gasoline-derived hydrocarbons have been measured in occupational settings. Thus, concentrations of up to 150 hydrocarbons have been reported in 15 job groups involving gasoline exposure (CONCAWE, 1987). Among those, components with independent toxic effects such as n-hexane, toluene, the xylenes and trimethylbenzenes were present in concentrations well below their respective established exposure limits. Exposure levels of 1,3-butadiene (see IARC, 1986a, 1987c) for various job groups are summarized in Table 10.

Table 10. Personal exposures (mg/m^3) to 1,3-butadiene associated with gasoline[a]

	Mean	Range	Exposure duration
Production on-site (refining)	0.3	ND[b]–11.4	8-h TWA
Production off-site (refining)	0.1	ND–1.6	8-h TWA
Loading ships (closed system)	6.4	ND–21.0	8-h TWA
Loading ships (open system)	1.1	ND–4.2	8-h TWA
Loading barges	2.6	ND–15.2	8-h TWA
Jettyman	2.6	ND–15.9	8-h TWA
Bulk loading road tankers			
Top loading <1 h	1.4	ND–32.3	<1–h TWA
Top loading >1 h	0.4	ND–4.7	8-h TWA
Bottom loading <1 h	0.2	ND–3.0	<1–h TWA
Bottom loading >1 h	0.4	ND–14.1	8-h TWA
Road tanker delivery (bulk plant to service station)	ND		
Railcar top loading	0.6	ND–6.2	8-h TWA
Drumming	ND		
Service station attendant (dispensing fuel)	0.3	ND–1.1	8-h TWA
Self-service station (filling tank)	1.6	ND–10.6	2-min TWA

[a]From CONCAWE (1987)
[b]ND, not detected

Concentrations of airborne tetraethyllead, tetramethyllead (see IARC, 1980, 1987a), ethylene dichloride (1,2-dichloroethane; see IARC, 1979, 1987d) and ethylene dibromide (1,2-dibromoethane; see IARC, 1977, 1987e), all additives in leaded gasoline, were found to be too low to be detected in the breathing zone of tank truck loaders (McDermott & Killiany, 1978). Additional data on exposure to tetraalkyllead compounds, 1,2-dibromoethane, 1,2-dichloroethane, *tert*-butyl alcohol and methyl-*tert*-butyl ether of gasoline-exposed workers inside and outside refineries are given in the monograph on occupational exposures in petroleum refining.

Table 11 summarizes various biological exposure measurements made on workers exposed to gasoline.

Table 11. Biological exposure measurements in workers exposed to gasoline

Matrix	Occupation (no. of workers)	Biological indicator	Concentration	Reference
Blood	Tank cleaner (3)	Tetramethyllead	0.01–0.027 µg/ml[a]	Andersson et al. (1984)
Blood	Pump attendant (6)	Tetramethyllead	0.005–0.006 µg/ml[a]	Andersson et al. (1984)
Blood	Service station attendant (8)	Benzene	<0.003–0.020 µg/ml[b]	Elster et al. (1978)
Blood	Service station attendant (8)	Toluene	0.010–0.045 µg/ml[b]	Elster et al. (1978)
Urine	Service station attendant (48)	Total thioethers	[c]	Stock & Priestly (1986)
Urine	Service station attendant (51)	Phenol	40 mg/l (mean)[d] >20 mg/l (88% of workers)	Pandya et al. (1975)
Urine	Top loading of rail tankers (3)	Phenol	12, 25 (loader) and 83 (weigher) mg/l[b]	Sherwood (1972)
Urine	Service station attendant (5)	Phenol	5–18 mg/l[b]	Parkinson (1971)
Urine	Loading rail tankers (2)	Phenol	ND[e]–10 mg/l[b]	Parkinson (1971)
Urine	Loading and discharging road tankers (7)	Phenol	4–48 mg/l[d,f]	Parkinson (1971)
Exhaled breath	Loading rail tankers (2)	Benzene	0.3–2.8 mg/m^3[b]	Parkinson (1971)
Exhaled breath	Top loading of rail tankers (3)	Benzene	0.44, 0.56 and 2.7 (weigher) mg/m^3[b]	Sherwood (1972)

[a]Expressed as lead; blood tetramethyllead concentration in reference group, <0.003 µg/ml

[b]Samples taken at end of work

[c]End of working day samples significantly higher than morning samples ($p < 0.001$); pump operators higher than self-service attendants.

[d]Gasoline contained 10–17% of benzene; hot weather conditions

[e]ND, not detected

[f]Gasoline contained 20–33% benzene

(b) *Environmental exposure*

Ground water contamination due to leaks from below-ground storage tanks has become a serious environmental problem. In New Jersey, USA, more than 1400 incidents were reported in 1978, resulting in spillage of 1.1 million gallons (4.2 million l) of petroleum compounds. The number of incidents reported has continued to rise and is approaching 2000 per year in New Jersey alone (Kramer, 1982).

Approximately 110 billion gallons (420 billion l) of gasoline are used in the USA each year. Nearly all gasoline used for transportation purposes is stored underground before it is used, but, of the estimated 1.4 million underground gasoline storage tanks in the USA, approximately 85% are made of steel and have no protection against corrosion. Following the rupture of a storage tank, gasoline travels down through the porous material towards the ground water table, adhering to soil particles along the way. If enough gasoline is spilled and the residual saturation requirement is satisfied, free gasoline then enters the water table. Since gasoline hydrocarbons are toxic at concentrations below solubility limits and saturated material can come into contact with fluctuating water tables and/or ground water recharge, saturated soil can pose a long-term threat to ground water supplies due to the relatively soluble aromatic constitutents (Hoag & Marley, 1986).

In a study by Kearney and Dunham (1986; see also Table 9), the concentration of total hydrocarbons measured when customers at a self-service station filled one tank was 3.9–63.5 mg/m^3 (12 samples; average sampling time, 10 min). Concentrations measured in the area of self-service and serviced pump islands and at the perimeter were 3.6–16.1 (three samples; average sampling time, 426 min), 0.9–9.9 (five; 408) and not detected-9.7 mg/m^3 (17; 416), respectively. The concentration of 1,2-dichloroethane during filling of gasoline tanks at self-service stations has been evaluated as 6 μg/m^3 for 2.2 h per year (Gold, 1980).

Accidental releases of gasoline in the recent past include the following. In 1968, a tank leak of 100 000–250 000 gallons (378 500–946 250 l) occurred in Los Angeles-Glendale, CA, USA (McKee *et al.*, 1972). In March 1978, 1900 tonnes of gasoline were released into the waters of Block Island Sound, RI, USA, after the grounding of *Ocean Barge 250* (Dimock *et al.*, 1980). Thirty tonnes of gasoline leaked from a barge near Queen Charlotte Islands, Canada, in March 1984 (McLaren, 1985)

2.3 Analysis

Since gasoline is composed of a complex mixture of hydrocarbons, there are few methods for the environmental analysis of 'gasoline' as an entity, but many methods are reported for the analysis of its component hydrocarbons. These methods are used to identify or 'fingerprint' the origin of a specific gasoline sample on the basis of the proportions of its component hydrocarbons. Selected methods for the quantitative determination of gasoline in air are listed in Table 12.

Four air sampling methods for unleaded gasoline have been tested and compared, two based on charcoal tubes of differing capacity and two on passive organic vapour monitors. The analytical method involves chlorobenzene desorption and capillary or packed column

Table 12. Methods for the determination of gasoline in air

Sample preparation	Assay procedure[a]	Limit of detection[b]	Remarks	Reference
Absorption (porous polymer and charcoal); thermal desorption (one or two stage)	GC/FID capillary column	0.03 mg/m³ THC	Applicable to THC and individual components[c]	CONCAWE (1986)
Absorption (charcoal); desorption (dichloromethane)	GC/FID capillary column	0.5 mg/m³[d] THC	Applicable to THC and individual components[e]	Kearney & Dunham (1986)

[a]GC/FID, gas chromatography/flame ionization detection

[b]THC, total hydrocarbon

[c]Method validated for 22 hydrocarbons (from propane to *n*-decane, including benzene, toluene and *ortho*-xylene); this method also allows the determination of additives such as methanol and methyl-*tert*-butyl ether.

[d]Lower limit of stated working range

[e]24 Aliphatic and aromatic hydrocarbons actually measured in a service station

separation with flame ionization detection. Samples were analysed for total hydrocarbons as well as for eight individual compounds. A dependence on humidity was found at high concentrations of total hydrocarbons (375 mg/m³) for all methods except those involving high-capacity charcoal tubes (American Petroleum Institute, 1984).

Benzene in exhaled air and phenol in urine have been measured by gas chromatographic methods as indices of exposure to gasoline (IARC, 1982; Fishbein & O'Neill, 1988).

3. Biological Data Relevant to the Evaluation of Carcinogenic Risk to Humans

3.1 Carcinogenicity studies in animals[1]

Studies on the carcinogenicity in experimental animals of light straight-run naphtha [3] and light catalytically cracked naphtha [22] refinery streams, which are components of automobile gasoline, have been described in the monograph on occupational exposures in petroleum refining.

Inhalation

Mouse: Groups of 100 male and 100 female B6C3F1 mice, six weeks of age, were exposed to 0, 67, 292 or 2056 ppm [0, ~ 200, 870 or 6170 mg/m³] totally volatilized

---

[1]The Working Group was aware of skin-painting studies in progress in mice using unleaded gasoline (IARC, 1986b).

unleaded gasoline (benzene content, 2%) by inhalation for 6 h per day on five days per week for 103–113 weeks. The sample was blended to conform to US specifications existing in 1976. Ten male and ten female mice from each group were killed at three, six, 12 and 18 months and the remainder at the end of the study. Survival in the groups of exposed female mice was not significantly different from that of controls [rates not reported]. That of the low- and medium-dose male mice was significantly higher than that in controls, although survival of high-dose males was lower than that of controls [rates not reported]. The incidences of hepatocellular adenomas and carcinomas were increased in exposed females. In mice killed at 18–24 months, the percentages of animals with liver tumours were: controls, 14%; low dose, 19%; medium dose, 21%; high dose, 48% [ratio of benign to malignant tumours unspecified]. The incidence of hepatocellular tumours was not increased in treated male mice. A renal adenoma occurred in one high-dose female and a bilateral renal tubular adenocarcinoma in another (MacFarland *et al.*, 1984). [The Working Group noted the inadequate reporting of the experimental data.]

Rat: Groups of 100 male and 100 female Fischer 344 rats, six weeks of age, were exposed to 0, 67, 292 or 2056 ppm [0, ~200, 870 or 6170 mg/m^3] totally volatilized unleaded gasoline (benzene content, 2%) by inhalation for 6 h per day on five days per week for 107 or 109 weeks. Ten males and ten females from each group were killed at three, six, 12 and 18 months and the remainder at the end of the study. Survival in the groups of exposed female rats was not significantly different from that of controls [rates not reported]. That of control male rats was significantly higher than that of any of the exposed groups after week 80 [rates not reported]. Increased incidences of renal tumours were observed in male rats: renal adenomas — controls, 0; low-dose, 0; medium-dose, 2; high-dose, 1; renal carcinomas — control, 0; low-dose, 1; medium-dose, 2; high-dose, 6. No renal adenoma or carcinoma was observed in female rats. Renal sarcomas occurred in one medium-dose male and in one medium-dose female (MacFarland, 1982; MacFarland *et al.*, 1984). [The Working Group noted the inadequate reporting of the experiment.]

3.2 Other relevant data

(*a*) *Experimental systems*

Absorption, distribution, excretion and metabolism
No data were available to the Working Group.

Toxic effects
Male albino [Wistar] rats given a single dose of 2.0 ml/kg bw gasoline (Indian Oil Corp.) by intraperitoneal injection showed increased lipid peroxidation in the liver after 24 h (Rao & Pandya, 1978). Female Wistar rats administered 1.0 ml/kg bw gasoline (Indian Oil Corp.) intraperitoneally had depressed activities of hepatic δ-aminolaevulinic acid synthetase and dehydratase within 20 h (Rao & Pandya, 1980).

Male Porton rats exposed in a chamber to gasoline vapour (50% super:50% standard) at a calculated concentration of 5 mg/l, for 8 h per day for three weeks, showed moderate increases in liver microsomal cytochrome P450 activities (Harman *et al.*, 1981).

In electroencephalographic studies with male Wistar rats given 10 ml/kg bw of either unleaded or leaded (1000 ppm (16.5 mg/kg bw) tetraethyllead) gasoline by intraperitoneal injection, animals given leaded gasoline showed excessive tension and excitement by day 6–7. Both unleaded and leaded gasoline decreased δ, θ and α waves after one to three days, whereas the electrocorticogram of rats given leaded gasoline showed marked α and θ waves after six to seven days (Saito, 1973).

Treatment of male Fischer 344 rats by gavage with 0.04–2.0 ml/kg bw unleaded gasoline daily for nine days markedly increased the number and size of hyaline droplets in cells of the renal proximal convoluted tubules. The renal content of the male rat-specific low molecular protein α_{2u}-globulin was increased up to 4.4 fold (Olson et al., 1987). A series of gavage screening studies using male Fischer 344 rats was conducted on components of gasoline to identify more clearly the major contributors to nephrotoxicity. The alkane components were found to be primarily responsible, and the degree of branching was related to the potency of the nephrotoxic response (Halder et al., 1985). An active nephrotoxic component of gasoline, 2,2,4-trimethylpentane, induced hyaline droplet accumulation, degeneration and necrosis in the renal proximal convoluted tubules after administration of 50–500 mg/kg bw daily by gavage for 21 days. In cell proliferation studies, 2,2,4-trimethylpentane led to a five- to six-fold increase in the labelling index of the P2 segment of the kidney tubule (Short et al., 1986). The extent and localization of cell proliferation elicited by 0.2–50 mg/kg bw 2,2,4-trimethylpentane given by gavage on five days per week for three weeks to male Fischer 344 rats closely paralleled the extent and severity of renal tubular accumulation of crystalloid hyaline droplets and single-cell necrosis. Similar cell proliferation, hyaline droplet accumulation and necrosis were seen in male rats exposed by inhalation to 2–2000 ppm [~6–6000 mg/m³] unleaded gasoline for 6 h per day on five days per week for three weeks (Short et al., 1987). A metabolite of 2,2,4-trimethylpentane, 2,4,4-trimethyl-2-pentanol, has been shown to accumulate in the male (but not in female) rat kidney and to bind reversibly to kidney α_{2u}-globulin (Charbonneau et al., 1987; Lock et al., 1987).

Female rats [strain unspecified] exposed to 100 ppm [~300 mg/m³] leaded gasoline vapour (octane rating, 98%; 0.45 g/l tetraethyllead) for 8 h per day, on five days per week up to 12 weeks, exhibited a high incidence of changes in the lung parenchyma characterized by interstitial fibrosis with associated alveolar collapse. Initial changes, appearing after six weeks, included degeneration of endothelium and interstitial fibroblasts followed by hypertrophy of type 2 pneumocytes (Lykke & Stewart, 1978; Lykke et al., 1979). Among female Wistar rats similarly exposed for up to 15 days, reduced levels of pulmonary surfactant, with no qualitative alteration in the phospholipid components, were observed. However, such treatment did not result in changes in RNA or DNA synthesis in lung tissue in vivo (Stewart et al., 1979).

Male and female Sprague-Dawley rats exposed to 29, 416 or 3316 ppm (0.11, 1.58 or 12.61 mg/l TWA) unleaded gasoline blend by inhalation for 6 h per day on five days per week for 21 days developed mild renal tubular degenerative and regenerative changes, including increased levels of hyaline droplet formation, necrosis and degeneration of the proximal convoluted tubule of the renal cortex in males only. When exposure was extended to 90 days at concentrations of 40, 379 or 3866 ppm (0.15, 1.44 or 14.70 mg/l), a concentration-related incidence of tubular dilatation and necrosis at the corticomedullary junction was observed in male rats only (Halder *et al.*, 1984). Similarly, in another study, male Sprague-Dawley rats exposed to 1552 ppm [~4650 mg/m^3] unleaded gasoline vapour for 6 h per day on five days per week for 90 days had regenerative epithelium and dilatation of kidney tubules. These effects were not seen in females and were not seen with leaded gasoline in animals of either sex (Kuna & Ulrich, 1984).

In a long-term study, groups of male and female Fischer 344 rats were exposed to 67, 292 or 2056 ppm [~200, 870 or 6170 mg/m^3] unleaded gasoline vapours for 6 h per day on five days per week for three, six, 12, 18 and 24 months. After three, six and 12 months at the highest doses, the males had increased foci of regenerative epithelium in the renal cortex and dilated tubules. Both exposed and control rats developed spontaneous chronic progressive nephropathy after 18 and 24 months' exposure. However, male rats exposed to 292 and 2056 ppm for 12, 18 and 24 months had linear mineral deposits in the renal medullae (Busey & Cockrell, 1984; MacFarland *et al.*, 1984).

Effects on reproduction and prenatal toxicity

As reported in a review of teratology studies of rats exposed to different fuels by inhalation, exposure of animals on days 6–15 of gestation for 6 h daily to 400 and 1600 ppm [~1200 and 4800 mg/m^3]) of unleaded gasoline resulted in no teratogenic effect (Schreiner, 1984). [The Working Group noted that details were not reported.]

Genetic and related effects

Unleaded gasoline (containing 2% benzene; boiling range, 31–192°C; 39% aromatics) did not induce mutation in *Salmonella typhimurium* TA1535, TA1537, TA1538, TA98 or TA100 in the presence or absence of an exogenous metabolic system from rat liver using either the plate incorporation (0.001–5 µl/plate) or suspension method (3.75–30 µl/ml; Conaway *et al.*, 1984). As reported in an abstract, unleaded gasoline, regular gasoline and two samples of aviation gasoline (one with an additive) did not induce mutation in *S. typhimurium* [strain unspecified] in the presence or absence of an exogenous metabolic system from Aroclor 1254-induced rat liver (Farrow *et al.*, 1983).

A dimethyl sulfoxide extract (5–200 µl/plate) and a residue from evaporation (50–10 000 µg/plate) of unleaded gasoline (American Petroleum Institute reference PS-6) were not mutagenic to *S. typhimurium* TA98 in the presence of an exogenous metabolic system from Aroclor 1254-induced rat and hamster liver, respectively (Dooley *et al.*, 1988).

A commercial leaded gasoline (with a maximum concentration of 0.04% lead and 2–4% v/v benzene) administered by larval feeding of 2.5% in the culture medium induced somatic mutations for eye pigmentation in *Drosophila melanogaster* (Nylander *et al.*, 1978).

Unleaded gasoline (PS-6 with 2% benzene w/w; same lot as used by MacFarland *et al.*, 1984, see p. 176) induced unscheduled DNA synthesis *in vitro* in hepatocytes from male Fischer-344/CrlBR rats (0.05 and 0.10% v/v), in hepatocytes from male B6C3F1/CrlBR mice (0.01% v/v) and in human hepatocytes (0.01% v/v; Loury *et al.*, 1986). Unleaded gasoline (PS-6; same lot as above) did not induce significant unscheduled DNA synthesis *in vitro* (0.005–0.010% v/v) in primary cultures of kidney cells from male Fischer-344/CrlBR rats (Loury *et al.*, 1987).

One sample of unleaded gasoline (containing 2% benzene; boiling range, 31–192°C; 39% aromatics) tested at a concentration of 0–1.0 μl/ml in the presence of an exogenous metabolic system from either rat or mouse liver (Conaway *et al.*, 1984) and another sample of unleaded gasoline (PS-6; with 2% benzene w/w) tested either in the presence (0.125–0.175 μl/ml) or absence (0.045–0.070 μl/ml) of an exogenous metabolic system from Aroclor 1254-induced rat liver did not induce mutation in cultured mouse lymphoma L5178Y $TK^{+/-}$ cells. However, mutation was induced in mouse lymphoma L5178Y $TK^{+/-}$ cells in a concentration-dependent manner by both a dimethyl sulfoxide extract of unleaded gasoline (PS-6; with 2% benzene w/w), only in the absence of an exogenous metabolic system from Aroclor 1254-induced rat liver, and a residue from the evaporation of the same unleaded gasoline, only in the presence of an exogenous metabolic system from Aroclor 1254-induced rat liver (Dooley *et al.*, 1988).

As reported in an abstract, unleaded gasoline, regular gasoline and two samples of aviation gasoline (one with an additive) induced mutations in mouse lymphoma L5178Y $TK^{+/-}$ cells but did not increase the frequency of sister chromatid exchange in cultured Chinese hamster ovary cells (Farrow *et al.*, 1983).

Unleaded gasoline (PS-6; with 2% benzene w/w) did not induce mutations at the thymidine kinase locus nor sister chromatid exchange in human lymphoblasts *in vitro* in the presence or absence of an exogenous metabolic system from Aroclor 1254-induced rat liver (Richardson *et al.*, 1986).

Unleaded gasoline (PS-6; with 2% benzene w/w) induced unscheduled DNA synthesis *in vivo* in hepatocytes from male and female B6C3F1/CrlBR mice 12 h after treatment with 2000 mg/kg bw by gavage. The percentage of S-phase cells in the hepatocytes of male, but not female, mice also increased. No increase was observed in unscheduled DNA synthesis *in vivo* in hepatocytes from male Fischer-344/CrlBR rats 2–48 h after gavage treatment at 100–5000 mg/kg bw. However, the percentage of S-phase cells was increased 24–48 h after treatment with 2000 mg/kg bw (Loury *et al.*, 1985, 1986). Unleaded gasoline (PS-6; with 2% benzene w/w) did not induce unscheduled DNA synthesis *in vivo* in kidney cells from male or female Fischer-344/CrlBR rats treated by inhalation at 2000 ppm [~6000 mg/m³] for four or 18 days (6 h per day) or 2–24 h after treatment by gavage (2000–5000 mg/kg bw single treatment or four daily treatments of 5000 mg/kg bw [male rats only]). The percentage of cells in S-phase increased in kidney cells from male rats exposed for 18 days by inhalation (2000 ppm [~6000 m³]; 6 h per day) or gavage (2000 mg/kg bw per day; Loury *et al.*, 1987).

Unleaded gasoline (containing 2% benzene; boiling range, 31–192°C; 39% aromatics) did not induce chromosomal aberrations in the bone marrow of male or female Sprague-Dawley CD rats in either of two protocols: 6–48 h after intraperitoneal injections of 0.03, 0.1 or 0.3 ml/rat; or after five daily intraperitoneal injections of 0.013, 0.04 or 0.13 ml/rat per day (Conaway *et al.*, 1984).

Similarly, in another experiment, unleaded gasoline (PS-6) did not induce chromosomal aberrations in the bone marrow of male Sprague-Dawley rats dosed orally with 500, 750 and 1000 mg/kg bw per day for five days (Dooley et al., 1988).

(b) *Humans*

Absorption, distribution excretion and metabolism

The more rapid absorption of gasoline via inhalation than by the oral route was suggested in an early review on the basis of experience of poisonings. Conclusive evidence that systemic gasoline poisoning arises solely due to skin absorption has not been documented (Machle, 1941).

After pregnant women working in a chemical industry were exposed to gasoline fumes, gasoline was found in fetal and neonatal tissues; neonatal blood concentrations of gasoline were about double the maternal blood concentrations (Lipovskii et al., 1979).

Urinary thioether excretion was increased in 35 gasoline service station attendants and in 13 workers in self-service stations when samples taken before and after work were compared. The difference between the samples was greater ($p < 0.001$) in persons working in attendant-operated service stations than in those in self-service outlets. Cigarette smokers, in general, excreted higher levels of thioethers in samples taken both before ($p < 0.005$) and after ($p < 0.001$) work (Stock & Priestly, 1986).

Toxic effects

It was stated in an early, extensive review of gasoline intoxications that single oral doses of approximately 7.5 g/kg bw are usually fatal to man; however, death had been caused by ingestion of as little as 10 g. Following inhalation of gasoline, acute intoxication is characterized primarily by severe symptoms in the central nervous system; signs and symptoms may include headache, blurred vision, vertigo, ataxia, tinnitus, nausea, anorexia, weakness, incoordination, restlessness, excitement, mental confusion, disorientation, disturbances of speech and of swallowing, delirium and coma (Machle, 1941).

Several cases of fatal intoxication have been reported. The major pathological findings and symptoms in the nervous system were cerebral oedema and petechial brain haemorrhages. The major pulmonary findings were oedema and haemorrhage. Skin burns and superficial epidermolysis were also reported, in addition to fatty infiltration of the liver (Helbling, 1950; Aidin, 1958; Ainsworth, 1960). Toxic nephrosis was reported in one child (Banner & Walson, 1983).

Eye irritation was the only significant effect reported among volunteers exposed for 30 min to gasoline vapour at concentrations of about 200, 500 and 1000 ppm [~600, 1500 and 3000 mg/m^3] in air; the highest concentrations had the most severe effects (Davis et al., 1960).

Young male volunteers were exposed in a chamber to a range of concentrations of vapour from commercial gasoline. Initial central nervous system symptoms started at concentrations between 700 (0.07%) and 2800 (0.28%) ppm [~2100 and 8400 mg/m^3]; exposure to 1000 ppm (0.1%) [~3000 mg/m^3] gasoline vapour caused serious central nervous system symptoms; and, at 10 000 ppm (1%) [~30 000 mg/m³], dizziness and drunkenness started after about 5 min of exposure (Drinker *et al.*, 1943).

Leukocytopenia (13%), thrombocytopenia (7%) and small-diameter erythrocytes were observed among 200 crewmen on gasoline tankers operating mainly in the Black Sea basin. A relationship was seen between length of service of sailors on tankers and the haematological changes (Kirjakov *et al.*, 1966). Haematological changes were also observed in a group of painters who used gasoline diluents for paints (Sterner, 1941).

Among 19 male gasoline station attendants in Australia, aged 16—50 years, all of whom had had more than one year's exposure and none of whom were taking drugs, shorter salivary antipyrine half-lives were observed compared to controls, indicating that occupational exposure to gasoline may result in enhanced microsomal drug metabolism. In these workers, the blood lead level was similar to that of an unexposed population (Harman *et al.*, 1981).

Chronic sniffing of leaded gasoline may cause a range of neurological effects including encephalopathy, ataxia and tremor. In clinical studies of 73 chronic sniffers of leaded gasoline (age range, four to 20 years), 69 showed definite neurological effects and had blood lead levels ranging between 30 and 344 µg/dl (Seshia *et al.*, 1978; Coulehan *et al.*, 1983). In those presenting with encephalopathy, the mean blood level was 95 µg/dl (Coulehan *et al.*, 1983). [The Working Group noted that tetraethyllead may cause hallucinations and behavioural changes, and it is not clear whether the clinical findings are due to the presence of aliphatic and aromatic hydrocarbons in gasoline or to tetraethyllead or to the action of both.]

Cardiac arrest has been suggested as one of the most important causes of sudden death in subjects who sniff gasoline vapour. Death often occurs in association with physical activity, such as running after sniffing or a stressful situation. The mechanism of this sudden death is not fully elucidated, but is likely to be caused by hydrocarbon-induced cardiac arrythmia. No measurement has been made of free norepinephrine at target cells at the time of stress (Bass, 1986).

Effects on reproduction and prenatal toxicity

Sixty-six men with disturbances of sexual function who had been exposed to leaded gasoline for four to eight years were investigated at a district sexological clinic in the USSR. Urological, neurological, endocrinological and psychiatric problems were ruled out as causes of the disturbances in these men. Erection disturbances and early ejaculation were the most common symptoms; investigations of ejaculates revealed low sperm-cell counts, with up to 20% immobile spermatozoa in 44 men. The 24-h urinary excretion of 17 α-ketosteroids was decreased in 16 men. After discontinuation of exposure and subsequent therapy, sexual function was restored or significantly improved in all but two of the men within one to two months; however, no improvement was seen in ejaculates. These effects were attributed to exposure to tetraethyllead (Neshkov, 1971).

Reproductive function and gynaecological disorders were studied in 360 women exposed to gasoline and some chlorinated hydrocarbons, in particular 1,2-dichloroethane and dichloromethane, in a plant manufacturing rubber articles for technical purposes. A control group of 616 women who had no contact with chemicals was also studied. The majority (78.9%) of exposed women were aged 20—40 years and 60.8% had been employed for three years or more. A higher percentage of exposed women (16.8% *versus* 8.4% of controls) had toxaemia of pregnancy and short gestation period (11.2% *versus* 4.2%), and perinatal mortality was reported to be increased (Mukhametova & Vozovaya, 1972). [The Working Group noted the complex exposure of the women in the rubber plant and the lack of control for potential confounding factors.]

Genetic and related effects

A group of 16 tank cleaners were studied for cytogenetic changes; a subgroup of four men who had cleaned gasoline tanks over the preceding ten months was also included. Micronuclei in bone-marrow cells and chromosomal aberrations in peripheral blood lymphocytes were reported to be significantly more prevalent in the whole group than in the control group (Högstedt *et al.*, 1981). [The Working Group noted that the results were not reported separately for the different subgroups of cleaners and that the workers would have been subjected to mixed exposures.]

3.3 Epidemiological and case report studies of carcinogenicity to humans

The studies considered in this section generally involved mixed exposures. In particular, exposure was often to both gasoline and diesel fuels, and it is not possible from the data to separate the effects of the two types of fuel. In the selection of papers for consideration, emphasis was placed on those which discussed exposure to the fuels themselves and not on those which concerned their combustion products, which are covered in Volume 46 of the *Monographs* series (IARC, 1989).

(a) Cohort studies

An analysis of the mortality of 23 306 men employed for at least one year between 1950 and 1975 at petroleum distribution centres in the UK was performed by Rushton and Alderson (1983). The dominant job titles were drivers (43%) and operators (20%), according to company records. No detailed exposure data were given. Only 0.2% of the men were not traced in a follow-up of the cohort until 1975. Causes of death (3926) were obtained from central registers; in comparison with male mortality rates for England and Wales, a significant ($p < 0.0001$) deficit in overall mortality (standardized mortality ratio (SMR), 0.85) was observed in the cohort, which was consistent for most malignant and nonmalignant causes of death. Mortality from neoplasms of the lymphatic and haematopoietic tissues was slightly increased overall (77 deaths; SMR, 1.1; $p = 0.3$), reaching significance for myelofibrosis only (SMR, 2.8; $p = 0.04$). Mortality was increased in some subgroups of the population defined primarily by company and job, but no consistent pattern emerged, suggesting that these were chance findings.

In a study of the risks for pancreatic cancer in various occupations, a record linkage was performed between the 1960 Swedish census and the Swedish cancer registry for 1961—79 (Norell *et al.*, 1986). Information on branch of industry was obtained from the census for about two million male employees aged 20—64 years, and the observed number of pancreatic cancer cases in certain occupational groups was compared with corresponding expected numbers based on cumulative incidence in the total cohort. Particular attention was paid to employment in the wood and paper industry, and to occupations involving potential exposure to metals or petroleum products. The observed number of cases was similar to those expected for the occupational groups studied, although a moderate excess in the incidence of pancreatic cancer was noted among gasoline station workers (SMR, 1.6; 90% confidence interval (CI), 1.1—2.3).

[The Working Group noted the lack of detailed exposure data and lack of control of potentially important confounding factors, which render the interpretation of these studies difficult.]

Information on occupation and cause of death from death records of a total of 429 926 men in Washington State, USA, from 1950—79 were used in a proportionate mortality ratio (PMR) analysis standardized for age and year of death (Milham, 1983). Three occupational groups in which exposure to gasoline may occur were studied: service station and garage owners and attendants; fuel oil dealers/workers and motor vehicle mechanics/repairmen. Considering all age groups during the total observation period, increased PMRs ($p < 0.05$) were found for cancer of the oesophagus, bronchus and lung and for non-Hodgkin's lymphomas in motor vehicle mechanics/repairmen. When specific decades were considered, elevated PMRs were also found for lymphatic leukaemia in motor vehicle mechanics/repairmen (1960—69; 8 cases; PMR, 2.8) and bladder cancer in service station and garage owners and attendants (1950—59; 9 cases; PMR, 2.2; and 1960—69; 11 cases; PMR, 1.9).

A PMR analysis was conducted of all white male deaths (37 426) occurring in the state of New Hampshire, USA, between 1975 and 1985 (Schwartz, 1987). Information on occupation, industry and cause of death was abstracted from death certificates, and expected numbers were calculated from the US general population. Total numbers of 453 and 134 deaths were recorded among motor vehicle mechanics and workers in the gasoline service industry, respectively. No significantly elevated PMR was noted for malignant neoplasms among motor vehicle mechanics, although there was a slight increase for leukaemias and aleukaemias (PMR, 1.8). For workers in service stations, the increase in PMR for leukaemia and aleukaemia was significant (PMR, 3.3; $p < 0.05$). Among nine cases of leukaemia observed, five were myeloid, two were lymphoid and two were unspecified.

[The Working Group noted the limitations inherent in PMR analysis. Furthermore, crude exposure information and lack of control for potentially important confounding factors weaken the possibility of causal interpretations.]

(b) Case-control studies

(i) Kidney

In a population-based case-control study, risk factors for renal-cell carcinoma, including occupational exposures, were investigated (McLaughlin *et al.*, 1984). A total of 506 cases diagnosed between 1974 and 1979 were identified from hospitals in the

Minneapolis/St Paul area of Minnesota, USA. An age- and sex-stratified sample of 714 population controls was taken from the same area. In addition, 495 deceased controls were frequency-matched on age at death and year of death to cases who were either deceased (237) or too ill to be interviewed directly (14). Information on smoking, diet and drug use as well as on medical, occupational and residential history was obtained from interviews of study subjects or next of kin. The response rate was 98%. Positive dose-response relationships were noted for smoking and some other exposures. In men, an elevated odds ratio adjusted for age and smoking was associated with occupational exposure to 'petroleum, tar, and pitch products' (1.7; 95% CI, 1.0—2.9). In a subsequent, more detailed analysis of this material (McLaughlin *et al.*, 1985), no clear association with petroleum-related occupations or with employment as a service station attendant was found, although a nonsignificant upward trend in risk with duration of employment was seen in the latter category.

A study was carried out of 92 white men, aged 30—89, with histologically confirmed renal-cell carcinoma and 1588 controls selected from among patients admitted to the same hospital in Buffalo, NY, USA, from 1957 to 1965 (Domiano *et al.*, 1985). Patients with neoplastic disease or with circulatory, respiratory, mental or urogenital disorders were excluded from the control group. Information on smoking habits, diet, occupational history and other variables had been obtained by interview at the time of admission. The age-adjusted odds ratio for the group exposed to gasoline was 0.53, based on four cases. The age-adjusted odds ratio associated with employment in service stations among men with over 20 pack-years of smoking was 1.6 [95% CI, 0.48—5.3].

A case-control study of cancer at many sites was performed in Montréal, Canada, to generate hypotheses on potential occupational carcinogens (Siemiatycki *et al.*, 1987a,b). Each cancer type constituted a case series. About 20 types of cancer were included and, for each cancer site analysed, controls were selected from among cases with cancer at other sites. Job histories and information on possible confounders were obtained by interview from 3726 men aged 35—70 years with cancer diagnosed at one of 19 participating hospitals between 1979 and 1985. The response rate was 82%. Each job was translated into a series of potential exposures by a team of chemists and hygienists using a check-list of 300 of the most common occupational exposures in Montréal. A separate analysis of risks associated with exposure to different petroleum-derived liquids was performed. Cumulative indices of exposure were estimated for a number of occupational exposures. Exposure below the median was considered to be 'nonsubstantial' and that above the median to be 'substantial'. Among men exposed to aviation gasoline, an increased risk was seen for kidney cancer only (adjusted odds ratio, 3.1; 90% CI, 1.5—6.5). Among subjects classified as having substantial exposure, the odds ratio was 3.9 (1.7—8.8) using a logistic regression analysis taking confounding factors detected in a preliminary analysis into consideration. There was overlap between groups exposed to aviation gasoline and groups exposed to jet fuel resulting from combined exposures (see also monograph on jet fuel).

(ii) *Lower urinary tract*

All residents, aged 20—89 years, of an area in eastern Massachusetts, USA, with newly diagnosed, histologically confirmed transitional- or squamous-cell malignancy of the lower urinary tract, including the renal pelvis, ureter, bladder or urethra, were ascertained for an 18-month period (Cole et al., 1972). Occupational risk factors were investigated for 461 of the patients with neoplasms and for 485 population controls living in the same area. Of the cases, 94% had a bladder tumour. Data on smoking and occupational histories were obtained by interview. Among men, an age- and smoking-adjusted odds ratio of 1.0 (95% CI, 0.75–1.3) was associated with employment in occupations with suspected exposure to 'petroleum products'; 81% of controls in this exposure category were 'machinists and mechanics'. Specific data on occupations with exposure to gasoline were not provided.

A Danish case-control study of bladder cancer and occupational risk factors consisted of 212 patients (165 men and 47 women), diagnosed in 1977–79 for men and 1979–80 for women at a hospital department serving a predominantly rural area, and 259 population controls (Mommsen et al., 1982, 1983; Mommsen & Aagaard, 1984). Controls were individually matched to cases (men, 1:1; women, 2:1) for sex, age, geographic area and degree of urbanization. Occupational histories were obtained by hospital interviews for cases and by telephone or by mailed questionnaire for controls. The authors compiled a list of occupations thought to involve exposure to oil or gasoline. An odds ratio of 2.7 (95% CI, 1.2–6.2), restricted to men, associated with 'oil or gasoline' work was estimated by logistic regression analysis, without adjustment for potential confounders. Among the exposed men, there were five mechanics, four 'semiskilled workers', three blacksmiths, two printers, two engineers and four workers in other occupations. [An odds ratio of 1.8 was estimated by the Working Group for work as a blacksmith or mechanic, adjusting for smoking habits, nocturia and previous venereal disease. The Working Group noted that information on exposure was obtained differently for cases and controls.]

In a population-based case-control study investigating risk factors for cancers of the renal pelvis, including occupational exposures, a total of 74 cases diagnosed between 1974 and 1979 were identified from hospitals in the Minneapolis/St Paul area of Minnesota, USA (McLaughlin et al., 1983). An age- and sex-stratified sample of 697 population controls was taken from the same area. Information on smoking, diet, drug use and occupational and residential history was obtained by interview with study subjects or next of kin. An age- and smoking-adjusted odds ratio of 2.4 (95% CI, 0.9–6.1) was associated with occupational exposure to 'petroleum, tar, or pitch products'. No further specification was given about exposures or occupations in this group.

As part of the US National Bladder Cancer Study, a population-based case-control study was carried out on occupation and cancer of the lower urinary tract in men in Detroit, MI, USA (Silverman et al., 1983). The cases were diagnosed in 1977–78, and 95% had urinary bladder specified as the primary site. Controls were selected from the general population of the study area in such a way that the age distribution corresponded to that of the case series. Following exclusion of non-whites, of subjects who had never held jobs during at least six months and of refusals, a total of 303 cases and 296 controls remained for analysis. Information on smoking, diet, occupation, residence and other items was obtained by home interviews. Workers in the gasoline service industry had a crude odds ratio of 1.6 (95% CI, 0.8–3.5); after adjustment for smoking, the odds ratio was 1.3. Mechanics and repairmen had an odds ratio of 1.0 (0.6–1.4).

Another part of the US National Bladder Cancer Study was based in New Jersey in 1978 (Schoenberg et al., 1984). The design was similar to that of the study described above and included 658 male incident cases and 1258 population controls. Home interviews with the study subjects provided information on a variety of personal and environmental risk factors. In a logistic regression analysis with adjustment for age and cigarette smoking, the odds ratio was 2.4 (95% CI, 1.5–3.8) for garage and/or service station workers. For motor vehicle mechanics, the odds ratio was 1.3 (0.87–1.8). There was no clear trend in risk in relation to latency since first exposure or duration among the garage and/or gasoline station workers.

A study based partly in New Jersey also used data from the US National Bladder Cancer Study during 1977–78 (Smith et al., 1985). An analysis of some occupational groups among 2108 male bladder cancer cases and 4046 controls frequency matched on age and sex revealed odds ratios for automobile and truck mechanics of 1.3 (95% CI, 0.77–2.3) and 1.2 (0.90–1.6) for nonsmokers and smokers, respectively. The corresponding odds ratios for 'chemically-related exposures' were 1.5 (1.1–2.1) and 0.99 (0.81–1.2). This occupational group included electrical and petroleum engineers, repairmen, mechanics and drivers, as well as garage and service station attendants.

[The Working Group noted that it was not possible to determine the degree of overlap of the two studies carried out in New Jersey.]

(iii) Other sites

Job titles and information on occupational exposure to motor fuels were recorded for all 50 male patients with acute nonlymphocytic leukaemia seen at a department of the University Hospital of Lund, Sweden, from 1969 to 1977 (Brandt et al., 1978). Three clinical groups served as controls: 100 outpatients treated for nonmalignant disorders, 100 treated for allergic diseases and 31 men treated for other types of leukaemias. Eighteen acute nonlymphocytic leukaemia patients, and ten, ten and three patients in the three control groups, respectively, had been occupationally exposed to petroleum products (e.g., as service station attendants and as bus or truck drivers). [The Working Group estimated an unadjusted odds ratio of 5.1 (95% CI, 2.6–9.8).] The authors suggested that benzene present in gasoline was a possible etiological factor, but detailed exposure data were not given. [The Working Group noted the inadequate description of the methodology used in this study.]

Case-control studies on some rare malignant neoplasms, including testicular cancer and cancer of the pancreas, were conducted in five metropolitan areas in the USA between 1972 and 1975 (Lin & Kessler, 1979, 1981). Eligible patients were identified from hospital records, and an equal number of controls was selected from among contemporary admissions to the participating hospitals for nonmalignant diseases and matched to the cases on age, sex, race and marital status. Occupational histories were obtained by interview. The 205 cases of testicular cancer were reported to be 'significantly more likely to be employed as truck drivers, gasoline station attendants, garage workers, firemen, smelter workers and metal heaters or to hold other jobs involving heat exposure'. No quantitative data were given. There seemed to be a positive association between occupational exposure to dry cleaning or gasoline (e.g., work in service stations and garages) among the 67 male pancreatic cancer cases. For men employed for more than ten years, the odds ratio was 5.1 [95% CI, 1.5–16.9].

A case-control study on occupational risk factors and liver cancer was performed in New Jersey on a total of 355 cases diagnosed from 1975 to 1980, identified from hospital records, the tumour registry and death certificates, and 530 controls selected from hospital records and death certificates and matched to the cases on vital status (Stemhagen et al., 1983). Information on smoking, alcohol consumption and occupation was obtained by home interviews; 96% of the interviews were performed with family members of deceased or incompetent study subjects. Among men, an odds ratio of 2.9 (95% CI, 1.2–6.9) was associated with employment for six months or more at service stations. When the analysis was restricted to hepatocellular carcinomas, the odds ratio increased to 4.2 (1.6–11.4). Other occupations with increased risks for men included farm labourer, wine maker, bartender and employment in laundries and dry-cleaning services.

In the Canadian study described above (p. 185; Siemiatycki et al., 1987b), among men exposed to automotive gasoline, the only significant increase in risk was seen for stomach cancer (odds ratio, 1.5; 90% CI, 1.2–1.9). There was also some evidence of a positive association with duration of exposure. Mechanics and repairmen, who constituted the largest group among those classified as exposed to gasoline, showed an odds ratio of 2.0 (1.1–3.5) in a logistic regression analysis taking into consideration confounding factors detected in a preliminary analysis.

[The Working Group noted that none of the case-control studies provided a detailed description of exposure to gasoline, and it is not clear to what extent exposure to other agents of etiological importance occurred in the occupations of interest. Other types of uncontrolled confounding may also be of relevance.]

(iv) *Childhood cancer*

There have been a number of epidemiological studies on cancer risks in children in relation to the occupations of their parents. Some of the studies have focused on occupations involving exposure to 'hydrocarbons'. As a rule, the classification of exposure to hydrocarbons was based on information on parental occupations; no data were available on exposure to specific compounds. Furthermore, the definitions of occupations involving exposure to hydrocarbons often differed between the studies, which makes it difficult to compare the results. In this section, only studies that provide data on occupations assumed to involve exposure to gasoline, e.g., motor vehicle mechanics and service station attendants, are included.

Fabia and Thuy (1974) conducted a study including children under the age of five years who had died of malignant diseases between 1965 and 1970 in Québec, Canada. The cases were identified from death certificates, hospital insurance data and hospital records. Birth records were found for 386 of the 402 patients ascertained. Two controls per case were selected from birth records matched on date of birth. Information on paternal occupation was obtained from birth certificates. An odds ratio of 2.1 [95% CI, 1.8–2.4] was associated with father's employment as a motor vehicle mechanic or service station attendant. The increased risks for this exposure group were seen for both leukaemias/lymphomas (16 cases) and tumours of the central nervous system (10 cases). [The Working Group could not judge whether the case series was representative of the general population on the basis of the data provided.]

In a similar study, Hakulinen et al. (1976) included all cases of childhood (<15 years old) cancer reported to the Finnish Cancer Registry during 1959–68. Controls were matched for date and district of birth. Information on fathers' occupations was obtained from records at maternity clinics. Following exclusions due to lack of exposure data and of twins, a total of 852 pairs remained for analysis. The odds ratio for cancer based on matched analysis was 1.2 (seven pairs) associated with father's employment as a motor vehicle mechanic. For children under five years of age, the odds ratio was 1.0.

Kantor et al. (1979) studied the occupations of the fathers of children with Wilms' tumour. All 149 patients with this tumour born in Connecticut, USA, and reported to the state tumour registry between 1935 and 1973 were included. An equal number of controls were individually matched for sex, race and year of birth using birth certificate files. Information on paternal occupation was also obtained from this source. An odds ratio of 2.4 (95% CI, 1.1–5.7) was associated with hydrocarbon-related occupations of the fathers. The excess was contributed largely by occupations involving exposure to gasoline and its combustion products, i.e., driver, motor vehicle mechanic and service station attendant.

A total of 692 children who had died from cancer before the age of 15 in Massachusetts, USA, and had been born during the years 1947–57 and 1963–67 were identified by Kwa and Fine (1980). Two controls were chosen for each case from birth registers, and parental occupations were extracted from birth certificates. The fathers of 5.1% of the cases (and 4.4% of the controls) had worked as motor vehicle mechanics or service station attendants. The percentage of exposed fathers for leukaemia/lymphoma cases was 4.9%, that for neurological tumours 4.5%, for urinary tract carcinomas 11.8%, and for other carcinomas 4.2%. 'Housewife' was listed as the occupation of the mother for 98% of both cases and controls.

Occupations of parents and step-parents were investigated for 296 children with cancer seen at the Texas Children's Hospital Research Hematology Clinic, Houston, TX, USA, in 1976 and 1977 (Zack et al., 1980). One control group included parents of 283 children with other diseases treated at the same clinic; a second control group contained 413 uncles and 425 aunts of the children in the case group. Neighbours with children were selected for a third control group (228 fathers and 237 mothers). Information including occupation, education and residence was obtained by interview. The percentage of fathers with hydrocarbon-related occupations was similar in the different groups. Among fathers of cases, uncles of cases, male neighbours and fathers of clinical controls, 1.0, 1.2, 0.4 and 1.8%, respectively, were motor vehicle mechanics or service station attendants. No association was seen with different types of cancer, for pre- or postnatal paternal occupation or for maternal occupation.

Information on the occupations of parents of children with leukaemia and brain tumours diagnosed in the Baltimore Standard Metropolitan Statistical Area from 1969 and 1965, respectively, to 1974 was obtained by interview of the mothers (Gold et al., 1982). Two control groups providing similar information were also included: one group consisted of children with no known malignant disease selected from birth certificates and the other of children with malignancies other than leukaemia or brain tumours. Both control groups were matched to the cases by sex, date of birth and race, giving a total of 43 and 70 triplets of cases and controls for leukaemias and brain tumours, respectively. For occupations related to motor vehicles (driver, motor vehicle mechanic, service station attendant and railroad worker/engineer) of the father before birth of the index child, the matched-pair odds ratio for leukaemia was 0.75 with normal controls; for cancer controls, the odds ratio could not be calculated: there were six pairs in which only the case had been exposed, and none in which only the control had been exposed ($p < 0.05$). Corresponding ratios for brain tumour patients were 0.33 and 0.5, respectively. Similar results were obtained when the occupations of the fathers between birth and diagnosis of the index child were considered. No meaningful analysis could be made of maternal occupations since most mothers had not worked outside the home.

Patients with Wilms' tumour diagnosed between 1950 and 1981 were identified through the Columbus Children's Hospital Tumor Registry in Ohio, USA, by Wilkins and Sinks (1984). Two control groups were selected from the Ohio birth certificate files and matched individually to the cases by sex, race and year of birth. One of the control groups was also matched with respect to mother's county of residence when the child was born. Information on paternal occupations could be obtained from the birth certificates for 62 of 105 matched triplets of cases and controls. An odds ratio of 1.4 (95% CI, 0.59–3.1) was associated with hydrocarbon-related occupations of the fathers, i.e., motor vehicle mechanic, service station attendant, driver/heavy equipment operator or metal worker/machinist. Only two fathers of cases and three of controls had worked as motor vehicle mechanics or service station attendants.

A study on possible etiological factors was performed in the Netherlands using cases identified from a nationwide register of childhood leukaemia between 1973 and 1980 (Van Steensel-Moll *et al.*, 1985). Controls were drawn from population registers and individually matched with cases according to age, sex and place of residence. Data on parental occupations, smoking habits, alcohol consumption and viral infections were obtained by a questionnaire mailed to the parents. The response rates were 88% and 66% for the cases and controls, respectively, giving a total of 519 patients with acute lymphocytic leukaemia and 507 controls for analysis. Seven mothers of cases and three mothers of controls reported having had hydrocarbon-related occupations during pregnancy (printer, dyer, service station attendant, pharmacist or chemical analyst), corresponding to an odds ratio of 2.5 (95% CI, 0.7–9.4). For maternal occupation as a petroleum or chemical industry worker, pharmacist or service station attendant one year before diagnosis of the index children, the odds ratio was 1.0 (three cases; 95% CI, 0.2–4.7). For father's occupation at time of pregnancy as a motor vehicle mechanic, machinist, service station attendant or miner, the odds ratio was 0.8 (18 cases; 0.4–1.5), with a corresponding odds ratio for paternal occupation one year before diagnosis of 0.8 (16 cases; 0.4–1.7). Inclusion of some confounding factors in logistic regression models did not materially change the odds ratios.

Occupations of fathers of children who had died from tumours of the nervous system between 1964 and 1980 in Texas, USA, were studied by Johnson *et al.* (1987). Controls were selected from birth registers and frequency-matched to cases by race, sex and year of birth. Information on paternal occupations was extracted from birth certificates. The final study group consisted of 499 cases with intracranial or spinal cord tumours and 998 controls. There was no consistent increase in risk for hydrocarbon-related occupations as defined in earlier studies. For father's occupation as motor vehicle mechanic or service station attendant, the odds ratio was 0.7 (95% CI, 0.3–1.5).

(c) *Correlation studies*

There was an increase in mortality from kidney cancer among US white men, but not women, between 1950 and 1977 which paralleled the increase in production per head of gasoline that had begun some decades earlier (Enterline & Viren, 1985). There was also an association between annual gasoline consumption per head and renal cancer mortality in both men and women in different countries.

(d) *Case reports*

Two Indian men developed carcinoma of the tongue or of the tongue and palate within a decade of exposure to petrol, diesel and other machine oils in the repair of agricultural pumps. The carcinomas developed at the site of contact with jet flow during sucking. Both patients were teetotalers, but one was a heavy smoker (Sengupta *et al.*, 1984).

4. Summary of Data Reported and Evaluation[1]

4.1 Exposure data

Gasoline is a complex mixture of volatile hydrocarbons, predominantly in the C_4–C_{12} range, with a boiling range of 50–200°C. Most automotive gasoline is produced by blending naphtha process streams, such as light straight-run [3], reformed [15], alkylate [13], isomerization [14] and thermally [28, 29] and catalytically cracked [22, 23] naphthas. Alkylate naphtha [13] is typically the main component used in the production of aviation gasoline. Saleable gasolines may contain numerous additives, such as alkyllead compounds, 1,2-dibromoethane (ethylene dibromide), 1,2-dichloroethane (ethylene dichloride), alkyl phosphates, phenols, alcohols and methyl-*tert*-butyl ether, in order to meet product specifications. Automotive gasoline may contain 0–7%, and typically contains 2–3%, benzene. Occupational exposure to gasoline vapours occurs during production in petroleum refineries and during transport and distribution to retailers. Exposures to vapours are in most cases principally to lighter hydrocarbons, C_6 or lower. Personal 8-h time-weighted average exposures of bulk and drum gasoline loaders and tank cleaners have been reported as 40–850 mg/m³ total hydrocarbons and 1–27 mg/m³ benzene, and for bulk loaders up to 6 mg/m³ 1,3-butadiene. Higher levels of exposure to benzene have been reported for gasoline rail-loading and for some gasoline storage tank cleaning operations. Service station attendants and customers are exposed to lower levels of gasoline vapours.

---

[1]The numbers in square brackets are those assigned to the major process streams of petroleum refining in Table 2 of the monograph on occupational exposures in petroleum refining (p. 44).

4.2 Experimental data

A sample of totally volatilized unleaded gasoline was tested for carcinogenicity in one strain of mice and in one strain of rats by inhalation, producing an increase in the incidence of hepatocellular adenomas and carcinomas in female mice; no such increase was observed in males. Exposure of male rats resulted in an increased incidence of adenomas and carcinomas of the kidney; no such tumour was found in females.

One sample of light straight-run naphtha [3] and one sample of light catalytically cracked naphtha [22] produced skin tumours in mice. (See the monograph on occupational exposures in petroleum refining.)

4.3 Human data

This section describes studies of occupations in which exposure to gasoline may occur, including service station attendants and motor vehicle mechanics. None of the studies provided detailed data concerning exposure to gasoline. Furthermore, it was not possible to distinguish the effects of the combustion products from those of gasoline itself.

In a large UK cohort study on oil distribution workers, some of whom had presumably had occupational exposure to gasoline, a lower total cancer mortality was found than expected on the basis of national rates, but there was a slightly elevated number of deaths from neoplasms of the lymphatic and haematopoietic tissues. A Swedish register-based cohort study on pancreatic cancer showed moderately increased incidence among service station workers.

Two US proportionate mortality studies showed some consistency regarding elevated risks for some types of lymphopoietic cancers in motor vehicle mechanics, although not all findings were significant. For service station workers, the proportionate mortality ratio for leukaemia and aleukaemia was increased in one study but not in another.

In a US case-control study on kidney cancer, there was some evidence of a positive trend in risk with duration of employment as a service station attendant. Another US study showed a nonsignificant deficit in risk for renal-cell carcinoma among people classified as exposed to gasoline, but an increase in risk was suggested among heavy smokers with employment in service stations. A case-control study of cancer at many sites in Canada revealed an elevated risk for kidney cancer in men exposed to aviation gasoline; there were indications of a dose-response relationship.

Several case-control studies have investigated risks for cancer of the lower urinary tract in different occupations with possible exposure to gasoline. An early study from the USA revealed no excess risk among workers in occupations involving exposure to petroleum products. In a Danish study on bladder cancer, an elevated risk was associated with 'oil or gasoline work'. Nonsignificantly increased risks were found in two US studies on bladder cancer among motor vehicle mechanics, while no increase was seen in a third study. There was a significantly elevated risk for bladder cancer among garage workers and service station attendants in one of these studies, and another showed a nonsignificant elevation in risk for workers in the gasoline service industry. A US study on cancer of the renal pelvis suggested an elevated risk for workers exposed to unspecified petroleum, tar or pitch products.

A Swedish study, similar in design to a case-control study, indicated an increased risk for acute nonlymphocytic leukaemia in men with occupational exposure to petroleum products. One hospital-based case-control study in the USA revealed an increased risk for testicular cancer in service station attendants and garage workers; another showed an increased risk for pancreatic cancer in men with occupational exposure to dry cleaning agents or gasoline. Another US case-control study demonstrated an increased risk for liver cancer in service station attendants, particularly for hepatocellular carcinoma. A case-control study of cancer at many sites in Canada revealed an elevated risk only for stomach cancer among men exposed to automotive gasoline.

Nine case-control studies from four countries provide data on paternal occupations involving exposure to hydrocarbons and the risk for cancer in children. There was no consistent association between father's occupation and risk for childhood cancer, although significant results appeared in a few of the studies. Only one study gave detailed data on maternal occupations involving exposure to hydrocarbons during pregnancy; this suggested an increased risk for leukaemia in their children. No study specifically assessed exposure to gasoline, but paternal occupations such as motor vehicle mechanic and service station attendant were not consistently associated with an increase in risk.

4.4 Other relevant data

Urinary thioether excretion was increased in samples taken from service station attendants after work. The half-life of antipyrine was reduced in such workers.

No report specifically designed to study genetic and related effects in humans following exposures to gasoline was available to the Working Group.

Male, but not female, rats developed nephropathy after exposure to unleaded gasoline, with hyaline droplet accumulation, necrosis and degeneration of proximal convoluted tubules. The extent and severity of hyaline droplet accumulation paralleled the extent and localization of renal tubular cell proliferation.

Two samples of unleaded gasoline (one described as PS-6, the other as having a boiling range of 31–192°C) were tested in a series of assays for genetic and related effects. Neither sample induced chromosomal aberrations in the bone marrow of rats treated *in vivo*. The PS-6 sample induced unscheduled DNA synthesis *in vivo* in male and female mouse hepatocytes, but not in male rat hepatocytes or in male or female rat kidney cells, nor did it induce sister chromatid exchange or mutation in cultured human lymphocytes. Neither sample induced mutation in cultured mammalian cells; however, an extract of and the residue from the evaporation of the PS-6 sample did induce mutation in cultured mammalian cells. The PS-6 sample induced unscheduled DNA synthesis *in vitro* in mouse, rat and human hepatocytes but not in rat kidney cells. A leaded gasoline induced somatic mutation in insects. The other sample of unleaded gasoline, an extract of the PS-6 sample and the residue from the evaporation of the PS-6 sample did not induce mutation in bacteria (see Appendix 1).

4.5 Evaluation[1]

There is *inadequate evidence* for the carcinogenicity in humans of gasoline.

There is *limited evidence* for the carcinogenicity in experimental animals of unleaded automotive gasoline.

In making the overall evaluation, the Working Group also took note of the following supporting evidence. Unleaded gasoline induces unscheduled DNA synthesis in hepatocytes from male and female mice treated *in vivo* and in cultured mouse, rat and human hepatocytes. There is *limited evidence* for the carcinogenicity in experimental animals of light straight-run naphtha and of light catalytically-cracked naphtha (see the monograph on occupational exposures in petroleum refining). Benzene is carcinogenic to humans (Group 1); for 1,3-butadiene, there is *inadequate evidence* for carcinogenicity in humans and *sufficient evidence* for carcinogenicity in experimental animals (Group 2B) (IARC, 1987).

Overall evaluation

Gasoline *is possibly carcinogenic to humans (Group 2B)*.

5. References

Aidin, R. (1958) Petrol-vapour poisoning. *Br. med. J.*, *ii*, 369–370

Ainsworth, R.W. (1960) Petrol-vapour poisoning. *Br. med. J.*, *i*, 1547–1548

American Conference of Governmental Industrial Hygienists (1987) *Threshold Limit Values and Biological Exposure Indices for 1987–1988*, Cincinnati, OH, p. 22

American Petroleum Institute (1981) *Standard Definitions for Petroleum Statistics (Technical Report No. 1)*, 3rd ed., Washington DC

American Petroleum Institute (1984) *Evaluation of Four Air Sampling Methods Used for Monitoring Worker Exposure to Gasoline Vapors (API med. Res. Publ. 32-30231)*, Washington DC

Andersson, K., Nilsson, C.-A. & Nygren, O. (1984) A new method for the analysis of tetramethyllead in blood. *Scand. J. Work Environ. Health*, *10*, 51–55

Arbetarskyddsstyrelsen (1981) *Rationale for the Exposure Limit, Benzene* (Swed.), Solna

Banner, W., Jr & Walson, P.D. (1983) Systemic toxicity following gasoline aspiration. *Am. J. Emergency Med.*, *3*, 292–294

Bass, M. (1986) Sniffing gasoline. *J. Am. med. Assoc.*, *255*, 2604–2605

Brandt, L., Nilsson, P.G. & Mitelman, F. (1978) Occupational exposure to petroleum products in men with acute non-lymphocytic leukaemia. *Br. med. J.*, *i*, 553

Busey, W.M. & Cockrell, B.Y. (1984) *Non-neoplastic exposure-related renal lesions in rats following inhalation of unleaded gasoline vapors*. In: Mehlman, M.A., Hemstreet, G.P., III, Thorpe, J.J. & Weaver, N.K., eds, *Advances in Modern Environmental Toxicology*, Vol. VII, *Renal Effects of Petroleum Hydrocarbons*, Princeton, NJ, Princeton Scientific Publishers, pp. 57–64

---

[1]For definition of the italicized terms, see Preamble, pp. 25–28.

Charbonneau, M., Lock, E.A., Strasser, J., Cox, M.G., Turner, M.J. & Bus, J.S. (1987) 2,2,4-Trimethylpentane-induced nephrotoxicity. I. Metabolic disposition of TMP in male and female Fischer 344 rats. *Toxicol. appl. Pharmacol.*, *91*, 171–181

Cole, P., Hoover, R. & Friedell, G.H. (1972) Occupation and cancer of the lower urinary tract. *Cancer*, *29*, 1250–1260

Conaway, C.C., Schreiner, C.A. & Cragg, S.T. (1984) *Mutagenicity evaluation of petroleum hydrocarbons*. In: MacFarland, H.N., Holdsworth, C.E., MacGregor, J.A., Call, R.W. & Lane, M.L., eds, *Advances in Modern Environmental Toxicology*, Vol. VI, *Applied Toxicology of Petroleum Hydrocarbons*, Princeton, NJ, Princeton Scientific Publishers, pp. 89–107

CONCAWE (1985) *Health Aspects of Petroleum Fuels. Potential Hazards and Precautions for Individual Classes of Fuels (Report No. 85/51)*, The Hague

CONCAWE (1986) *Method for Monitoring Exposure to Gasoline Vapour in Air (Report No. 8/86)*, The Hague

CONCAWE (1987) *A Survey of Exposures to Gasoline Vapour (Report No. 4/87)*, The Hague

CONCAWE (1988) *Trends in Motor Vehicle Emission and Fuel Consumption Regulations — 1988 Update (Report No. 4/88)*, The Hague

Coulehan, J.L., Hirsch, W., Brillman, J., Sanandria, J., Welty, T.K., Colaiaco, P., Koros, A. & Lober, A. (1983) Gasoline sniffing and lead toxicity in Navajo adolescents. *Pediatrics*, *71*, 113–117

Council of the European Communities (1987) Council Directive of 21 July 1987 amending Directive 85/210/EEC on the approximation of the laws of the Member States concerning the lead content of petrol. *Off. J. Eur. Communities*, *L225*, 33–34

CRCS (1985) *Information Review — Unleaded Gasoline*, Rockville, MD

Davis, A., Schafer, L.J. & Bell, Z.G. (1960) The effects on human volunteers of exposure to air containing gasoline vapor. *Arch. environ. Health*, *1*, 548–554

Dimock, C.W., Lake, J.L., Norwood, C.B., Bowen, R.D., Hoffman, E.J., Kyle, B. & Quinn, J.G. (1980) Field and laboratory methods for investigating a marine gasoline spill. *Environ. Sci. Technol.*, *14*, 1472–1475

Domiano, S.F., Vena, J.E. & Swanson, M.K. (1985) Gasoline exposure, smoking, and kidney cancer. *J. occup. Med.*, *27*, 398–399

Dooley, J.F., Skinner, M.J., Roy, T.A., Blackburn, G.R., Schreiner, C.A. & MacKerer, C.R. (1988) *Evaluation of the genotoxicity of API reference unleaded gasoline*. In: Cooke, M. & Dennis, A.D., eds, *Proceedings of the 10th Annual Symposium on Polynuclear Aromatic Hydrocarbons: A Decade of Progress*, Columbia, OH, Battelle Press, pp. 179–194

Drinker, P., Yaglou, C.P. & Warren, M.F. (1943) The threshold toxicity of gasoline vapor. *J. ind. Hyg. Toxicol.*, *25*, 225–232

Elster, I., Bencsáth, F.A., Drysch, K. & Häfele, H. (1978) Benzene intoxication in service station attendants (Ger.). *Sicherheitsingenieur*, *78*, 36–39

Enterline, P.E. & Viren, J. (1985) Epidemiologic evidence for an association between gasoline and kidney cancer. *Environ. Health Perspect.*, *62*, 303–312

Fabia, J. & Thuy, T.D. (1974) Occupation of father at time of birth of children dying of malignant diseases. *Br. J. prev. soc. Med.*, *28*, 98–100

Farrow, M.G., McCarroll, N., Cortina, T., Draus, M., Munson, A., Steinberg, M., Kirwin, C. & Thomas, W. (1983) In vitro mutagenicity and genotoxicity of fuels and paraffinic hydrocarbons in the Ames, sister chromatid exchange, and mouse lymphoma assays (Abstract No. 144). *Toxicologist*, *3*, 36

Fishbein, L. & O'Neill, I.K., eds (1988) *Environmental Carcinogens: Methods of Analysis and Exposure Measurement*, Vol. 10, *Benzene and Alkylated Benzenes* (*IARC Scientific Publications No. 85*), Lyon, International Agency for Research on Cancer

Gold, E.B., Diener, M.D. & Szklo, M. (1982) Parental occupations and cancer in children. A case-control study and review of the methodologic issues. *J. occup. Med.*, *24*, 578–584

Gold, L.S. (1980) *Human exposures to ethylene dichloride*. In: Ames, B., Infante, P. & Reitz, R., eds, *Ethylene Dichloride: A Potential Health Risk?* (*Banbury Report 5*), Cold Spring Harbor, NY, CSH Press, p. 216

Guthrie, V.B., ed. (1960) *Petroleum Products Handbook*, New York, McGraw-Hill, pp. 4-2 – 4-4

Hakulinen, T., Salonen, T. & Teppo, L. (1976) Cancer in the offspring of fathers in hydrocarbon-related occupations. *Br. J. prev. soc. Med.*, *30*, 138–140

Halder, C.A., Warne, T.M. & Hatoum, N.S. (1984) *Renal toxicity of gasoline and related petroleum naphthas in male rats*. In: Mehlman, M.A., Hemstreet, G.P., III, Thorpe, J.J. & Weaver, N.K., eds, *Advances in Modern Environmental Toxicology*, Vol. VII, *Renal Effects of Petroleum Hydrocarbons*, Princeton, NJ, Princeton Scientific Publishers, pp. 73–88

Halder, C.A., Holdsworth, C.E., Cockrell, B.Y. & Piccirillo, V.J. (1985) Hydrocarbon nephropathy in male rats: identification of the nephrotoxic components of unleaded gasoline. *Toxicol. ind. Health*, *1*, 67–87

Halder, C.A., Van Gorp, G.S., Hatoum, N.S. & Warne, T.M. (1986) Gasoline vapor exposures. Part I. Characterization of workplace exposures. *Am. ind. Hyg. Assoc. J.*, *47*, 164–172

Harman, A.W., Frewin, D.B. & Priestly, B.G. (1981) Induction of microsomal drug metabolism in man and in the rat by exposure to petroleum. *Br. J. ind. Med.*, *38*, 91–97

Helbling, V. (1950) One case of acute percutaneous and inhalation exposure to gasoline followed by death (Ger.). *Z. Unfallmed. Berufskr.*, *43*, 218–228

Hoag, G.E. & Marley, M.C. (1986) Gasoline residual saturation in unsaturated uniform aquifer materials. *J. Environ. Eng.*, *112*, 586–604

Hoffman, H.L. (1982) *Petroleum (products)*. In: Grayson, M., ed., *Kirk-Othmer Encyclopedia of Chemical Technology*, 3rd ed., Vol. 17, New York, John Wiley & Sons, pp. 257–271

Högstedt, B., Gullberg, B., Mark-Vendel, E., Mitelman, F. & Skerfving, S. (1981) Micronuclei and chromosome aberrations in bone marrow cells and lymphocytes of humans exposed mainly to petroleum vapors. *Hereditas*, *94*, 179–187

Holmberg, B. & Lundberg, P. (1985) Benzene: standards, occurrence, and exposure. *Am. J. ind. Med.*, *7*, 375–383

Huddle, J.G. (1983) *Petroleum Refining and Motor Gasoline Blending*, Washington DC, American Petroleum Institute

IARC (1977) *IARC Monographs on the Evaluation of the Carcinogenic Risk of Chemicals to Man*, Vol. 15, *Some Fumigants, The Herbicides 2,4-D and 2,4,5-T, Chlorinated Dibenzodioxins and Miscellaneous Industrial Chemicals*, Lyon, pp. 195–209

IARC (1979) *IARC Monographs on the Evaluation of the Carcinogenic Risk of Chemicals to Humans*, Vol. 20, *Some Halogenated Hydrocarbons*, Lyon, pp. 429–448

IARC (1980) *IARC Monographs on the Evaluation of the Carcinogenic Risk of Chemicals to Humans*, Vol. 23, *Some Metals and Metallic Compounds*, Lyon, pp. 39-141, 325–415

IARC (1982) *IARC Monographs on the Evaluation of the Carcinogenic Risk of Chemicals to Humans*, Vol. 29, *Some Industrial Chemicals and Dyestuffs*, Lyon, pp. 93–148, 391–398

IARC (1986a) *IARC Monographs on the Evaluation of the Carcinogenic Risk of Chemicals to Humans*, Vol. 39, *Some Chemicals Used in Plastics and Elastomers*, Lyon, pp. 155–179

IARC (1986b) *Information Bulletin on the Survey of Chemicals Being Tested for Carcinogenicity*, No. 12, Lyon, p. 289

IARC (1987a) *IARC Monographs on the Evaluation of Carcinogenic Risks to Humans*, Suppl. 7, *Overall Evaluations of Carcinogenicity: An Updating of* IARC Monographs *Volumes 1 to 42*, Lyon, pp. 230–232

IARC (1987b) *IARC Monographs on the Evaluation of Carcinogenic Risks to Humans*, Suppl. 7, *Overall Evaluations of Carcinogenicity: An Updating of* IARC Monographs *Volumes 1 to 42*, Lyon, pp. 120–122

IARC (1987c) *IARC Monographs on the Evaluation of Carcinogenic Risks to Humans*, Suppl. 7, *Overall Evaluations of Carcinogenicity: An Updating of* IARC Monographs *Volumes 1 to 42*, Lyon, pp. 136–137

IARC (1987d) *IARC Monographs on the Evaluation of Carcinogenic Risks to Humans*, Suppl. 7, *Overall Evaluations of Carcinogenicity: An Updating of* IARC Monographs *Volumes 1 to 42*, Lyon, p. 62

IARC (1987e) *IARC Monographs on the Evaluation of Carcinogenic Risks to Humans*, Suppl. 7, *Overall Evaluations of Carcinogenicity: An Updating of* IARC Monographs *Volumes 1 to 42*, Lyon, pp. 204–205

IARC (1989) *IARC Monographs on the Evaluation of Carcinogenic Risks to Humans*, Vol. 46, *Diesel and Gasoline Engine Exhausts and Some Nitroarenes*, Lyon (in press)

International Energy Agency (1987) *Energy Statistics 1970-1985*, Vols I and II, Paris, Organisation for Economic Cooperation and Development

Irving, W.S., Jr & Grumbles, T.G. (1979) Benzene exposures during gasoline loading at bulk marketing terminals. *Am. ind. Hyg. Assoc. J.*, 40, 468–473

Johnson, C.C., Annegers, J.F., Frankowski, R.F., Spitz, M.R. & Buffler, P.A. (1987) Childhood nervous system tumors — an evaluation of the association with paternal occupational exposure to hydrocarbons. *Am. J. Epidemiol.*, 126, 605–613

Kantor, A.F., McCrea Curnen, M.G., Meigs, J.W. & Flannery, J.T. (1979) Occupations of fathers of patients with Wilms' tumour. *J. Epidemiol. Commun. Health.*, 33, 253–256

Kearney, C.A. & Dunham, D.B. (1986) Gasoline vapor exposures at a high volume service station. *Am. ind. Hyg. Assoc. J.*, 47, 535–539

Kirjakov, K., Kolkovskij, P., Petrov, P., Dojcinov, A., Rajceva, V. & Nikov, G. (1966) Occupational petroleum intoxication among tanker fleet crews. *Bull. Inst. Mar. Med. Gdansk*, 17, 249–254

Kramer, W.H. (1982) Ground-water pollution from gasoline. *Ground Water Monit. Rev.*, 2, 18–22

Kuna, R.A. & Ulrich, C.E. (1984) Subchronic inhalation toxicity of two motor fuels. *J. Am. Coll. Toxicol.*, 3, 217–229

Kwa, S.-L. & Fine, L.J. (1980) The association between parental occupation and childhood malignancy. *J. occup. Med.*, 22, 792–794

Ladefoged, O. & Prior, M.B. (1984) *Nordic Expert Groups for TLVs Documentation. 46. Automotive Gasoline* (Swed.) (*Arbete och Hälsa 1984:7*), Solna, Arbetarskyddsstyrelsen, p. 10

Lane, J.C. (1980) Gasoline and other motor fuels. In: Grayson, M., ed., *Kirk-Othmer Encyclopedia of Chemical Technology*, Vol. 11, 3rd ed., New York, John Wiley & Sons, pp. 652–695

Langdon, W.M. (1986) *Gasoline*. In: *World Book Encyclopedia*, Chicago, A. Scott Fetzer Co., pp. 61–62

Lin, R.S. & Kessler, I.I. (1979) Epidemiologic findings in testicular cancer (Abstract). *Am. J. Epidemiol., 110*, 357

Lin, R.S. & Kessler, I.I. (1981) A multifactorial model for pancreatic cancer in man. Epidemiologic evidence. *J. Am. med. Assoc., 245*, 147–152

Lipovskii, S.M., Tomayeva, L.V., Varfolomeyev, D.I., Fedoseyev, Y.E. & Karganova, E.V. (1979) Deposition of petrol in the tissues and organs of pregnant woman (employed in the chemical industry), their fetuses and in pregnant rats primed with petrol (Russ.). *Gig. Tr. prof. Zabol., 3*, 25–28

Lock, E.A., Charbonneau, M., Strasser, J., Swenberg, J.A. & Bus, J.S. (1987) 2,4,4-Trimethylpentane-induced nephrotoxicity. II. The reversible binding of a TMP metabolite to a renal protein fraction containing alpha$_{2u}$-globulin. *Toxicol. appl. Pharmacol., 91*, 182–192

Loury, D.J., Smith-Oliver, T. & Butterworth, B.E. (1985) Measurements of DNA repair and cell replication in hepatocytes from rats exposed to 2,2,4-trimethylpentane or unleaded gasoline (Abstract). *Environ. Mutagenesis, 7 (Suppl. 3)*, 70

Loury, D.J., Smith-Oliver, T., Strom, S., Jirtle, R., Michalopoulos, G. & Butterworth, B.E. (1986) Assessment of unscheduled and replicative DNA synthesis in hepatocytes treated *in vivo* and *in vitro* with unleaded gasoline or 2,2,4-trimethylpentane. *Toxicol. appl. Pharmacol., 85*, 11–23

Loury, D.J., Smith-Oliver, T. & Butterworth, B.E. (1987) Assessment of unscheduled and replicative DNA synthesis in rat kidney cells exposed *in vitro* or *in vivo* to unleaded gasoline. *Toxicol. appl. Pharmacol., 87*, 127–140

Lykke, A.W.J. & Stewart, B.W. (1978) Fibrosing alveolitis (pulmonary interstitial fibrosis) evoked by experimental inhalation of gasoline vapours. *Experientia, 34*, 498

Lykke, A.W.J., Stewart, B.W., O'Connell, P.J. & Le Mesurier, S.M. (1979) Pulmonary responses to atmospheric pollutants. I. An ultrastructural study of fibrosing alveolitis evoked by petrol vapour. *Pathology, 11*, 71–80

MacFarland, H.N. (1982) *Chronic gasoline toxicity*. In: MacFarland, H.N., Holdsworth, C.E., MacGregor, J.A., Call, R.W. & Kane, M.L., eds, *Proceedings of a Symposium, The Toxicology of Petroleum Hydrocarbons*, Washington DC, American Petroleum Institute, pp. 78–86

MacFarland, H.N., Ulrich, C.E., Holdsworth, C.E., Kitchen, D.N., Halliwell, W.H. & Blum, S.C. (1984) A chronic inhalation study of unleaded gasoline vapor. *J. Am. Coll. Toxicol., 3*, 231–248

Machle, W. (1941) Gasoline intoxication. *J. Am. med. Assoc., 117*, 1965–1971

McDermott, H.J. & Killiany, S.E., Jr (1978) Quest for a gasoline TLV. *Am. ind. Hyg. Assoc. J., 39*, 110–117

McDermott, H.J. & Vos, G.A. (1979) Service station attendants' exposure to benzene and gasoline vapors. *Am. ind. Hyg. Assoc. J., 40*, 315–321

McKee, J.E., Laverty, F.B. & Hertel, R.M. (1972) Gasoline in groundwater. *J. Water Pollut. Control Fed., 44*, 293–302

McLaren, P. (1985) Behaviour of diesel fuel on a high energy beach. *Mar. Pollut. Bull., 16*, 191–196

McLaughlin, J.K., Blot, W.J., Mandel, J.S., Schuman, L.M., Mehl, E.S. & Fraumeni, J.F., Jr (1983) Etiology of cancer of the renal pelvis. *J. natl Cancer Inst.*, *71*, 287–291

McLaughlin, J.K., Mandel, J.S., Blot, W.J., Schuman, L.M., Mehl, E.S. & Fraumeni, J.F., Jr (1984) A population-based case-control study of renal cell carcinoma. *J. natl Cancer Inst.*, *72*, 275–284

McLaughlin, J.K., Blot, W.J., Mehl, E.S., Stewart, P.A., Venable, F.S. & Fraumeni, J.F., Jr (1985) Petroleum-related employment and renal cell cancer. *J. occup. Med.*, *27*, 672–674

Milham, S. (1983) *Occupational Mortality in Washington State 1950-1979 (DHSS (NIOSH) Publication No. 83-116)*, Cincinnati, OH, National Institute for Occupational Safety and Health

Mommsen, S. & Aagaard, J. (1984) Occupational exposure as risk indicator of male bladder carcinoma in a predominantly rural area. *Acta radiol. oncol.*, *23*, 147–152

Mommsen, S., Aagaard, J. & Sell, A. (1982) An epidemiological case-control study of bladder cancer in males from a predominantly rural district. *Eur. J. Cancer clin. Oncol.*, *18*, 1205–1210

Mommsen, S., Aagaard, J. & Sell, A. (1983) An epidemiological study of bladder cancer in a predominantly rural district. *Scand. J. Urol. Nephrol.*, *17*, 307–312

Mukkametova, G.M. & Vozovaya, M.A. (1972) Reproductive power and incidence of gynecological affections among female workers exposed to a combined effect of gasoline and chlorinated hydrocarbons (Russ.). *Gig. Tr. prof. Zabol.*, *16*, 6–9

Neshkov, N.S. (1971) The effect of chronic poisoning with ethylated gasoline on spermatogenesis and sexual function in males (Russ.). *Gig. Tr. prof. Zabol.*, *15*, 45–46

Norell, S., Ahlbom, A., Olin, R., Erwald, R., Jacobson, G., Lindberg-Navier, I. & Wiechel, K.-L. (1986) Occupational factors and pancreatic cancer. *Br. J. ind. Med.*, *43*, 775–778

Nylander, P.-O., Olofsson, H., Rasmuson, B. & Svahlin, H. (1978) Mutagenic effects of petrol in *Drosophila melanogaster*. I. Effects of benzene and 1,2-dichloroethane. *Mutat. Res.*, *57*, 163–167

Olson, M.J., Garg, B.D., Murty, C.V.R. & Roy, A.K. (1987) Accumulation of $alpha_{2u}$-globulin in the renal proximal tubules of male rats exposed to unleaded gasoline. *Toxicol. appl. Pharmacol.*, *90*, 43–51

Pandya, K.P., Rao, G.S., Dhasmana, A. & Zaidi, S.H. (1975) Occupational exposure of petrol pump workers. *Ann. occup. Hyg.*, *18*, 363–364

Parkinson, G.S. (1971) Benzene in motor gasoline — an investigation into possible health hazards in and around filling stations and in normal transport operations. *Ann. occup. Hyg.*, *14*, 145–153

Phillips, C.F. & Jones, R.K. (1978) Gasoline vapor exposure during bulk handling operations. *Am. ind. Hyg. Assoc. J.*, *39*, 118–128

Purdy, G.A. (1958) *Petroleum. Prehistoric to Petrochemicals*, New York, McGraw-Hill, pp. 152–164

Rao, G.S. & Pandya, K.P. (1978) Toxicity of petroleum products: effects on alkaline phosphatase and lipid peroxidation. *Environ. Res.*, *16*, 174–178

Rao, G.S. & Pandya, K.P. (1980) Hepatic metabolism of heme in rats after exposure to benzene, gasoline and kerosene. *Arch. Toxicol.*, *46*, 313–317

Rappaport, S.M., Selvin, S. & Waters, M.A. (1987) Exposures to hydrocarbon components of gasoline in the petroleum industry. *Appl. ind. Hyg.*, *2*, 148–154

Richardson, K.A., Wilmer, J.L., Smith-Simpson, D. & Skopek, T.R. (1986) Assessment of the genotoxic potential of unleaded gasoline and 2,2,4-trimethylpentane in human lymphoblasts *in vitro*. *Toxicol. appl. Pharmacol.*, *82*, 316–322

Royal Dutch/Shell Group of Companies (1983) *The Petroleum Handbook*, 6th ed., Amsterdam, Elsevier, p. 399

Runion, H.E. & Scott, L.M. (1985) Benzene exposure in the United States 1978–1983: an overview. *Am. J. ind. Med.*, *7*, 385–393

Rushton, L. & Alderson, M.R. (1983) Epidemiological survey of oil distribution centres in Britain. *Br. J. ind. Med.*, *40*, 330–339

Saito, K. (1973) Electroencephalographic studies on petrol intoxication: comparison between nonleaded and leaded white petrol. *Br. J. ind. Med.*, *30*, 352–358

Schoenberg, J.B., Stemhagen, A., Mogielnicki, A.P., Altman, R., Abe, T. & Mason, T.J. (1984) Case-control study of bladder cancer in New Jersey. I. Occupational exposures in white males. *J. natl Cancer Inst.*, *72*, 973–981

Schreiner, C.A. (1984) *Petroleum and petroleum products: a brief review of studies to evaluate reproductive effects*. In: Christian, M.S., Galbraith, W.M., Voytek, P. & Mehlman, M.A., eds, *Advances in Modern Environmental Toxicology*, Vol. III, *Assessment of Reproductive and Teratogenic Hazards*, Princeton, NJ, Princeton Scientific Publishers, pp. 29–45

Schwartz, E. (1987) Proportionate mortality ratio analysis of automobile mechanics and gasoline service station workers in New Hampshire. *Am. J. ind. Med.*, *12*, 91–99

Sengupta, P., Ray, D.N. & Poddar, S.P. (1984) Cancer of the tongue and palate following occupational exposure to petroleum products. *J. Indian med. Assoc.*, *82*, 59–61

Seshia, S.S., Rajani, K.R., Boeckx, R.L. & Chow, P.N. (1978) The neurological manifestations of chronic inhalation of leaded gasoline. *Dev. Med. Child Neurol.*, *20*, 323–334

Sherwood, R.J. (1972) Evaluation of exposure to benzene vapour during the loading of petrol. *Br. J. ind. Med.*, *29*, 65–69

Short, B.G., Burnett, V.L. & Swenberg, J.A. (1986) Histopathology and cell proliferation induced by 2,2,4-trimethylpentane in the male rat kidney. *Toxicol. Pathol.*, *14*, 194–203

Short, B.G., Burnett, V.L., Cox, M.G., Bus, J.S. & Swenberg, J.A. (1987) Site-specific renal cytotoxicity and cell proliferation in male rats exposed to petroleum hydrocarbons. *Lab. Invest.*, *57*, 564–577

Siemiatycki, J., Wacholder, S., Richardson, L., Dewar, R. & Gérin, M. (1987a) Discovering carcinogens in the occupational environment. Methods of data collection and analysis of a large case-referent monitoring system. *Scand. J. Work Environ. Health*, *13*, 486–492

Siemiatycki, J., Dewar, R., Nadon, L., Gérin, M., Richardson, L. & Wacholder, S. (1987b) Associations between several sites of cancer and twelve petroleum-derived liquids. Results from a case-referent study in Montreal. *Scand. J. Work Environ. Health*, *13*, 493–504

Silverman, D.T., Hoover, R.N., Albert, S. & Graff, K.M. (1983) Occupation and cancer of the lower urinary tract in Detroit. *J. natl Cancer Inst.*, *70*, 237–245

Smith, E.M., Miller, E.R., Woolson, R.F. & Brown, C.K. (1985) Bladder cancer risk among auto and truck mechanics and chemically related occupations. *Am. J. publ. Health*, *75*, 881–883

Stemhagen, A., Slade, J., Altman, R. & Bill, J. (1983) Occupational risk factors and liver cancer. A retrospective case-control study of primary liver cancer in New Jersey. *Am. J. Epidemiol.*, *117*, 443–454

Sterner, J.H. (1941) Study of hazards in spray painting with gasoline as diluent. *J. ind. Hyg. Toxicol.*, *23*, 437–448

Stewart, B.W., Le Mesurier, S.M. & Lykke, A.W.J. (1979) Correlation of biochemical and morphological changes induced by chemical injury to the lung. *Chem.-biol. Interactions*, *26*, 321–338

Stock, J.K. & Priestly, B.G. (1986) Urinary thioether output as an index of occupational chemical exposure in petroleum retailers. *Br. J. ind. Med.*, *43*, 718–720

Van Steensel-Moll, H.A., Valkenburg, H.A. & Van Zanen, G.E. (1985) Childhood leukemia and parental occupation. A register-based case-control study. *Am. J. Epidemiol.*, *121*, 216–224

Verwilghen, R.L., Van Dorpe, A. & Veulemans, H. (1975) Dangers of petrol used as a solvent. *Lancet*, *ii*, 1156

Ward, C.C. (1984) *Gasoline*. In: Holland, D., ed., *Encyclopedia Americana*, Danbury, CT, Grolier, Inc., pp. 337–338

Wilkins, J.R., III & Sinks, T.H., Jr (1984) Paternal occupation and Wilms' tumour in offspring. *J. Epidemiol. Commun. Health*, *38*, 7–11

Zack, M., Cannon, S., Loyd, D., Heath, C.W., Jr, Falletta, J.M., Jones, B., Housworth, J. & Crowley, S. (1980) Cancer in children of parents exposed to hydrocarbon-related industries and occupations. *Am. J. Epidemiol.*, *111*, 329–336

JET FUEL

1. Chemical and Physical Data

1.1 Synonyms and trade names

Chem. Abstr. Services Reg. No.: not assigned (kerosene, 8008-20-6)
Chem. Abstr. Name: not assigned
Synonyms: Aviation kerosene; AVCAT (JP-5); AVTAG (JP-4); AVTUR (JP-8); Jet A; Jet A-1; Jet B; jet kerosine; JP-7; kerosine; turbo fuel A; turbo fuel A-1; wide-cut jet fuel

1.2 Description

Many commercial jet fuels have basically the same composition as kerosene, but they are made under more stringent specifications than those for kerosene. Other commercial and military jet fuels are referred to as wide-cut fuels and are usually made by blending kerosene fractions with lower boiling streams to include more volatile hydrocarbons. Because the chemical composition of kerosene and most jet fuels is approximately similar, except for the additives, kerosene used for aviation purposes is described in this monograph. The other uses of kerosene, e.g., as a fuel oil or lamp oil, are described in the monograph on fuel oils (Fuel Oil No. 1).

Readily available commercial illuminating kerosene was the fuel chosen for early jet engines, largely because its use would not interfere with needs for gasoline, which was in short supply during wartime. The development of commercial jet aircraft following the Second World War centred primarily on the use of kerosene-type fuels. High-altitude flying requires fuel with a very low freezing-point; also, the fuel must be extremely clean (free of foreign matter), have a very low moisture content, burn cleanly (essentially free of smoke) and not cause corrosion of engine parts in prolonged service. Different types of engines used for different types of service require fuels with specific chemical and physical properties, and individual specifications have evolved to meet these needs. As international jet service increased, fuels with similar characteristics had to be available worldwide. Thus, steps were taken to meet these needs, although some variation in specifications still exists among different countries. Specifications of several common jet fuels are given in Table 1 (Dukek, 1978).

Table 1. Selected specification properties of aviation gas turbine fuels[a]

Characteristic	Civil ASTM D 1655		Military[b]				
	Jet A kerosene	Jet B wide-cut	Mil-T-5624-K		Mil-T-38219	Mil-T-83133	
			JP-4 wide-cut USAF	JP-5 kerosene USN	JP-7[c] kerosene USAF	JP-8 kerosene USAF	
Composition							
aromatics, vol. % max	20[d]	20[d]	25	25	5	25	
sulfur, wt % max	0.3	0.3	0.4	0.4	0.1	0.4	
Volatility							
distillation temperature max °C 10% received	204		190	205	196	205	
distillation temperature max °C 50% received		188					
endpoint	300		270	290	288	300	
flash-point, °C min	38			60	60	38	
vapour pressure at 38°C kPa max (psi)		21 (3)	14–21 (2–3)				
density at 15°C, kg/m³	775–840	751–802	751–802	788–845	779–806	775–840	
Fluidity							
freezing-point, °C max	–40[e]	–50	–58	–46	–43	–50	
viscosity at –20°C, mm³/s max (= cSt)	8.0			8.5	8.0	8.0	
Combustion							
heat content, MJ/kg, min	42.8	42.8	42.8	42.6	43.5	42.8	
smoke point, mm, min	20[f]	20[f]	20	19	35[c]	20	
H₂ content, wt % min			13.6	13.5	14.2[c]	13.6	
Stability							
test temperature[g], °C min	245	245	260	260	350[b]	260	

[a]From Dukek (1978); full specification requires other tests.
[b]USAF, US Air Force; USN, US Navy
[c]Estimated properties for advanced supersonic fuel
[d]Fuel up to 25 vol % aromatics may be supplied on notification (22 vol % for Jet A-1, Jet B).
[e]International airlines use Jet A-1 with –50°C freeze-point.
[f]Fuel with 18 smoke point may be supplied on notification (19 for Jet A-1, Jet B).
[g]Thermal stability test by D3241 to meet 3.3 kPa (25 mm Hg) pressure drop and Code 3 deposit rating

The early development of jet fuels differed in Europe and the USA. The wide-range distillate-type turbine fuel originated in the USA and evolved to the current jet propulsion, JP-4 military fuel; readily available gasoline fractions were used to supplement the basic kerosene type of fuel. In Europe, however, where gasoline was less readily available, kerosene was used to help conserve gasoline, particularly for the gasoline-fuelled aircraft used in the Second World War. In the postwar years, and particularly in the interests of standardization under the North Atlantic Treaty Organization (NATO), the British AVTAG wide-cut fuel has been brought closely in line with JP-4 (Boldt & Hall, 1977). A recent development with NATO forces in Europe has been the decision to convert military aircraft fuel completely from JP-4 to JP-8 kerosene fuel. The conversion is scheduled to be completed by 1990.

Naval aircraft have somewhat different requirements from those for land-based planes. Less volatile, higher flash-point fuels are needed to minimize vapour exposure of personnel and to reduce fire risk, particularly in enclosed areas below decks. This led to the development of JP-5, a 60°C minimum flash-point kerosene-type fuel for use in shipboard service. Supersonic aircraft also have certain special fuel needs, including low volatility and greater thermal stability than conventional kerosene. JP-7 has been developed to meet these needs. Smaller volumes of these special low-volatility fuels are produced than of the more conventional kerosene-type fuels.

1.3 Chemical composition and physical properties of technical products

The basic component of kerosene used for aviation is the straight-run kerosene stream [5] (refer to Table 2 and Figure 1 of the monograph on occupational exposures in petroleum refining) which consists of hydrocarbons with carbon numbers predominantly in the range of C_9-C_{16} (C_4-C_{16} for wide-cut fuels) and which boil in the range of approximately 150–290°C (CONCAWE, 1985). In the early 1980s, the final boiling-point specification was raised to 300°C maximum in order to allow increased availability of kerosene for jet fuel use (American Society for Testing and Materials (ASTM) D 3699).

Kerosene and jet fuels may actually be blends of heavy straight-run naphtha [4], derived from atmospheric distillation as a more volatile fraction than straight-run kerosene, plus one or more kerosene fractions, such as chemically neutralized kerosene [5C], hydrodesulfurized kerosene [5B] or hydrotreated kerosene [5A]. Some kerosene is made by including hydrocracked fractions which have a very low sulfur content and are otherwise suitable to be made a part of the kerosene product. Such blending permits the refiner increased flexibility in tailoring products to meet a variety of requirements. A net result of the special requirements of jet fuel is that nearly all of it is derived from treated stocks.

The chemical composition of kerosene depends upon the source of crude oil or blend streams from which it is derived. It consists of a complex combination of hydrocarbons, including alkanes (paraffins) and cycloalkanes (naphthenes), aromatics and small amounts of olefins (CONCAWE, 1985).

Alkanes and cycloalkanes are saturated with respect to hydrogen and are chemically stable, clean-burning components, which, together, constitute the major part of kerosene.

Aromatics are also present and represent usually anywhere from about 10% to 20% of the product, depending on the source of crude oil (Dickson & Woodward, 1987). While aromatics are a good source of energy, they tend to smoke when burned and also contribute to the odour of the product. Kerosene in the C_9-C_{16} range normally has a boiling range well above the boiling-point of benzene; accordingly, the benzene (see IARC, 1982, 1987) content of such kerosenes is normally below 0.02%. However, wide-cut products (45–280°C), such as those used for JP-4 and Jet B, are usually made by blending and may contain more benzene, normally <0.5% (CONCAWE, 1985). Dinuclear aromatic naphthalenes, with two benzene rings in a condensed structure, are also likely to be present in kerosene, at concentrations ranging from 0.1% to 3%, depending on the source of crude oil (Dickson & Woodward, 1987); however, the maximum final boiling range of approximately 300°C tends to exclude the presence of high-boiling polycyclic aromatic hydrocarbons such as the three- to seven-ring condensed aromatic structures (Dukek, 1978)

Olefins are normally present in straight-run kerosene at concentrations of about 1% or less (CONCAWE, 1985). Olefins are essentially eliminated by the hydrotreating processes used in finishing kerosene.

In the USA, the National Institute for Petroleum and Energy Research conducts annual surveys for the American Petroleum Institute and the US Department of Energy on various products, including aviation turbine fuels. The reports provide limited data on composition but include mercaptans, total sulfur, aromatic content and olefin content for JP-4 (wide-cut product) and JP-5 (60°C minimum flash-point) military jet fuels. In addition, the report for Jet A commercial jet fuel includes naphthalene content. These data, together with additional data gathered in the survey for 1986 are given in Table 2 (Dickson & Woodward, 1987). The composition data for commercial Jet A can be considered generally representative of kerosene in the USA, and the data in Table 2 for commercial Jet A-1 are typical of the European product.

ASTM standard D 1655 lists a number of additives that may be used with jet fuels, as agreed by the supplier and purchaser (ASTM D 1655). The International Air Transport Association recommendations require the addition of antioxidant immediately after processing for fuel which has been finished by hydrotreating.

Jet fuels are often transported through pipelines to terminals from which further distribution is made. Because of the risk of loss of some of the additives to pipeline surfaces in entrained water in these systems, some or most of the additives are added at terminals or final distribution centres to ensure correct concentrations in the product delivered to aircraft. The antioxidants approved under ASTM D 1655 for addition to jet fuels at concentrations not exceeding 24.0 mg/l are, e.g., 75% min 2,6-di-*tert*-butylphenol plus 25% max *tert*- and tri-*tert*-butylphenols; 72% min 2,4-dimethyl-6-*tert*-butylphenol plus 28% max monomethyl- and dimethyl-*tert*-butylphenols; and 55% min 2,4-dimethyl-6-*tert*-butylphenol plus 45% max mixed *tert*- and di-*tert*-butylphenols. Metal deactivators — such as *N,N*-disalicylidene-1,2-propanediamine, which is approved under ASTM D 1655 — may be added at concentrations not exceeding 5.7 mg/l. Electrical conductivity additives permitted as antistatic additives are ASA-3 (a Shell product) at concentrations up to 1 mg/l and 'Stadis' 450 (a DuPont product) at concentrations up to 3 mg/l (American Society for

Table 2. Physical properties and composition of various samples of jet fuels

Property and composition	USA[a]			Europe[b]
	Military aviation turbine fuel JP-4 (wide-cut)[c]	Military aviation turbine fuel JP-5	Commercial Jet fuel A	Commercial Jet fuel A-1
Gravity, °API	54.8	41.0	42.3	45.2
Distillation temperature				
10% evaporated, °C	92	198	188	169
50% evaporated, °C	138	215	213	194
90% evaporated, °C	198	242	246	236
Reid vapour pressure, psi [atm]	2.6 [0.18]	–	–	–
Freezing-point, °C	−61	−49	−45	−52
Viscosity, kinematic, −20°C, cSt	–	–	5.48	3.85
Aniline point, °C	53	59	60	–
Aniline-gravity product, no.	7007	5646	5976	6141
Water tolerance, ml	0.6	–	0.7	–
Sulfur: total wt %	0.018	0.020	0.035	0.054
mercaptan, wt %	0.000	–	0.001	0.001
Naphthalenes, wt %	–	–	1.59	1.74
Aromatic content, vol. %	13.4	19.1	18.5	18.5
Olefin content, vol. %	0.7	0.8	1.0	0.5
Smoke point, mm	25.6	21.2	22.6	24.2
Gum, mg/100 ml at 232°C	0.8	1.0	1.0	1.0
Heat of combustion, net, kJ/kg	43 024	42 564	42 709	42 757
Thermal stability:				
pressure drop, in mm Hg	0.2	0.0	0.2	–
Water separometer index no.	90	95	97	94

[a]From Dickson & Woodward (1987), based on analysis of samples collected in 1986
[b]Data provided by CONCAWE
[c]Similar to Jet B, with special additives

Testing and Materials, 1986). A fuel system icing inhibitor may also be added; ethylene glycol monomethyl ether, which conforms to ASTM specification D 4171 may be used in concentrations of 0.1–0.15 vol %.

In addition to those approved under ASTM D 1655, other special-purpose additives may be used, such as corrosion inhibitors (American Society for Testing and Materials, 1986), lubrication improvers, biocides (Dukek, 1978) and thermal stability improvers. The use and concentrations of such additives are agreed upon by the supplier and purchaser.

2. Production, Use, Occurrence and Analysis

2.1 Production and use

(a) Production

Kerosene is derived from crude oil, normally as the third product stream category from an atmospheric distillation tower, following removal of gases, light ends and naphtha streams (see Figure 1, monograph on occupational exposures in petroleum refining). Any need for further processing at this point depends on the type of crude oil from which the kerosene stream is derived. The principal impurities are generally nitrogen and sulfur compounds, which affect odour and overall product quality. The olefin and aromatic content is also an important consideration for some applications, particularly where the end use is as jet fuel. Kerosene derived from sweet crude oils (very low nitrogen and sulfur content) may be used without further treatment for noncritical applications; however, because the major use of kerosene is as jet fuel, most refiners sweeten the stream chemically, such as by caustic washing or other caustic or chemical treatments. Kerosene from sour crude oils, i.e., with higher sulfur content, is often hydrotreated, which markedly lowers the nitrogen and sulfur contents and saturates any olefins that may be present (Dukek, 1978).

When kerosene is finished by a hydrotreating process, it normally contains an oxidation inhibitor; use of further additives is usually agreed between the refiner and purchaser. Some years ago, addition of small amounts of blue dyes was sometimes used to enhance or 'brighten' the appearance of the product, but this practice is seldom used today, if at all. Additives may be required more extensively in jet fuels, in both kerosene types and wide-cut types.

The demand for kerosene, which had earlier been a major petroleum product, has gradually declined with time, whereas that for jet fuels has steadily increased. As a result of trends in demand, many refiners have found it more economical in recent years to produce Jet A-1 as the basic product and simply divert a portion of the product for marketing as kerosene.

Data on production and consumption of jet fuels, including both the kerosene-type and wide-cut fuels, for the USA and for the 24 countries included in the Organisation for Economic Cooperation and Development (OECD) combined for the period 1970–85 are presented in Table 3 (International Energy Agency, 1987), from which the appreciable increase in volumes of jet fuels are evident. Data on production and consumption of jet fuel for 1985 are given by geographical area or organization in Table 4.

(b) Use

A British patent application filed in 1930 for a turbojet engine resulted in an acceptable working model by 1937 (Dukek, 1978); however, Germans working from the British concept are credited with the first successful test flight of a jet plane that same year. Jet-powered aircraft came into only limited use during the Second World War; however, both military

Table 3. Production and consumption (in thousands of tonnes) of jet fuel in the USA and countries of the Organisation for Economic Cooperation and Development (OECD), 1970–85[a]

Area	Production/consumption	1970	1975	1980	1985
OECD	Production	57 659	68 002	81 217	90 280
	Consumption	61 810	70 557	79 748	88 880
USA	Production	37 636	41 690	48 580	56 939
	Consumption	43 950	46 497	51 020	58 179

[a]From International Energy Agency (1987)

Table 4. Production and consumption (in thousands of tonnes) of jet fuel by geographical area, 1985[a]

Region/organization	Production	Consumption
North America	60 460	61 616
USA	56 939	58 179
Canada	3 521	3 437
OECD[b] (Europe)	24 376	22 787
European Economic Community	22 438	20 199
Pacific[c]	5 444	4 447
OECD (All)	90 280	88 880

[a]From International Energy Agency (1987)
[b]Organisation for Economic Cooperation and Development
[c]Australia, Japan, New Zealand

and commercial development accelerated in the ensuing years to the point that jet engines began to dominate power sources for aircraft in the 1960s. In turbojet aircraft, the exhaust gases drive the compressor and create the thrust to power the aircraft. In turboprop aircraft, turbine power is used to drive a propeller.

Jet fuels A, A-1 and B (wide-cut) are generally used in civil aviation and jet fuels JP-4–JP-8 in military aviation.

(c) *Regulatory status and guidelines*

In Sweden, the occupational exposure limit (1984) for jet fuel has been set at 380 mg/m³ (8-h time-weighted average (TWA)) and 500 mg/m³ (15-min short-term exposure limit (STEL)) (Holm *et al.*, 1987). In the USA, a recommendation has been issued on an 8-h TWA limit of 100 mg/m³ for kerosene (National Institute for Occupational Safety and Health, 1977). Recommended values of 700 mg/m³ (8-h TWA) and 1050 mg/m³ (15-min STEL) for wide-cut jet fuels, evaluated as total hydrocarbon and expressed as *n*-hexane, have been developed by the US Air Force (Bishop *et al.*, 1983).

2.2 Occurrence

(a) Occupational exposure

Potential exposure to jet fuel in the work environment has been reported in association with the following operations: manually handled filling and discharge, including fuel filling of airplanes (CONCAWE, 1985; Døssing *et al.*, 1985; Holm *et al.*, 1987); tank dipping, pipeline pump repairs and filter cleaning in refineries, distribution terminals and depots (CONCAWE, 1985); maintenance, inspection and cleaning of jet fuel storage tanks, servicing of pump units (Fardell & Houghton, 1975/76; CONCAWE, 1985; Holm *et al.*, 1987); production and installation of aircraft fuel systems (Knave *et al.*, 1976); component testing and engine testing in a jet motor factory (Knave *et al.*, 1978); maintenance and service of aircraft fuel tanks, fuel systems and engines (Thomas & Richardson, 1981; CONCAWE, 1985; Holm *et al.*, 1987); routine sampling and laboratory analysis of jet fuel (CONCAWE, 1985); and use of high-pressure kerosene sprays for washing engines and other parts during maintenance or repairs (CONCAWE, 1985).

Available quantitative exposure data are summarized in Table 5. Those data refer mostly to exposure to wide-cut aviation turbine fuel, which, by its more volatile nature, is more likely to give rise to high vapour concentrations than regular kerosene jet fuel types. Inspection and maintenance of aircraft wing fuel tanks may, as a result of the confined working space, present opportunities for much higher exposures to jet fuel than most of the other operations listed above. Wide-cut jet fuel vapours may contain small concentrations of benzene and *n*-hexane (CONCAWE, 1985). Maximal overall 8-h TWA values of 16 and 4 mg/m³ for *n*-hexane and benzene, respectively, have been measured for aircraft unit personnel in Sweden (Holm *et al.*, 1987), with maximal 15-min STEL values at about 157 and 39 mg/m³ for these same two compounds.

(b) Environmental occurrence

An accidental spill of more than 14 tonnes of JP-5 jet fuel mixed with No. 2 fuel oil from a storage facility in Searsport, ME, USA, in March–June 1971 was reported (Dow *et al.*, 1975). In October 1975, 83 000 gallons [314 000 l] of JP-4 jet fuel were spilled in Charleston, SC, USA (Talts *et al.*, 1977). It is also noted that it is common practice for aircraft to jettison excess fuel in the air under some conditions.

2.3 Analysis

Since jet fuel or kerosene is composed of a complex mixture of hydrocarbons, there are few methods for the environmental analysis of 'jet fuel' or 'kerosene' as an entity, but many

Table 5. Concentrations of jet fuel vapours in various operations and occupations (personal samples)

Operation or occupation	Type of fuel	Duration of sampling (no. of samples)	Mean/median concentration (mg/m³)	Reference
Fuel filling attendants	Unspecified (military)	Several hours (69)	31 (median) 1–1020 (range)	Døssing et al. (1985)
Fuel systems component testing (jet motor factory)	Wide-cut	19–97 min (9)	423 mg/m³ (average of means)[a] 85–925 (range of means)	Knave et al. (1978)
Engine testing (jet motor factory)	Wide-cut	30–54 min (3)	128 mg/m³ (average of means)[a] 110–147 (range of means)	Knave et al. (1978)
Mechanics (jet motor factory)	Wide-cut	10–55 min (4)	149–974 (range of means)[a]	Knave et al., 1978
Inspection and repair of aircraft fuel tanks	Wide-cut (JP-4)	0.5–4 h (21)	<0.3–3014 (range)[b]	Thomas & Richardson (1981)
Jet fuel handling	Wide-cut (MC-77) military	8 h (12) 15 min (6)	0.9 GM[c] 2.7 GSD[d] 6.0 GM 6.9 GSD	Holm et al. (1987)
Flight service	Wide-cut	8 h (56) 15 min (28)	3.3 GM 5.0 GSD 9.3 GM 10.0 GSD	Holm et al. (1987)
Workshop service	Wide-cut	8 h (24) 15 min (12)	2.1 GM 5.3 GSD 5.8 GM 12.3 GSD	Holm et al. (1987)

[a]Time-weighted average of time-integrated means corresponding to measurements performed during various tasks involving exposure. These tasks cover ~50% of workers' time in testing activities and 35% for mechanics.
[b]Charcoal tube samples analysed by gas chromatography only. Nine samples above 800 mg/m³
[c]GM, geometric mean
[d]GSD, geometric standard deviation

methods are reported for the analysis of its component hydrocarbons. These methods are used to identify or 'fingerprint' the origin of a specific jet fuel or kerosene sample on the basis of the proportions of its component hydrocarbons. For a further discussion of analytical methods for component hydrocarbons of petroleum and petroleum products in environmental samples, see section 2.3 of the monograph on crude oil.

Selected methods applicable to the analysis of jet fuel are identified in Table 6.

Table 6. Methods applicable to the analysis of jet fuel in air

Sample preparation	Assay procedure[a]	Limit of detection	Remarks	Reference
Adsorb (charcoal); desorb (carbon disulfide); inject aliquot	GC/FID	5 mg/m³	Applies to kerosene vapours	Eller (1984)
Adsorb (charcoal or passive organic vapour monitor); desorb	IR	0.4 mg/m³	Applies to JP-4	Thomas & Richardson (1981)

[a]GC/FID, gas chromatography/flame ionization detection; IR, infra-red spectrophotometry

3. Biological Data Relevant to the Evaluation of Carcinogenic Risk to Humans

3.1 Carcinogenicity studies in animals

Studies on straight-run [5] and hydrotreated kerosene [5A], which are components of jet fuel, are described in the monograph on occupational exposures in petroleum refining, p. 72.

Skin application

Mouse: Groups of 50 male and 50 female B6C3F1 mice, eight weeks old, were given applications of 0, 250 or 500 mg/kg bw JP-5 navy fuel (52.8% cycloalkanes, 30.8% paraffins, 15.9% aromatics and 0.5% olefins) in 0.1 ml acetone on the skin on five days per week for 103 weeks. High-dose females were killed after 90 weeks because of the occurrence of non-neoplastic skin lesions. Survival at 105 weeks was: males — controls, 36/50; low-dose, 33/50; high-dose, 28/50; females — controls, 44/50, low-dose, 33/50; high dose, 17/50 (90 weeks). No neoplasm of the skin occurred at the application site in treated or vehicle-control mice of either sex. Carcinomas of the skin at the inguinal site occurred in one low-dose male, one high-dose male and one high-dose female. One papilloma of the skin occurred in a low-dose male. The incidence of malignant lymphomas was increased in low-dose female mice: controls, 7/48; low-dose, 19/49; high-dose, 5/47 (National Toxicology Program,

1986). [The Working Group noted that the incidence of lymphomas in low-dose female mice was within the range for historical untreated control female B6C3F1 mice in this laboratory.]

3.2 Other relevant data

(a) Experimental systems

Absorption, distribution, excretion and metabolism

No data were available to the Working Group.

Toxic effects

The oral LD_{50} in male Sprague-Dawley rats of jet propulsion fuel (JP-5) was >60 ml/kg bw. Male Sprague-Dawley rats treated with a single dose of 24 ml/kg bw JP-5 by gavage showed moderate renal and hepatic functional alterations, renal hyaline droplet formation, and renal and hepatic fatty change one to three days later (Parker *et al.*, 1981). Slight behavioural disturbances were observed after single oral administration of 1, 3 or 5 ml/kg bw JP-5 by gavage to male Sprague-Dawley rats 2.5–6 h after dosing (Bogo *et al.*, 1984).

Exposure of C57Bl/6 mice to 500 and 1000 mg/m³ JP-4 for 90 days caused centrilobular fatty change in the livers of females (MacNaughton & Uddin, 1984). Male Fischer 344 rats exposed continuously to JP-4 fuel vapour (500 and 1000 mg/m³) or JP-5 vapour (150 and 750 mg/m³) for 90 days developed dose-related nephropathy with cytoplasmic hyaline droplets, necrosis of proximal tubular cells and accumulation of intratubular necrotic debris (Bruner, 1984; Gaworski *et al.*, 1984). Rats held for life after the 90-day exposure to JP-5 showed abundant renal mineralized casts, papillary hyperplasia of pelvic urothelium and tubular degeneration (Bruner, 1984).

Male and female $C3H_f/Bd_f$ mice developed renal lesions after receiving dermal applications of 50 µl JP-5 and JP-8 jet fuel on their clipped backs thrice weekly for 60 weeks; atrophied and degenerating nephrons, as well as papillary necrosis, were observed (Easley *et al.*, 1982). Groups of male and female B6C3F1 mice were administered 0, 250 or 500 mg/kg bw JP-5 in acetone by dermal application on five days per week for 103 weeks (90 weeks for high-dose females due to ulceration of the skin). A marked increase in the incidence of ulceration, inflammation and epithelial hyperplasia was observed. No nephrotoxicity was seen, but the high-dose males and females had amyloidosis in multiple organs, possibly in response to the dermal ulcerations (National Toxicology Program, 1986).

Effects on reproduction and prenatal toxicity

No embryotoxic, fetotoxic or teratogenic effect was observed following exposure of Charles River CD rats by inhalation from day 6 to 15 of gestation for 6 h per day to 100 and 400 ppm jet fuel A (Beliles & Mecler, 1982). No toxic effect was detected on duck embryos after an application on the shell surface of weathered or unweathered aviation kerosene (1–20 µl per egg) on day 6 of incubation (Albers & Gay, 1982).

Genetic and related effects

Jet fuel A (boiling range, 163–282°C; 17.9% aromatics) was not mutagenic to *Salmonella typhimurium* TA1535, TA1537, TA1538, TA98 or TA100 [0.25–40 mg/plate] in the presence or absence of an exogenous metabolic system from rat liver (Conaway *et al.*, 1984). Similarly, jet fuel JP-5 was not mutagenic to *S. typhimurium* TA1535, TA97, TA98 or TA100 (100–10 000 µg/plate) in the presence or absence of an Aroclor 1254-induced rat or hamster liver preparation (National Toxicology Program, 1986). Jet fuel A induced mutation in mouse lymphoma L5178Y $TK^{+/-}$ cells only in the presence of an exogenous metabolic system from either rat or mouse liver. It induced chromosomal aberrations in the bone marrow of male and female Sprague-Dawley CD rats exposed by dynamic inhalation for 20 days to 100 ppm or for five days to 400 ppm (Conaway *et al.*, 1984).

(*b*) *Humans*

Absorption, distribution, excretion and metabolism
No data were available to the Working Group.

Toxic effects

Exposure to jet fuel vapours has been reported to cause a number of neurobehavioural symptoms, including dizziness, headache, nausea and fatigue (Davies, 1964; Knave *et al.*, 1976, 1978, 1979).

In a cross-sectional study of 30 workers exposed to jet fuel vapour (average, 300 mg/m^3; mean employment, 17 years) and 30 or 60 unexposed controls, a higher prevalence of psychiatric symptoms, poorer performance in some psychological tests and reduced sensorimotor speed were reported among the exposed group (Knave *et al.*, 1978, 1979).

Among 91 jet fuel-filling attendants in Denmark (exposure, 1–1020 mg/m^3; median, 31 mg/m^3), antipyrine clearance was higher during exposure than after an exposure-free period of two or four weeks; a similar, but smaller effect was reported in a control group of office workers (Døssing *et al.*, 1985). [The Working Group noted that no conclusion with respect to exposure to jet fuel can be made.]

Effects on reproduction and prenatal toxicity
No data were available to the Working Group.

Genetic and related effects
No data were available to the Working Group.

3.3 Epidemiological studies and case reports of carcinogenicity to humans

A cohort of 2182 men exposed to jet fuel in the Swedish armed forces was established in 1974 (Seldén & Ahlborg, 1986). Most of the men (86%) were employed in the Air Force, where exposure had been primarily to aviation kerosene, jet fuel, isopropyl nitrate (a starter fuel) and aviation gasoline (for piston engines). Measurements of jet fuel in air at some work places in 1975 and 1976 showed concentrations exceeding 350 mg/m^3. Cancer morbidity and mortality in the cohort were followed until 1981 and 1982, respectively, in central registers, with loss to follow-up of less than 0.2%. For Air Force personnel, there was significantly lower total mortality than expected on the basis of national rates (44 observed, 81.1 expected), due to low mortality from cardiovascular diseases. There were 25 malignant neoplasms compared with 29.4 expected. No clear increase in the frequency of cancers at specific sites was seen, even when duration of employment, latency, occupation or type of exposure were taken into consideration. These results were confirmed when the follow-up was continued for a further two years (Seldén & Ahlborg, 1987). [The Working Group noted the short duration of follow-up.]

In a case-control study of cancer at many sites in Montréal, Québec, Canada, which is described in detail in the monograph on gasoline (p. 185), among men exposed to jet fuel (kerosene-type and wide-cut), an increased risk was seen for kidney cancer only (adjusted odds ratio, 3.1; 90% confidence interval, 1.5–6.6) (Siemiatycki et al., 1987). In subjects in jobs which were estimated to result in substantial exposure, the adjusted odds ratio was 3.4 (1.5–7.6). Aircraft mechanics and repairmen constituted the largest occupational group, and there was an overlap between groups exposed to aviation gasoline and jet fuel, resulting from combined exposures.

4. Summary of Data Reported and Evaluation[1]

4.1 Exposure data

Jet fuels are produced mainly from straight-run [5] and hydrotreated kerosene [5A] or kerosene blended with heavy naphtha streams [4 and derived streams] from the atmospheric distillation of crude oil. Jet fuels are composed mainly of aliphatic and aromatic hydrocarbons with boiling ranges of 150–300°C (kerosene type) and 45–280°C (wide-cut type). The formulated products are used in turbine engines of civil and military aircraft. Exposures to jet fuel may occur during its production, transport and storage as well as during refuelling and maintenance of aircraft. Heavier exposures may occur during inspection and repair of aircraft wing tanks owing to the confined working space.

4.2 Experimental data[2]

One sample of jet fuel was tested by skin application in one experiment in male and female mice. No skin tumour occurred at the application site.

Two samples of straight-run kerosene [5] and one sample of hydrotreated kerosene [5A] produced skin tumours in mice. (See the monograph on occupational exposures in petroleum refining.)

---

[1]The numbers in square brackets are those assigned to the major process streams of petroleum refining in Table 2 of the monograph on occupational exposures in petroleum refining (p. 44).
[2]Subsequent to the meeting, the Secretariat became aware of a study in which skin tumours were reported in mice after application to the skin of jet fuel A [kerosene type] and JP-4 [wide-cut type] (Clark et al., 1988).

4.3 Human data

A cohort of men exposed to jet fuel, aviation kerosene and other fuels in the Swedish Air Force had no increased cancer risk during ten years of follow-up. A case-control study of cancer at many sites in Canada revealed an elevated risk for kidney cancer, with some indication of a positive dose-response relationship, in men exposed to jet fuel.

4.4 Other relevant data

In single studies, one sample of jet fuel induced chromosomal aberrations in bone-marrow cells of rats and mutations in cultured mammalian cells in the presence of an exogenous metabolic system but did not induce mutation in bacteria. A further sample was also not mutagenic to bacteria. (See Appendix 1.)

4.5 Evaluation[1]

There is *inadequate evidence* for the carcinogenicity in humans of jet fuel.

There is *inadequate evidence* for the carcinogenicity in experimental animals of jet fuel.

In formulating the overall evaluation, the Working Group also took note of the following supporting evidence from the monograph on occupational exposures in petroleum refining. There is *limited evidence* for the carcinogenicity in experimental animals of straight-run kerosene and of hydrotreated kerosene.

Overall evaluation

Jet fuel *is not classifiable as to its carcinogenicity to humans (Group 3)*.

5. References

Albers, P.H. & Gay, M.L. (1982) Unweathered and weathered aviation kerosine: chemical characterization and effects on hatching success of duck eggs. *Bull. environ. Contam. Toxicol.*, 28, 430–434

American Society for Testing and Materials (1986) *Annual Book of ASTM Standards*, Vol. 05.01, Philadelphia, pp. 835–844

Beliles, R.P. & Mecler, F.J. (1982) *Inhalation teratology of jet fuel A, fuel oil and petroleum naphtha in rats.* In: MacFarland, H.N., Holdsworth, C.E., MacGregor, J.A., Call, R.W. & Lane, M.L., eds, *Proceedings of a Symposium. The Toxicology of Petroleum Hydrocarbons*, Washington DC, American Petroleum Institute, pp. 233–238

Bishop, E.C., MacNaughton, M.G., deTreville, R.T.P. & Drawbaugh, R.B. (1983) *Rationale for a Threshold Limit Value (TLV®) for JP-4/Jet B Wide Cut Aviation Turbine Fuel (Report No. 83-128 EH 111 DGA)*, Brooks, TX, US Air Force Occupational and Environmental Health Laboratory

---

[1]For definition of the italicized terms, see Preamble, pp. 25–28.

Bogo, V., Young, R.W., Hill, T.A., Cartledge, R.M., Nold, J. & Parker, G.A. (1984) *Neurobehavioral toxicology of petroleum- and shale-derived jet propulsion fuel No. 5 (JP5).* In: MacFarland, H.N., Holdsworth, C.E., MacGregor, J.A., Call, R.W. & Lane, M.L., eds, *Advances in Modern Environmental Toxicology*, Vol. VI, *Applied Toxicology of Petroleum Hydrocarbons*, Princeton, NJ, Princeton Scientific Publishers, pp. 17–32

Boldt, K. & Hall, B.R., eds (1977) *Significance of Tests for Petroleum Products (ASTM Special Technical Publication 7C)*, Philadelphia, PA, American Society for Testing and Materials

Bruner, R.H. (1984) *Pathologic findings in laboratory animals exposed to hydrocarbon fuels of military interest.* In: Mehlman, M.A., Hemstreet, G.P., III, Thorpe, J.J. & Weaver, N.K., eds, *Advances in Modern Environmental Toxicology*, Vol. VII, *Renal Effects of Petroleum Hydrocarbons*, Princeton, NJ, Princeton Scientific Publishers, pp. 133–140

Clark, C.R., Walter, M.K., Ferguson, P.W. & Katchen, M. (1988) Comparative dermal carcinogenesis of shale and petroleum-derived distillates. *Toxicol. ind. Health*, 4, 11–22

Conaway, C.C., Schreiner, C.A. & Cragg, S.T. (1984) *Mutagenicity evaluation of petroleum hydrocarbons.* In: MacFarland, H.N., Holdsworth, C.E., MacGregor, J.A., Call, R.W. & Lane, M.L., eds, *Advances in Modern Environmental Toxicology*, Vol. VI, *Applied Toxicology of Petroleum Hydrocarbons*, Princeton, NJ, Princeton Scientific, pp. 89–107

CONCAWE (1985) *Health Aspects of Petroleum Fuels. Potential Hazards and Precautions for Individual Classes of Fuels (Report No. 85/51)*, The Hague, pp. 16–22

Davies, N.E. (1964) Jet fuel intoxication. *Aerospace Med.*, 35, 481–482

Dickson, C.L. & Woodward, P.W. (1987) *Aviation Turbine Fuels, 1986 (NIPER 149 PPS)*, Batesville, OK, National Institute for Petroleum and Energy Research

Døssing, M., Loft, S. & Schroeder, E. (1985) Jet fuel and liver function. *Scand. J. Work Environ. Health*, 11, 433–437

Dow, R.L., Hurst, J.W., Jr, Mayo, D.W., Cogger, C.G., Donovan, D.J., Gambardella, R.A., Jiang, L.C., Quan, J., Barry, M. & Yevich, P.P. (1975) The ecological, chemical and histopathological evaluation of an oil spill site. *Mar. Pollut. Bull.*, 6, 164–173

Dukek, W.G. (1978) *Aviation and other gas turbine fuels.* In: Grayson, M., ed., *Kirk-Othmer Encyclopedia of Chemical Technology*, 3rd ed., Vol. 3, New York, John Wiley & Sons, pp. 328–351

Easley, J.R., Holland, J.M., Gipson, L.C. & Whitaker, M.J. (1982) Renal toxicity of middle distillates of shale oil and petroleum in mice. *Toxicol. appl. Pharmacol.*, 65, 84–91

Eller, P.M. (1984) *NIOSH Manual of Analytical Methods*, 3rd ed., Vol. 2 *(DHHS (NIOSH) Publ. No. 84-100)*, Washington DC, US Government Printing Office, pp. 1550-1 — 1550-5

Fardell, P.J. & Houghton, B.W. (1975/76) The evaluation of an improved method of gas-freeing an aviation fuel storage tank. *J. hazardous Mater.*, 1, 237–251

Gaworski, C.L., MacEwen, J.D., Vernot, E.H., Bruner, R.H. & Cowan, M.J., Jr (1984) *Comparison of the subchronic inhalation toxicity of petroleum and oil shale JP-5 jet fuels.* In: McFarland, H.N., Holdsworth, C.E., MacGregor, J.A., Call, R.W. & Lane, M.L., eds, *Advances in Modern Environmental Toxicology*, Vol. VI, *Applied Toxicology of Petroleum Hydrocarbons*, Princeton, NJ, Princeton Scientific Publishers, pp. 33–47

Holm, S., Norbäck, D., Frenning, B. & Göthe, C.-J. (1987) Hydrocarbon exposure from handling jet fuel at some Swedish aircraft units. *Scand. J. Work Environ. Health*, 13, 438–444

IARC (1982) *IARC Monographs on the Evaluation of the Carcinogenic Risk of Chemicals to Humans*, Vol. 29, *Some Industrial Chemicals and Dyestuffs*, Lyon, pp. 93–148, 391–398

IARC (1987) *IARC Monographs on the Evaluation of Carcinogenic Risks to Humans*, Suppl. 7, *Overall Evaluations of Carcinogenicity: An Updating of* IARC Monographs *Volumes 1 to 42*, Lyon, pp. 120–122

International Energy Agency (1987) *Energy Statistics 1970-1985*, Vols I and II, Paris, Organisation for Economic Cooperation and Development

Knave, B., Persson, H.E., Goldberg, J.M. & Westerholm, P. (1976) Long-term exposure to jet fuel. An investigation on occupationally exposed workers with special reference to the nervous system. *Scand. J. Work Environ. Health, 3*, 152–164

Knave, B., Olson, B.A., Elofsson, S., Gamberale, F., Isaksson, A., Mindus, P., Persson, H.E., Struwe, G., Wennberg, A. & Westerholm, P. (1978) Long-term exposure to jet fuel. II. A cross-sectional epidemiologic investigation on occupationally exposed industrial workers with special reference to the nervous system. *Scand. J. Work Environ. Health, 4*, 19–45

Knave, B., Mindus, P. & Struwe, G. (1979) Neurasthenic symptoms in workers occupationally exposed to jet fuel. *Acta psychiatr. scand., 60*, 39–49

MacNaughton, M.G. & Uddin, D.E. (1984) *Toxicology of mixed distillate and high-energy synthetic fuels*. In: Mehlman, M.A., Hemstreet, G.P., III, Thorpe, T.J. & Weaver, N.K., eds, *Advances in Modern Environmental Toxicology*, Vol. VII, *Renal Effects of Petroleum Hydrocarbons*, Princeton, NJ, Princeton Scientific Publishers, pp. 121–132

National Institute for Occupational Safety and Health (1977) *Criteria for a Recommended Standard. Occupational Exposure to Refined Petroleum Solvents (DHEW (NIOSH) Publ. No. 77-192)*, Washington DC, US Government Printing Office, p. 193

National Toxicology Program (1986) *Toxicology and Carcinogenesis Studies of Marine Diesel Fuel and JP-5 Navy Fuel (CAS No. 8008-20-6) in B6C3F1 Mice (Dermal Studies) (Technical Report Series No. 310)*, Research Triangle Park, NC, US Department of Health and Human Services

Parker, G.A., Bogo, V. & Young, R.W. (1981) Acute toxicity of conventional versus shale-derived JP5 jet fuel: light microscopic, hematologic and serum chemistry studies. *Toxicol. appl. Pharmacol., 57*, 302–317

Seldén, A. & Ahlborg, G., Jr (1986) *Causes of Death and Cancer Morbidity at Exposure to Aviation Fuels in the Swedish Armed Forces* (Swed.) *(ASF Project 84-0308)*, Örebro, Department of Occupational Medicine

Seldén, A. & Ahlborg, G., Jr (1987) *Causes of Death and Cancer Morbidity at Exposure to Aviation Fuels in the Swedish Armed Forces. An Update* (Swed.), Örebro, Department of Occupational Medicine

Siemiatycki, J., Dewar, R., Nadon, L., Gérin, M., Richardson, L. & Wacholder, S. (1987) Associations between several sites of cancer and twelve petroleum-derived liquids: results from a case-control study in Montreal. *Scand. J. Work Environ. Health, 13*, 493–504

Talts, A., Bauer, J., Martin, C. & Reeves, D. (1977) *Discovery, containment and recovery of a jet fuel storage tank leak: a case history*. In: *Proceedings of the 1977 Oil Spill Conference, New Orleans, LA, March 8-10 1977*, Washington DC, American Petroleum Institute, pp. 259–263

Thomas, T.C. & Richardson, A., III (1981) *An infrared analysis method for the determination of hydrocarbons collected on charcoal tubes*. In: Choudhary, G., ed., *Chemical Hazards in the Workplace (ACS Symposium Series 149)*, Washington DC, American Chemical Society, pp. 37–48

DIESEL FUELS

1. Chemical and Physical Data

1.1 Synonyms and trade names

Diesel fuel (general)

    Chem. Abstr. Services Reg. No.: 68334-30-5
    Chem. Abstr. Name: Diesel oil
    IUPAC Systematic Name: —
    Synonyms: Auto diesel; automotive diesel oil (ADO); derv; diesel; diesel fuel oil; diesel oil; gas oil

Diesel fuel No. 1

    Chem. Abstr. Services Reg. No.: not assigned (essentially equivalent to kerosene, 8008-20-6)
    Synonyms: Diesel fuel oil No. 1; diesel oil No. 1; No. 1 diesel (These designations are not used in European terminology. Where fuels similar to US diesel fuel No. 1 are available in Europe (Scandinavia), they are commonly referred to as kerosine or Arctic diesel. In some cases, non-descriptive terminology applies, e.g., dipolar in Sweden for special kerosene fuels used in urban areas.)

Diesel fuel No. 2

    Chem. Abstr. Services Reg. No.: 68476-34-6 (applicable for specific viscosity limits)
    Chem. Abstr. Name: No. 2 diesel fuel
    Synonyms: Diesel fuel; diesel fuel oil No. 2; diesel oil No. 2; No. 2 diesel (term not used in Europe) In the UK, distillate fuels are frequently categorized as Class A1 (road diesel) and A2 (off-highway diesel).

Diesel fuel No. 4

    Chem. Abstr. Services Reg. No.: not assigned
    Synonyms: Marine diesel fuel; distillate marine diesel fuel

1.2 Description

The diesel engine and diesel fuel which provides the energy to run the engine derive their names from Rudolf Diesel, the German engineer who patented the engine design in 1892 (Anon., 1966). He operated his first successful engine in 1897 (Lane, 1980).

In its early history, the diesel engine was exploited for its versatility and ability to use a variety of cheap fuels. More recently, the requirements of efficiency and economics have prompted the development of fuel standards to meet desired performance characteristics, particularly for transportation service. Diesel fuels are appreciably less volatile than gasoline. They are classed as middle distillates and are more dense than gasoline, thus providing more energy per unit volume than gasoline. The product definition for diesel oil in the US Chemical Substances Inventory under the Toxic Substances Control Act is:

> *Diesel Oil* (CAS No. 68334-30-5) — A complex combination of hydrocarbons produced by the distillation of crude oil. It consists of hydrocarbons having carbon numbers predominantly in the range of C_9-C_{20} and boiling in the range of approximately 163–357°C.

In Europe, carbon numbers up to 28 and final boiling-points up to 390°C can be found for automotive diesel oil (CONCAWE, 1985).

The US definition encompasses both diesel fuel No. 1 and diesel fuel No. 2. There is no US Chemical Substances Inventory description for diesel fuel No. 1 or the equivalent European kerosene grade; however, in practice, this product is generally a straight-run petroleum distillate with a boiling range consistent with that of kerosene [5] (refer to Table 2 and Figure 1 of the monograph on occupational exposures in petroleum refining and to the monograph on jet fuel for the processing history of kerosene). Kerosene, and hence diesel fuel No. 1, consists of hydrocarbons with carbon numbers predominantly in the range of C_9-C_{16} and boiling in the range of approximately 150-300°C. Fuel oil No. 1 (heating) and kerosene used in Europe for heating applications have similar boiling ranges and are described in the monograph on fuel oils.

Diesel fuel No. 2 manufactured in the USA is generally a blend of straight-run and catalytically cracked streams, including straight-run kerosene [5], straight-run middle distillate [6], hydrodesulfurized middle distillate [6A] and light catalytically [24] and thermally cracked [30] distillates. The boiling range is generally approximately 160–360°C. The major component streams in European diesel fuels are presented in Table 1.

Diesel fuel No. 4 for low- and medium-speed engines, also characterized as a marine diesel fuel, is approximately similar to fuel oil No. 4 (CAS No. 68476-31-3), discussed in the monograph on fuel oils. As indicated in Table 2, American Society for Testing and Materials (ASTM) No. 4-D grade is more viscous than diesel fuel No. 2 and allows higher levels of ash and sulfur in the product. A No. 4 grade oil is generally classed as a residual fuel. It may be made either as a refinery stream which contains high boiling material classed as residual oil [8, 21, 31] or by blending residual fuel oil with a lighter material such as diesel fuel No. 2. In either case, it normally contains up to 15% residual oil components (CONCAWE, 1985). Some engines have been designed to operate on two different fuels,

Table 1. Major component streams of European automotive diesel oil (diesel fuel No. 2) and distillate marine diesel fuel (diesel fuel No. 4)[a]

TSCA Inventory name and identification number[b]	Refinery process stream (nomenclature used in Europe)	Automotive diesel oil (vol. %)	Distillate marine diesel fuel (vol. %)
	Straight-run (atmospheric) gas oil		
Straight-run middle distillate [6]	– light	40–100	40–100
Straight-run gas oil [7]	– heavy	0–3	0–50
Light vacuum distillate [19]	Vacuum gas oil	0–10	0–20
Light thermally cracked distillate [30]	Thermally cracked gas oil	0–20	0–30
Light catalytically cracked distillate [24]	Light catalytically cracked gas oil (cycle oil)	0–25	0–40

[a]From CONCAWE (1985)
[b]See Table 2 and Figure 1 in the monograph on occupational exposures in petroleum refining

with diesel fuel No. 2 used for idle and intermittent service and a No. 4 grade used for high-load, sustained operations (Guthrie, 1960).

Residual oil components are readily available at lower cost than distillate fuels and provide more energy per unit volume of product. These fuels are used in the same ways.

In general, the higher the content of straight-chain paraffins and paraffin side-chains in diesel fuels, the lower the autoignition temperature, and the higher the cetane number. However, waxy components tend to cause flow problems in very cold weather. Accordingly, more kerosene is often blended into winter grades of diesel fuel No. 2 to improve the flow properties. Diesel fuels are generally dried by passing through salt driers or water coalescers and filtered to remove rust and dirt.

1.3 Chemical composition and physical properties of technical products

Diesel fuel No. 1 is essentially equivalent to kerosene, the composition and properties of which are discussed in the monographs on jet fuel and fuel oils. It contains normal and branched-chain alkanes (paraffins), cycloalkanes (naphthenes), aromatics and mixed aromatic cycloalkanes. Normal alkanes usually predominate, resulting in a clean-burning diesel fuel with a relatively high cetane number. Cetane (n-hexadecane) gives excellent performance in diesel engines and was arbitrarily assigned the value of 100 in the cetane number scale (see Glossary); α-methylnaphthalene gives poor diesel engine performance and was assigned a value of zero (Lane, 1980).

The boiling range of diesel fuel No. 1 largely excludes the presence of benzene and polycyclic aromatic hydrocarbons. No direct data on concentrations were available to the

Table 2. Detailed requirements for diesel fuel oils (ASTM specification D 975[a])

Grade of diesel fuel oil	Flash-point °C (min)	Water and sediment vol. % (max)	Carbon residue on 10% residue % (max)	Ash weight % (max)	Distillation temperatures °C (90% point)		Viscosity				Sulfur weight % (max)	Copper strip corrosion	Cetane number (min)
							Kinematic cSt t 40°C (max)		Seybolt universal sec at 38°C[b]				
					min	max	min	max	min	max			
No. 1-D A volatile distillate fuel oil for engines in service requiring frequent speed and load changes	38	0.05	0.15	0.01	–	288	1.3	2.4	–	34.4	0.50	No. 3	40
No. 2-D A distillate fuel oil of lower volatility for engines in industrial and heavy mobile service	52	0.05	0.35	0.01	282	338[b]	1.9	4.1	32.6	40.1	0.50	No. 3	40
No. 4-D A fuel oil for low- and medium-speed engines	55	0.50	–	0.10	–	–	5.5	24.0	45.0	125.0	2.0	–	30

[a] Adapted from Lane (1980) and Hoffman (1982)
[b] Provided by American Petroleum Institute

Working Group, but kerosene which is approximately equivalent to diesel fuel No. 1 normally contains less than 0.02% benzene (CONCAWE, 1985; see IARC, 1982, 1987) and very low levels of three- to seven-ring polycyclic aromatic hydrocarbons (Dukek, 1978).

Because of the similarity of chemical composition, the discussion on fuel oil No. 2, in a separate monograph, is also generally applicable to diesel fuel No. 2 and European automotive diesel fuels. It contains normal and branched-chain alkanes (paraffins), cycloalkanes (naphthenes), aromatics and mixed aromatic cycloalkanes. Because it is likely to contain cracked stocks as one or more of the blend streams, it also contains olefins and mixed aromatic olefin types such as styrenes. Because of its more complex composition and lower percentage of straight-run fractions, diesel fuel No. 2 tends to have a lower cetane number than the No. 1 grade; however, cetane numbers can be improved by the use of additives.

Diesel fuel No. 2, when it consists predominantly of atmospheric distillate streams, contains possibly less than 5% of three- to seven-membered, condensed ring aromatic hydrocarbons (measured by the dimethyl sulfoxide extraction method of the Institute of Petroleum). In fuels that contain high proportions of heavy atmospheric, vacuum and light cracked distillates, the level may be as high as 10% (CONCAWE, 1985). Levels of some individual polycyclic aromatics in fuel oil No. 2 (which is approximately equivalent to diesel fuel No. 2) are given in Table 3 of the monograph on fuel oils. Some marine diesel fuels may contain more than 10% polycyclic aromatic hydrocarbons (CONCAWE, 1985; see also the monograph on fuel oils). Diesel fuels may also contain minor amount of constituents such as n-hexane (below 0.1%), benzene (below 0.02%), toluene, xylenes and ethyl benzene (0.25–0.5%).

Refiners normally select blend stocks to ensure easy starting and smooth engine performance. Sulfur, nitrogen and oxygen compounds are present as impurities in these streams, but their presence can be limited by hydrotreating and other processes. Because No. 2 diesel fuel, and European automotive diesel fuels in particular, normally contains minor quantities of olefins, the stability of the product in storage is of concern. Fuel degradation products formed during long-term storage can result in troublesome contamination. High temperatures and oil-soluble metal compounds (particularly those containing copper) can hasten degradation. Storage in the presence of water promotes bacterial growth which can result in sludge. Refiners generally prefer not to use additives in diesel fuel, although they can improve and preserve its quality.

Cetane improvers, such as organic nitrates, can be added to improve the ignition quality of the product. Oxidation inhibitors are added to prevent product degradation; corrosion inhibitors and metal deactivators can be added as required. Biocides are sometimes used when bacterial growth in storage may be a problem, and rust inhibitors can be added to minimize corrosion, particularly in storage facilities. Additives such as cetane improvers and oxidation inhibitors are usually added to normal production volumes by refiners; the use and concentration of other additives may be agreed by the supplier and the purchaser. A wide range of additives may be employed to assure satisfactory technical performance; examples are shown in Table 3. Military specifications for diesel fuels include many additives (US Navy, 1985).

Table 3. Examples of additives used in diesel fuels[a]

Flow improvers: ethylene/vinyl acetate polymers — about 500 ppm max
- long-chain polyester derived from acetic acid and unsaturated C_{16} alcohol
- polyolefin ester derived from 2-ethylhexyl acrylate

Antistatics: used typically at 1–5 ppm
- Cr and Ca salts of mono- and di-alkyl salicylic and dodecyl sulfosuccinic acids
- toluene, alkyl benzene sulfonate, high mol. wt polysulfone, polyamine
- polyamide, carboxylate, carboxylic acid in aromatic oil

Other additives:

Antioxidant	2,4-Dimethyl-6-*tert*-butylphenol	9–25 ppm
Stability improver	Polymethacrylate, polyisobutene, alkanolamine, amide, carboxylate	50 ppm
Ash modifier	Zinc diaryl dithiophosphate, phenols, carboxylate	300 ppm
Ignition (cetane) improver	Organic nitrates (e.g., isopropyl nitrate)	200–800 ppm
Multi-purpose	Styrene/ester copolymer	20–200 ppm
Antiwear	Polymeric ester	0.1 vol%
Lubricity improver	Phosphate ester amide, neutralized with long chain amine	0.03 wt%
Metal deactivator	N,N'-Disalicylidene-1,2-propanediamine	5.8 mg/l
Biocides	Thiazine derivatives	

[a]Provided by CONCAWE

Performance requirements for diesel fuels are defined primarily in terms of physical tests rather than chemical composition. Table 2 lists the ASTM D 975 test specifications for diesel fuels; Tables 4 and 5 (compiled by CONCAWE) give a summary of the European national standards by country, including kerosene standards (similar to ASTM No. 1).

The discussions here and in the monograph on fuel oils regarding composition and processing of fuel oils are generally applicable to gas turbine fuel oils, except in those instances where the inclusion of residual components is permitted.

Table 4. Compilation of national industrial standards and regulatory requirements for kerosene (1986)

Country	National Standards Reference (date)	Flash-point IP 170[a] °C (min)	Flash-point D56[b] °C (max)	Smoke point mm (min)	Wick char °C (min)	Density at 15°C kg/m³ (max)	Kinematic viscosity at 40°C mm²/sec	Sulfur mass % (max)	Distillation
Germany, Federal Republic of	DIN 51 636A		40			830		0.07	initial boiling-point, 130°C min 10% max at 150°C 95% min at 280°C
Italy	UNI 6579 (1977)		21			770–820		0.25	90% max at 210°C 65% min at 250°C
United Kingdom	BS 2869 C2 (1983)	38		20	20		1.0–2.0	0.20	15% min at 200°C final boiling-point, 300°C max

[a] UK Institute of Petroleum Method IP 170
[b] ASTM method D56

Table 5. National industrial standards and regulatory requirements for automotive diesel fuel (1986)

	Austria	Belgium & Luxembourg	France	Germany, F.R.	Ireland	Italy	Netherlands[a]	Norway	Switzerland	United Kingdom	
National Standard reference (date)	ONORM C1104[b] (1986)	NBN 52-501[c] (1969)	CSR 0.9-1 (1986)	DIN 51.601 (1986)	IS 251 (1981)	NC 630 01[b] (1985)	No national standard	No national standard	SNV 181160/1 (1985)	BS 2869 A1[d]	A2[e]
Cetane no.	45	–	50[f]	45	–	47	–	–	48[g]	50	45
Cetane index (min)	–	–	–	–	–	48	–	–	48[g]	–	–
Cloud-point W (S)[h] °C (max)	–	–	0 (–)	–	0 (–)	–	–	–	–6 (–6)[g]	–	–
Pour-point W (S) °C (max)	–	–6 (–)	–12 (–7)	–	–	–6 (–6)	–	–	–15 (–9)	–	–
Cold filter plugging point W (S) °C (max)	–15 (+5)	–	–12 (0)[i]	–15(0)	–9 (–)[j]	–10 (–)	–	–	–15 (–8)[g]	–9 (0)	–12 (–4)
Density at 15°C (kg/m³)	Report	–	810–890	820–860	810–860	805–865	–	–	815–860	–	–
Flash-point PM[k] °C (min)	55	50	55–120	55	55	55	55	60[l]	55	56	56
Kinematic viscosity											
at 20°C (mm²/sec)	3.0–8.0	7.4 max	9.5 max	2.0–8.0	–	2.0–5.35	–	–	3.0–6.0	1.5–5.0	1.5–5.5
at 40°C (mm²/sec)	–	–	–	–	1.5–6.0	–	–	–	–	–	–
Sulfur mass % (max)	0.15	0.3	0.3	0.3[m]	0.5	0.3[b]	0.3	0.5[n]	0.3[o]	0.3	0.5[p]
Distillation	90% min at 350°C	65% max at 250°C 85% min at 350°C	65% max at 250°C 85% min at 350°C	65% max at 250°C 85% min at 250°C	Initial boiling-point, 170°C min Final boiling-point, 380°C max	2% max at 150°C 65% max at 250°C 85% min at 350°C	65% min at 250°C 85% max at 350°C	–	90% max at 360°C	85% min at 350°C	85% min at 350°C
Water (max)	–	–	Trace	0.05 mass %	0.04 mass %	–	–	–	–	0.05 vol %	0.05 vol %
Sediment (max)	–	–	Nil	–	–	–	–	–	–	0.01 mass %	0.01 mass %
Water and sediment (max)	–	0.10	–	–	–	0.05 vol %	–	–	Nil	–	–
Ash mass % (max)	0.01	–	Trace	0.02	–	0.01	–	–	0.005	0.01	0.01

Table 5 (contd)

	Austria	Belgium & Luxembourg	France	Germany, F.R.	Ireland	Italy	Nether-lands[a]	Norway	Switzer-land	United Kingdom	
Carbon residue[q] Mass % (max) 10% bottoms mass % (max)	0.25 (C)	—	—	—	—	0.15 (C)	—	—	0.05 (C)	A1 0.2 (R)	A2 0.2 (R)
Strong acid no.	—	—	Nil	—	—	—	—	—	—	—	—
Copper strip corrosion rating	1b max (3 h at 100°C)	—	—	—	—	2 max (3 h at 50°C)	—	—	—	1 max (3 h at 100°C)	1 max (3 h at 100°C)
Neutralization no. mg KOH/g (max)	0.15	—	—	—	—	—	—	—	—	—	—
Dyes and markers	None	None	None	None	None	None	None	None	None	None	Red dye and quinzarin

[a] Industrial and EEC customs standards
[b] Revised standard
[c] New standard under discussion
[d] A1 for automotive use (BS2869, 1983); revision under review
[e] A2 for stationary units (BS2869, revised 1986); revised standard
[f] 50 min summer, 48 min winter; revision to 48 min all year under review, with further relaxation to 45 under study
[g] Alternative standard
[h] W, winter; S, summer
[i] −18°C capability with additional flow improver
[j] Alternative is −7°C max cloud-point
[k] Pensky-Martens method
[l] Government regulation
[m] Reduction to 0.1-0.15 mass % likely around 1988
[n] By agreement
[o] 0.2 mass % max from July 1987
[p] 0.3 mass % expected around 1988
[q] C, Conradson; R, Ramsbottom method of measurement

2. Production, Use, Occurrence and Analysis

2.1 Production and use

(a) Production and consumption

As the product name suggests, diesel fuels are designed for use as fuels in diesel engines. The No. 1 grade is the more volatile of the two principal grades and gives good performance in engines requiring frequent changes in speed and load, such as city buses. It is also the cleaner burning of the two grades. The No. 2 grade has a higher specific gravity, providing more energy per unit volume of fuel, which is an important economic factor in industrial and heavy transportation service such as railroads, trucks and river boats. Hence the major growth in consumption has been in the No. 2 grade. Diesel fuel No. 4 is a special grade of fuel oil for low- and medium-speed engines that can use a more viscous fuel oil with a relatively high sulfur content (max, 2.0 wt %; Lane, 1980).

The conversion of railroads to diesel engines accelerated in the 1940s and continued after the Second World War, after which time there was a rapid conversion of trucks to diesel service. Today, most heavy duty transportation is powered by diesel engines. Although the conversion of automobiles to diesel service has been very limited in the USA, cars powered by diesel engines are used extensively in Europe, where diesel car registrations accounted for 3.8% of new passenger cars in 1977, 6.9% in 1980 and 17.5% in 1986 (data provided by CONCAWE).

Production and consumption of diesel fuels combined as one class of product for the USA and for the 24 countries included in the Organisation for Economic Cooperation and Development (OECD) combined are presented in Table 6, and cover the period 1970-1985 in five-year increments (International Energy Agency, 1987). Continued growth in demand for diesel fuel is reflected by the data until 1980.

Table 6. Production and consumption (in thousands of tonnes) of diesel fuel[a] in the USA and in countries of the Organisation for Economic Cooperation and Development (OECD) for 1970-85[b]

Area	Production/ consumption	1970	1975	1980	1985
USA	Production	120 254	134 967	138 323	135 181
	Consumption	120 151	133 300	136 161	130 297
OECD	Production	336 688	370 240	408 848	372 728
	Consumption	336 678	380 181	403 642	386 081

[a]Including gas oils in Europe
[b]From International Energy Agency (1987)

Data on production and consumption of diesel fuels for 1985 are listed by geographical area in Table 7.

Table 7. Production and consumption (in thousands of tonnes of diesel fuel[a] by geographical area, 1985[b]

Region or organization	Production	Consumption
North America	154 368	149 427
USA	135 181	130 297
Canada	19 187	19 130
OECD (Europe)	173 474	190 960
European Economic Community	152 091	163 132
Pacific[c]	44 886	45 694
OECD (All)	372 728	386 081

[a]Including gas oils in Europe
[b]From International Energy Agency (1987)
[c]Australia, Japan, New Zealand

(b) Use

Diesel Fuel No. 4 is used in railroads, to move river barges and for stationary engines in continuous, high-load service. In addition to their principal use as transportation fuels, diesel fuels are used in stationary gas turbines, for example, to generate electic power during peak load periods. Distillate fuel oils defined by ASTM Specification D 396 (see monograph on fuel oils) are also used in stationary gas turbines. While the respective basic grades of fuel oils and diesel fuel are similar, there are specific requirements that are important for gas turbine service.

(c) Regulatory status and guidelines

No data were available on occupational exposure limits for diesel fuel.

2.2 Occurrence

(a) Occupational exposure

Occupational exposure to diesel fuel (diesel oil) has been associated with the following operations (CONCAWE, 1985): manually handled filling and discharge; marine diesel bunkering involving the manual handling of discharge lines; retailing through filling stations; tank dipping, pipeline and pump repairs, filter cleaning in refineries, distribution terminals and depots; tank inspection, cleaning and repairing; manufacture, repair, servicing and testing of diesel engines or equipment and injection and fuel systems; routine sampling and laboratory handling of diesel oils; and practices in which diesel oils are used as cleaning agents or solvents.

Because of their low volatility, at normal temperatures diesel fuels should generate vapours at only low concentrations, except in confined spaces. High operating temperatures could result in significant vapour concentrations and, as in the case of residual fuel oils, in the evolution of hydrogen sulfide gas (CONCAWE, 1985). No published quantitative data on exposure levels to diesel fuel were available to the Working Group.

(b) Environmental exposure

Table 8 lists some accidental releases of diesel fuel that have been reported in the recent past.

Table 8. Examples of major accidental releases of diesel fuel

Place	Date	Type	Quantity	Reference
Spitzbergen, Norway	April–May 1978	Rupture of diesel fuel storage tank	130 m^3	Carstens & Sendstad (1979)
Queen Charlotte Islands, Canada	March 1984	Barge spill	130 tonnes	McLaren (1985)
Yaquina Bay, OR, USA	November 1983	Diesel fuel and bunker C fuel oil from wreck of tanker, *Blue Magpie*	284 000 l	Kemp *et al.* (1986)
Floreffe, PA, USA	December 1987	Rupture of diesel fuel storage tank	3 million gallons (11.4 million l)	MacKerron & Kiesche (1988)

2.3 Analysis

Since diesel fuel is composed of a complex mixture of hydrocarbons, there are few methods for the environmental analysis of 'diesel fuel' as an entity, but many methods are reported for the analysis of its component hydrocarbons. These methods are used to identify or 'fingerprint' the origin of a specific diesel fuel sample on the basis of the proportions of its component hydrocarbons. No specific method for the sampling and analysis of diesel fuel vapours was available.

3. Biological Data Relevant to the Evaluation of Carcinogenic Risk to Humans

3.1 Carcinogenicity studies in animals

Studies on the carcinogenicity in experimental animals of straight-run kerosene [5], which is a component of diesel fuel Nos 1 and 2, and of light catalytically cracked distillates [24] and light vacuum distillate [19], which are used in diesel oil Nos 2 and 4, are described in the monograph on occupational exposures in petroleum refining. Studies on residues of thermally cracked oils [31], which may be used in diesel fuel No. 4, are also described in that monograph.

Skin application

Mouse: Groups of 49 or 50 male and 50 female B6C3F1 mice, eight weeks old, were administered 250 or 500 mg/kg bw marine diesel fuel in 0.1 ml acetone by application to clipped interscapular dorsal skin on five days per week for 103 weeks or 84 weeks (high-dose group terminated due to severe ulceration of the skin), respectively. A control group received the vehicle only. The diesel fuel was a mixture of petroleum-derived hydrocarbons containing 12.7% paraffins and 87.3% aromatic compounds. Survival at 84 weeks was 26/50 and 29/50 among high-dose males and females, respectively; at 104 weeks, survival was 20/49 and 12/50 in low-dose males and females, and 30/50 and 40/50 among vehicle-control males and females, respectively. There was a significant increase in the incidence of squamous-cell papillomas and carcinomas at the application site in males (controls, 0/49; low-dose, 0/49; high-dose, 3/49 (two carcinomas; $p = 0.019$). The incidences of these tumours at the adjacent inguinal site in males were: controls, 1/50 (papilloma); low-dose, 2/49 (carcinomas); high-dose, 0/50. The incidences of squamous-cell carcinomas at the application site in females were: controls, 0/50; low-dose, 1/45; high-dose, 2/48; no papilloma occurred, and no tumour was found at the adjacent inguinal region. Although no data on historical controls were available for acetone-treated animals of this strain, the background rate for skin neoplasms among untreated mice is quite low (<1%). The incidences of hepatocellular adenomas in males were: control, 5/50; low-dose, 10/48; high-dose, 10/49. The total numbers of male mice with hepatocellular tumours (adenomas and carcinomas combined) were: controls, 9/50; low-dose, 17/48; high-dose, 14/49 ($p = 0.035$). The incidence of hepatocellular tumours did not differ significantly from that in historical controls (540/1784; 30 ± 8%; National Toxicology Program, 1986).

3.2 Other relevant data

(a) *Experimental systems*

Absorption, distribution, excretion and metabolism

No data on the absorption, distribution, excretion and metabolism of diesel fuel in laboratory animals were available to the Working Group. One study has been reported on gulls and ducks (McEwan & Whitehead, 1980).

Toxic effects

The oral LD_{50} of diesel fuel [unspecified] in rats was 7.5 g/kg bw. No mortality was induced in acute dermal toxicity studies in rats dosed at 5 g/kg bw (Beck *et al.*, 1984).

Groups of male and female B6C3F1 mice were administered 2000-40 000 mg/kg bw 100% marine diesel fuel by dermal application for 14 consecutive days. No animal treated with 20 000 or 40 000 mg/kg survived. Skin lesions were similar in all dosed groups —

moderate acanthosis, parakeratosis and hyperkeratosis, accompanied by mixed cellular inflammatory infiltrate in the upper dermis (National Toxicology Program, 1986).

Groups of male and female B6C3F1 mice were administered 250–2000 mg/kg bw marine diesel fuel in acetone or 4000 mg/kg 100% marine diesel fuel by dermal application on five days per week for 13 weeks; no treatment-related death occurred. An increased severity of mild chronic active dermatitis at the site of application was observed in the high-dose group (National Toxicology Program, 1986).

Groups of male and female B6C3F1 mice were administered 250 or 500 mg/kg bw marine diesel fuel in acetone by dermal application on five days per week for 103 weeks (84 weeks for high-dose groups; early termination was due to ulceration of the skin). Increases in haematopoiesis were found in the spleen in animals of each sex and in the liver in females. Increases in plasmacytosis occurred in lymph nodes in females and in high-dose males. Ulcers and chronic dermatitis were observed at increased rates at the site of dermal application and in the inguinal region of the skin (National Toxicology Program, 1986).

Effects on reproduction and prenatal toxicity

As reported in a review of teratology studies in rats exposed to different fuels by inhalation, exposure of animals on days 6–15 of gestation for 6 h per day to 100 and 400 ppm diesel fuel [unspecified] resulted in no teratogenic effect (Schreiner, 1984). [The Working Group noted that details were not reported.]

Genetic and related effects

Diesel fuel (boiling range, 186–357°C; 24% aromatics) was found to be weakly mutagenic to *Salmonella typhimurium* TA98 using the suspension method (3.38–25 μl/ml) but not using the plate incorporation method (0.001–5 μl/plate), in the presence and absence of an exogenous metabolic system from rat liver (Conaway *et al.*, 1984). Diesel 25 [not further specified] was not mutagenic to *S. typhimurium* TA1535, TA1538, TA98 or TA100 (plate test; Vandermeulen *et al.*, 1985), or to *Chlamydomonas reinhardtii* in a forward mutation assay (streptomycin resistance; Vandermeulen & Lee, 1986). Marine diesel fuel was not mutagenic to *S. typhimurium* TA1935, TA1937, TA98 or TA100 in the presence or absence of Aroclor 1254-induced rat or hamster liver microsomes (National Toxicology Program, 1986).

Neither aliphatic nor aromatic fractions separated from diesel fuel No. 7911 [not further specified] by dimethyl sulfoxide induced mutation in *S. typhimurium* TA100 (Henderson *et al.*, 1981).

Diesel fuel (boiling range, 186–375°C; 24% aromatics) was not mutagenic to L5178Y $TK^{+/-}$ mouse lymphoma cells either in the presence or absence of an exogenous metabolic system from either rat or mouse liver. Undiluted diesel fuel increased the frequency of chromosomal aberrations in the bone marrow of Sprague-Dawley rats 6–48 h after a single intraperitoneal injection of 2 or 6 ml/kg bw or after five daily intraperitoneal injections of 2 or 6 ml/kg bw per day (Conaway *et al.*, 1984).

(b) *Humans*

Absorption, distribution, excretion and metabolism

Absorption was assumed to have occurred mainly through the skin of a 28-year-old sailor who developed symptoms of intoxication after using diesel fuel as a shampoo (Barrientos *et al.*, 1977).

Toxic effects

Anuria, renal failure and gastrointestinal symptoms developed several hours after the incident described above; the sailor recovered after dialysis. A renal biopsy on the second day showed tubular dilatation with casts, flattening of epithelial cells, mitosis and vacuolization (Barrientos *et al.*, 1977).

A man who cleaned his hands and arms with diesel fuel over several weeks developed renal failure over about three months. Renal biopsy showed acute tubular damage, with patchy degeneration and necrosis of proximal and distal tubular epithelium and preservation of basement membranes (Crisp *et al.*, 1979).

Cutaneous hyperkeratosis has been described in engine drivers exposed occupationally to diesel fuel (Gusein-Zade, 1974).

A young woman who claimed to have ingested a large amount of diesel fuel (1.5 l) in a suicidal attempt developed toxic lung disease over the next few days, with fever, dry cough and basal opacities on chest X-ray. The condition resolved over the following four months (Boudet *et al.*, 1983).

A woman aged 28 years who accidentally inhaled diesel fuel immediately began to cough, became dyspnoeic and cyanosed and lost consciousness for 1 h. A productive cough with sputum smelling of diesel fuel persisted for 37 days. Chest X-ray showed diffuse shadowing, most prominent at the lung bases, which resolved slowly with treatment but was still present at day 37. Blood biochemistry indicated slight hepatotoxic effects but with no clinical problem (Perez Rodriguez *et al.*, 1976).

Effects on reproduction and prenatal toxicity

No data were available to the Working Group.

Genetic and related effects

A group of 12 diesel vehicle drivers (six smokers and six nonsmokers) exposed to vehicle exhausts and to fuel, among other agents, was studied for cytogenetic changes. The nonsmoking drivers were reported to have more chromosomal aberrations (mean, 3.6% aberrant cells) than nonsmoking gasoline-vehicle drivers and nonsmoking unexposed controls (mean, 1.4% aberrant cells). [The Working Group noted that a 72-h culture time was used in this study.] No difference between the groups was noted in the frequency of sister chromatid exchange, although smokers in all groups had significantly higher mean frequencies than nonsmokers (Fredga *et al.*, 1982). [The Working Group noted the small size of the group and the mixed exposure of the workers.]

3.3 Epidemiological studies and case reports of carcinogenicity to humans

The studies reviewed in the monograph on gasoline often involved subjects or occupational groups with mixed exposures, particularly to gasoline and diesel fuel. It was often not possible to separate the effects of the two types of fuel. Studies that primarily addressed the risk associated with exposure to combustion products of diesel fuel are not considered here but are the subject of *IARC Monographs* Vol. 46 (IARC, 1989).

In a case-control study of cancer at many sites in Montréal, Canada, described in detail in the monograph on gasoline (p. 185), an increased risk for cancer of the prostate, with an adjusted odds ratio of 1.9 (90% confidence interval (CI), 1.2–3.0), was observed among men exposed to diesel fuel; however, there was no evidence of a positive dose-response relationship (Siemiatycki *et al.*, 1987). There was an increased risk for squamous-cell carcinoma of the lung in men exposed to diesel fuel (adjusted odds ratio (including smoking), 1.6; 90% CI, 1.0–2.6); for men with estimated 'nonsubstantial' exposure, the odds ratio was 1.0 (0.4–2.0), and for those with 'substantial' exposure, it was 2.5 (1.3–4.7). Mechanics and repairmen, who constituted the largest group exposed to diesel fuel, had an adjusted odds ratio of 2.0 (0.9–4.2). [The Working Group noted that, in the interpretation of the lung cancer risks, no attempt was made to separate the effects of exposure to combustion products from those of exposure to the liquid itself.]

4. Summary of Data Reported and Evaluation[1]

4.1 Exposure data

Diesel fuels are complex mixtures of alkanes, cycloalkanes and aromatic hydrocarbons with carbon numbers in the range of C_9-C_{28} and with a boiling-range of 150–390°C. Kerosene-type diesel fuel (diesel fuel No. 1) is manufactured from straight-run petroleum distillates [5]. Automotive and railroad diesel fuel (diesel fuel No. 2) contains straight-run middle distillate [6], often blended with straight-run kerosene [5], straight-run gas oil [7], light vacuum distillate [19] and light thermally cracked [30] or light catalytically cracked distillates [24]. Some blended marine diesel fuels also contain heavy residues from distillation [8, 21] and thermal cracking [31] operations. In diesel fuel consisting mainly of atmospheric distillates, the content of three- to seven-ring polycyclic aromatic hydrocarbons is generally less than 5%; in diesel fuel that contains high proportions of heavy atmospheric, vacuum and light cracked distillates, the content of such polycyclic aromatic hydrocarbons may be as high as 10%. Some marine diesel fuels may contain higher levels. Saleable diesel fuel may also contain a variety of additives, such as organic nitrates, amines, phenols and polymeric substances. Exposure to diesel fuel through the skin and by inhalation may occur during its production, storage, distribution and use as well as during maintenance of diesel engines.

---

[1]The numbers in square brackets are those assigned to the major process streams of petroleum refining in Table 2 of the monograph on occupational exposures in petroleum refining (p. 44).

4.2 Experimental data[1]

One sample of marine diesel fuel was tested for carcinogenicity in one strain of mice by skin application, producing a few squamous-cell carcinomas and papillomas at the application site in animals of each sex and a few carcinomas at the adjacent inguinal region in males.

Two samples of straight-run kerosene [5], one sample of light vacuum distillate [19] and three samples of light catalytically cracked distillate [24] produced skin tumours in mice. Some residues from thermal cracking [31] produced benign and malignant skin tumours in mice. (See the monograph on occupational exposures in petroleum refining.)

4.3 Human data

In a case-control study of cancer at many sites, there was evidence of an increased risk for squamous-cell carcinoma of the lung in men estimated to have had substantial exposure to diesel fuel. There was also an indication of an increased risk for cancer of the prostate. No attempt was made to separate the effects of combustion products from those of exposure to diesel fuel itself.

4.4 Other relevant data

Inhalation or ingestion of diesel fuel resulted in acute and persistent lung damage in humans.

No report specifically designed to study genetic and related effects in humans following exposure to diesel fuel was available to the Working Group.

Application of marine diesel fuel to the skin of mice resulted in ulceration.

In a single study, diesel fuel induced chromosomal aberrations in bone-marrow cells of rats; it did not induce mutation in cultured mammalian cells but was weakly mutagenic to bacteria. Another sample did not induce mutation in bacteria or algae; a sample of marine diesel fuel and aliphatic and aromatic fractions of an unspecified diesel fuel were also not mutagenic to bacteria. (See Appendix 1.)

4.5 Evaluation[2]

There is *inadequate evidence* for the carcinogenicity in humans of diesel fuels.

There is *limited evidence* for the carcinogenicity in experimental animals of marine diesel fuel.

---

[1]Subsequent to the meeting, the secretariat became aware of a study in which skin tumours were reported in mice after application to the skin of petroleum diesel (boiling range, 198–343°C) [corresponding to diesel fuel No. 2] (Clark *et al.*, 1988).

[2]For definitions of the italicized terms, see Preamble, pp. 24–28.

In formulating the overall evaluation, the Working Group also took note of the following supporting evidence reported in the monograph on occupational exposures in petroleum refining. There is *limited evidence* for the carcinogenicity in experimental animals of straight-run kerosene and *sufficient evidence* for the carcinogenicity in experimental animals of light vacuum distillates, of light catalytically cracked distillates and of cracked residues derived from the refining of crude oil.

Overall evaluation

Marine diesel fuel *is possibly carcinogenic to humans (Group 2B)*.

Distillate (light) diesel fuels *are not classifiable as to their carcinogenicity to humans (Group 3)*.

5. References

Anon. (1966) *Encyclopaedia Britannica*, Vol. 7, London, William Benton, p. 396

Barrientos, A., Ortuño, M.T., Morales, J.M., Martinez Tello, F. & Rodicio, J.L. (1977) Acute renal failure after use of diesel fuel as shampoo. *Arch. intern. Med.*, *137*, 1217

Beck, L.S., Hepler, D.I. & Hansen, K.L. (1984) *The acute toxicology of selected petroleum hydrocarbons.* In: MacFarland, H.N., Holdsworth, C.E., MacGregor, J.A., Call, R.W. & Lane, M.L., eds, *Advances in Modern Environmental Toxicology*, Vol. VI, *Applied Toxicology of Petroleum Hydrocarbons*, Princeton, NJ, Princeton Scientific Publishers, pp. 1–16

Boudet, F., Fabre, M., Boe, M., Delon, M., Ruiz, J. & Lareng, L. (1983) Toxic lung disease after voluntary ingestion of a litre and a half of diesel fuel (Fr.). *Toxicol. Eur. Res.*, *5*, 247–249

Carstens, T. & Sendstad, E. (1979) *Oil spill on the shore of an ice-covered fjord in Spitsbergen.* In: *Proceedings of the 79th International Conference on Port and Ocean Engineering Under Arctic Conditions, August 13-18, Trondheim*, University of Trondheim, Norwegian Institute of Technology, pp. 1227–1242

Clark, C.R., Walter, M.K., Ferguson, P.W. & Katchen, M. (1988) Comparative dermal carcinogenesis of shale and petroleum-derived distillates. *Toxicol. ind. Health*, *4*, 11–22

Conaway, C.C., Schreiner, C.A. & Cragg, S.T. (1984) *Mutagenicity evaluation of petroleum hydrocarbons.* In: MacFarland, H.N., Holdsworth, C.E., MacGregor, J.A., Call, R.W. & Lane, M.L., eds, *Advances in Modern Environmental Toxicology*, Vol. VI, *Applied Toxicology of Petroleum Hydrocarbons*, Princeton, NJ, Princeton Scientific Publishers, pp. 89–106

CONCAWE (1985) *Health Aspects of Petroleum Fuels. Potential Hazards and Precautions for Individual Classes of Fuels* (Report No. 85/51), The Hague, pp. 23–29, 47

Crisp, A.J., Bhalla, A.K. & Hoffbrand, B.I. (1979) Acute tubular necrosis after exposure to diesel oil. *Br. med. J.*, *ii*, 177

Dukek, W.G. (1978) *Aviation and other gas turbine fuels.* In: Grayson, M., ed., *Kirk-Othmer Encyclopedia of Chemical Technology*, 3rd ed., Vol. 3, New York, John Wiley & Sons, pp. 328–351

Fredga, K., Dävring, L., Sunner, M., Bengtsson, B.O., Elinder, C.-G., Sigtryggsson, P. & Berlin, M. (1982) Chromosome changes in workers (smokers and nonsmokers) exposed to automobile fuels and exhaust gases. *Scand. J. Work Environ. Health*, *8*, 209–221

Gusein-Zade, K.M. (1974) The results of dermatological examinations of engine drivers working in oil fields of Apsheron (Russ.). *Vestn. Dermatol. Venereol., 10,* 47–49

Guthrie, V.B., ed. (1960) *Petroleum Products Handbook,* New York, McGraw-Hill, pp. 1–17

Henderson, T.R., Li, A.P., Royer, R.E. & Clark, C.R. (1981) Increased cytotoxicity and mutagenicity of diesel fuel after reaction with NO_2. *Environ. Mutagenesis, 3,* 211–220

Hoffman, H.L. (1982) *Petroleum (products).* In: Grayson, M., ed., *Kirk-Othmer Encyclopedia of Chemical Technology,* 3rd ed., Vol. 17, New York, John Wiley & Sons, pp. 257–271

IARC (1982) *IARC Monographs on the Evaluation of the Carcinogenic Risk of Chemicals to Humans,* Vol. 29, *Some Industrial Chemicals and Dyestuffs,* Lyon, pp. 93–148, 391–398

IARC (1987) *IARC Monographs on the Evaluation of Carcinogenic Risks to Humans,* Suppl. 7, *Overall Evaluations of Carcinogenicity: An Updating of* IARC Monographs *Volumes 1 to 42,* Lyon, pp. 120–122

IARC (1989) *IARC Monographs on the Evaluation of Carcinogenic Risks to Humans,* Vol. 46, *Diesel and Gasoline Engine Exhausts and Some Nitroarenes,* Lyon (in press)

International Energy Agency (1987) *Energy Statistics 1970-1985,* Vols I and II, Paris, Organisation for Economic Cooperation and Development

Kemp, P.F., Swartz, R.C. & Lamberson, J.O. (1986) Response of the phoxocephalid amphipod, *Rhepoxynius abronius,* to a small oil spill in Yaquina Bay, Oregon. *Estuaries, 9,* 340–347

Lane, J.C. (1980) *Gasoline and other motor fuels.* In: Grayson, M., ed., *Kirk-Othmer Encyclopedia of Chemical Technology,* 3rd ed., Vol. 11, New York, John Wiley & Sons, pp. 652–695

MacKerron, C.B. & Kiesche, E. (1988) After the Ashland spill, more regulations? *Chem. Week, 142,* 19–20

McEwan, E.H. & Whitehead, P.M. (1980) Uptake and clearance of petroleum hydrocarbons by the glaucous-winged gull (*Laras glaucescens*) and the mallard duck (*Anas platyrhynchos*). *Can. J. Zool., 58,* 723–726

McLaren, P. (1985) Behaviour of diesel fuel on a high energy beach. *Mar. Pollut. Bull., 16,* 191–196

National Toxicology Program (1986) *Toxicology and Carcinogenesis Studies of Marine Diesel Fuel and JP-5 Navy Fuel (CAS No. 8008-20-6) in B6C3F1 Mice (Dermal Studies) (Technical Report Series No. 310),* Research Triangle Park, NC, US Department of Health and Human Services

Perez Rodriguez, E., Latour Perez, J., Aller Alvarez, J.L., Alix, J. & Alix, Y. (1976) Diesel fuel pneumonia. Presentation of a case (Sp.). *Rev. clin. esp., 143,* 397–400

Schreiner, C.A. (1984) *Petroleum and petroleum products: a brief review of studies to evaluate reproductive effects.* In: Christian, M.S., Galbraith, W.M., Voytek, P. & Mehlman, M.A., eds, *Advances in Modern Environmental Toxicology,* Vol. III, *Assessment of Reproductive and Teratogenic Hazards,* Princeton, NJ, Princeton Scientific Publishers, pp. 29–45

Siemiatycki, J., Dewar, R., Nadon, L., Gérin, M., Richardson, L. & Wacholder, S. (1987) Associations between several sites of cancer and twelve petroleum-derived liquids: results from a case-referent study in Montreal. *Scand. J. Work Environ. Health, 13,* 493–504

US Navy (1985) *Military Specification. Fuel, Naval Distillate (MIL-F-16884H),* Washington DC, US Government Printing Office

Vandermeulen, J.H. & Lee, R.W. (1986) Lack of mutagenic activity of crude and refined oils in the unicellular alga *Chlamydomonas reinhardtii. Bull. environ. Contam. Toxicol., 36,* 250–253

Vandermeulen, J.H., Foda, A. & Stuttard, C. (1985) Toxicity vs mutagenicity of some crude oils, distillates and their water soluble fractions. *Water Res., 19,* 1283–1289

FUEL OILS (HEATING OILS)

1. Chemical and Physical Data

1.1 Synonyms and trade names

Distillate fuel oils (light fuel oils)

Chemically-neutralized light distillate (CAS No. 64742-31-0); domestic fuel oil; domestic heating oil; fuel oil No. 1 (USA); fuel oil No. 2 (USA) (CAS No. 68476-30-2); furnace oil No. 1; furnace oil No. 2; heating oil; home heating oil; hydrotreated light distillate (CAS No. 64742-47-8); kerosene; kerosene, straight run [5][1] (CAS No. 8008-20-6); kerosine; lamp oil; light heating oil; paraffin oil (UK); petroleum distillate; rotary burner fuel; stove oil

Residual fuel oils (heavy fuel oils)

Bunker C; bunker C fuel oil; bunker fuel oil; bunker oil; fuel oil lourd; fuel oil No. 4 (USA) (CAS No. 68476-31-3); fuel oil No. 5 (USA); fuel oil No. 6 (USA) (CAS No. 68553-00-4); fuel oil, residual (CAS No. 68476-33-5); industrial fuel oil; marine boiler fuels; power station fuel oil; residual fuel oil grade 4; residual fuel oil grade 5; residual fuel oil grade 6

1.2 Description

The fuel oils discussed in this monograph are used as burner fuel for domestic and industrial heating, and for raising steam for electricity generation and marine propulsion.

Because of the methods employed in their production, fuel oils fall into two broad classifications: distillates and residuals. The distillates consist of distilled process streams [5, 6, 6A, 7, 19, 24, 30]. The residual fuel oils are residues remaining after distillation [8, 21] or cracking [27, 31] and blends of these residues with distillates. In American Society for Testing and Materials (ASTM) Specification D 396 (Table 1), grades No. 1 and No. 2 are distillates and grades No. 4 to No. 6 are usually residual, although some heavy distillates [20, 26] may be sold as grade No. 4 (Hoffman, 1982).

---

[1]See Table 2 and Figure 1 of the monograph on occupational exposures in petroleum refining

Table 1. Detailed requirements for fuel oils[a] (ASTM specification D396[b])

Grade descriptions	No. 1	No. 2	No. 4 (Light)	No. 4	No. 5 (Light)	No. 5 (Heavy)	No. 6
Specific gravity, 15/15°C (°API)							
max	0.8499 (35 min)	0.8762 (30 min)	0.8762[c] (30 max)	—	—	—	—
min	—	—	—	—	—	—	—
Flash-point, °C min	38	38	38	55	55	55	60
Pour-point, °C max	−18[d]	−6[d]	−6[d]	−6[d]	—	—	—[e]
Kinematic viscosity, mm²/s (cSt)[f]							
At 38°C min	1.4	2.0[d]	2.0	5.8	—	—	—
max	2.2	3.6	5.8	26.4[g]	—	—	—
At 40°C min	1.3	1.9[d]	—	5.5	>26.4	>65	—
max	2.1	3.4	—	24/0[g]	65[g]	194[g]	—
At 100°C min	—	—	—	—	>24.0	>58	15.0
max	—	—	—	—	(58)[g]	(168)[g]	50.0
Saybolt viscosity[f]					5.0	9.0	
Universal at 38°C min	—	(32.6)	(32.6)	(45)	8.9[g]	14.9[g]	
max	—	(37.9)	(45)	(125)	(>125)	(>300)	(>900)
Furol at 50°C min	—	—	—	—	(300)	(900)	(9000)
max	—	—	—	—	—	(23)	(>45)
						(40)	(300)
Distillation temperature, °C							
10% point max	215	—	—	—	—	—	—
90% point min	—	282[d]	—	—	—	—	—
max	288	338	—	—	—	—	—
Sulfur content, mass %, max	0.5	0.5[h]	—	—	—	—	—
Corrosion copper strip, max	3	3	—	—	—	—	—

Table 1 (contd)

Grade descriptions	No. 1	No. 2	No. 4 (Light)	No. 4	No. 5 (Light)	No. 5 (Heavy)	No. 6
Ash, % mass, max	—	—	0.05	0.10	0.15	0.15	—
Carbon residue, 10% bottoms, mass %, max	0.15	0.35	—	—	—	—	—
Water and sediment, vol %, max	0.05	0.05	$(0.50)^i$	$(0.50)^i$	$(1.00)^i$	$(1.00)^i$	$(2.00)^i$

[a] Failure to meet any requirement of a given grade does not automatically place an oil in the next lower grade unless in fact it meets all requirements of the lower grade. No. 1, a distillate oil intended for vaporizing pot-type burners and other burners requiring this grade of fuel; No. 2, a distillate oil for general purpose heating for use in burners not requiring No. 1 fuel oil; No. 4 (light) and No. 4, preheating not usually required for handling or burning; No. 5 (light), preheating may be required depending on climate and equipment; No. 5 (heavy), preheating may be required for burning and, in cold climates, for handling; No. 6, preheating required for handling and burning equipment.

[b] From American Society for Testing and Materials (1986)

[c] This limit guarantees a minimum heating value and also prevents misrepresentation and misapplication of this product as grade No. 2.

[d] Lower or higher pour-points may be specified whenever required by conditions of storage or use. When pour-point less than −18°C is specified, the minimum viscosity for grade No. 2 shall be 1.7 cSt (31.5 SUS) and the minimum 90% point shall be waived.

[e] Where low-sulfur fuel oil is required, a grade 6 fuel oil will be classified as low pour +15°C (max or high pour (no max)). Low pour fuel oil should be used unless all tanks and lines are heated.

[f] Viscosity values in parentheses are for information only and not necessarily limiting.

[g] Where low-sulfur fuel oil is required, fuel oil falling in the viscosity range of a lower numbered grade down to and including No. 4 may be supplied by agreement between purchaser and supplier. The viscosity range of the initial shipment shall be identified and advance notice shall be required when changing from one viscosity range to another. This notice shall be in sufficient time to permit the user to make the necessary adjustments.

[h] In countries outside the USA, other sulfur limits may apply.

[i] The amount of water by distillation plus the sediment by extraction shall not exceed the value shown in the table. For grade No. 6 fuel oil, the amount of sediment by extraction shall not exceed 0.50 wt %, and a deduction in quantity shall be made for all water and sediment in excess of 1.0 wt %.

(a) *Distillate fuel oils*

Specifications for both middle distillate heating fuels and transportation fuels are similar; as a consequence, it is often possible for refiners to satisfy the performance requirements of both applications with the same process stream or blend of process streams. The final products will have been treated (sweetened, dried, clay filtered, etc.) as required for a particular application, and may contain additives that are specific for the intended use, but they are otherwise virtually indistinguishable on the basis of their gross physical or chemical properties.

(i) *Fuel oil No. 1 (kerosene)*

The development of fuel oil No. 1 (kerosene) as a product can be traced back to Abraham Gesner, a Canadian doctor and geologist, who patented a distillation process for refining petroleum in 1854 (Anon., 1966). Gesner produced an improved illuminating oil which he called kerosene, derived from the Greek word *keros*, which means wax. The spelling is still widely used in industry, although the Chemical Abstracts preferred spelling is kerosine. Gesner first refined the oil from coal; thus, for many years, the product was widely known as 'coal oil', although the predominant source of the product changed from coal to petroleum crude oil. Kerosene remained the principal refined product of petroleum refiners for more than 50 years (Guthrie, 1960).

Fuel oil No. 1 is a light distillate intended for use in burners of the vaporizing type in which the oil is converted to a vapour by contact with a heated surface or by radiation. High volatility is necessary to ensure that evaporation proceeds with a minimum of residue.

Fuel oil No. 1 is generally a straight-run distillate with a boiling range consistent with the specifications shown in Table 1. (Refer to Table 2 and Figure 1 of the monograph on occupational exposures in petroleum refining for the processing history and generic definitions of refinery process streams.) Less often, it may consist of a blend of kerosene and light hydrocracked distillate and/or light catalytically cracked distillate [24]. Fuel oil No. 1 is not normally sweetened but usually contains an antioxidant additive.

(ii) *Fuel oil No. 2*

Fuel oil No. 2 is a heavier distillate than fuel oil No. 1. It is intended for use in atomizing-type burners, which spray the oil into a combustion chamber where the droplets burn while in suspension. This grade of oil is used in most home heating installations and in many medium-capacity commercial or industrial burners.

Fuel oil No. 2 is generally a blend of straight-run and catalytically cracked distillates. Typically, straight-run kerosene [5], straight-run middle distillate [6], hydrodesulfurized middle distillate [6A], straight-run gas oil [7], light catalytically cracked distillate [24], light vacuum distillate [19] and light thermally cracked distillate [30] are all candidates for blending into fuel oil No. 2. The streams and proportions used depend upon the nature of the refinery crude oil mix and the influence of the individual blend stocks on the specification properties set forth in ASTM D 396. Fuel oil No. 2 is generally dried by passage through salt driers and filtered to remove rust and dirt. Additives include antioxidants, dispersants and corrosion inhibitors. US distillate fuels contain a higher proportion of cracked stocks and exhibit a narrower boiling range than those in most other parts of the world because of the greater degree of conversion carried out in order to maximize the yield of gasoline. The properties of a typical European distillate fuel oil for domestic or industrial use are given in Table 2.

Table 2. Typical properties of European fuel oil[a]

Property	Distillate (domestic/industrial heating oil)	Residual		
		Light	Medium	Heavy
Kinematic viscosity at 50°C				
(cSt) − inland	2−7 (at 20°C)	20−30	30−180	180−600
− marine	−	20−30	30−180	180−600
Sulphur (wt %) − inland	0.5	<-----	0.3−5.0	----->
− marine	−	<-----	0.2−4.5	----->
Boiling range (°C)	160−400	−	−	−
Ash wt %	−	0.1	0.15	0.15
Water and sediment	−	<-----	1% max	----->

[a]From CONCAWE (1985)

(b) Residual fuel oils

The most important specifications for residual fuel oils are the viscosity and sulfur content, although limits for flash-point, pour-point, water and sediment, and ash are included in ASTM D 396 (Table 1). Sulfur limits for the heavy fuels are controlled by federal, state and municipal regulation in the USA and consequently depend upon the location of use. For the heavier grades of industrial and bunker fuels, viscosity is of major importance. The imposition of viscosity limits ensures that adequate preheating facilities can be provided to permit transfer to the burner and atomization of the fuel. In addition, the maximal viscosity of fuel under storage conditions must be low enough to allow it to be pumped from the storage tank to the preheater. The properties of typical European residual fuel oils are shown in Table 2.

The principal manufacturing operation generally involves the addition of low viscosity blending stocks to high viscosity distillation residues in the proportions necessary to meet the viscosity specifications desired. The residues are typically atmospheric tower residue [8], vacuum residue [21] or thermally cracked residue [31]. Other residues, such as propane-precipitated bitumen, steam-cracked residue [34] (pyrolysis fuel oil) and solvent extracts of lubricant oils, are used infrequently. The blending stocks may be distillates or residues. Those frequently used are catalytically cracked clarified oil [27], heavy vacuum distillate [20] and heavy catalytically cracked distillate [26]. The specific refinery streams and the proportions in which the bottoms and the blending stock are combined depend upon market economics and on the viscosity specifications of the fuels being manufactured. In some cases, the viscosity of the residue is such that no blending is required. In a refinery where the character of the crude oil and the nature of the processing units is such that both low and high sulfur residues are generated, these streams are generally segregated so that both low and high sulfur heavy fuels can be produced. Residual fuels blended from bottoms containing high levels of vanadium may require desalting in hot water to reduce the sodium content, since the presence of high levels of both sodium and vanadium results in undesirably high ash contents.

(i) *Fuel oil No. 4*

Fuel oil No. 4 is usually a 'light' residual, but it sometimes is, or contains, a heavy distillate. It is intended for use in burners equipped with devices that atomize oils of higher viscosity than domestic burners can handle. Its permissible viscosity range allows it to be pumped and atomized at relatively low storage temperatures. Consequently, in all but extremely cold weather, it requires no preheating for handling.

(ii) *Fuel oil No. 5*

Fuel oil No. 5 (light) is a residual fuel of intermediate viscosity for burners capable of handling fuel more viscous than fuel oil No. 4 without preheating. Fuel oil No. 5 (heavy) is a residual fuel more viscous than fuel oil No. 5 (light) and is intended for use in similar service. Preheating of fuel oil No. 5 may be necessary in some types of equipment for burning and in colder climates for handling.

(iii) *Fuel oil No. 6 (Bunker fuel)*

Fuel oil No. 6, sometimes referred to as 'bunker fuel' or 'bunker C', is a high viscosity oil used mostly as a boiler fuel and in commercial and industrial heating. It requires preheating in storage tanks to permit pumping and additional preheating at the burner to permit atomizing. The extra equipment and maintenance required to handle this fuel usually preclude its use in small installations.

1.3 Chemical composition and physical properties of technical products

Descriptions of the chemical composition and physical properties of fuel oils are available (Rossini *et al.*, 1953; Royal Dutch/Shell Group of Companies, 1983).

(*a*) *Distillate fuel oils*

Distillate fuel oils are complex mixtures of hydrocarbons that also contain minor amounts of sulfur-, nitrogen- and oxygen-containing molecules. They contain normal and branched alkanes, cycloalkanes (naphthenes), partially reduced aromatics and aromatics. If they have been blended in part with cracked stocks, they will also contain significant amounts of normal, branched and cyclic olefins, and aromatic olefins, such as styrenes and indenes. Fuel oil No. 1 spans the carbon number range about C_9-C_{16}; fuel oil No. 2 spans the range about $C_{11}-C_{20}$. Although the complexity of the fuel oils precludes analysis of individual compounds, a number of studies of the composition of petroleum have provided knowledge of the structures that predominate within a given broad hydrocarbon class and have shed some light on the relative abundance of isomers.

The normal alkanes occur in substantially all straight-run fractions with boiling ranges typical of those exhibited by distillate fuels, but their total concentration is dependent on the crude oil used. Branched alkanes also contribute significantly to the composition of distillates in this boiling range. Single-branched isomers predominate; the concentrations of double-branched isomers are an order of magnitude less than those with a single branch, and those of the triple-branched isomers two orders of magnitude lower. The cycloalkanes constitute a substantial portion of the saturated hydrocarbons in distillate fuels. Although the five- and six-membered-ring monocycloalkanes predominate in the lower-boiling fractions, bi- and tricycloalkanes have become increasingly important constituents in the 200–400°C boiling range. The majority of multi-ring cycloalkanes have five- and/or six-membered condensed ring systems. As a general rule in alkyl substitution, the derivatives of the parent ring system with alkyl substituents containing the smallest number of carbon atoms predominate over structures with longer chains.

The mononuclear aromatics consist largely of alkylbenzenes; however, the proportion of alkyl indanes and alkyl tetralins becomes larger as the average carbon number increases. Alkylnaphthalenes are the most abundant dinuclear aromatics. Although the condensed aromatic ring system predominates, small quantities of alkylbiphenyls, fluorenes and acenaphthenes are also present. As in the case of cycloalkanes, for which there are several possibilities for alkyl substitution, the predominant isomers are generally those containing substituents with the smallest number of carbon atoms. Phenanthrenes are the predominant trinuclear aromatic type. Generally, when three aromatic rings occur in the same molecule, they are usually condensed angularly rather than linearly. The boiling range of the distillate fuel oils precludes the presence of appreciable quantities of aromatics containing four or more condensed rings (Mair, 1964; Pancirov & Brown, 1975).

While these generalizations characterize the molecular structures that predominate within a broad hydrocarbon class, the proportions of each of the major classes can differ from one crude oil to another. Consequently, there may be appreciable variation in the hydrocarbon composition of distillate fuels; however, the differences are ordinarily not as large as might be anticipated because the specifications that must be met restrict the levels of several physical properties related to the composition. Detailed analyses of several samples of fuel oil No. 1 and fuel oil No. 2 are given in Table 3. Differences due to type of crude oil and process are discernible and are most evident in the distribution of saturated hydrocarbon types; nonetheless, the gross compositions are not remarkably divergent. The presence of catalytically cracked stocks does not result in the introduction of large quantities of olefins; even when the blended product contains 50% catalytic stock, the olefin content is below 10%. The use of catalytically cracked blend stocks generally results in fuels with some olefin content, reduced cycloalkane content and somewhat increased aromatic content, but which otherwise do not differ substantially from straight-run distillates.

Distillate fuels contain minor amounts of sulfur-, nitrogen- and oxygen-containing compounds, which in general are undesirable but can be tolerated at sufficiently low levels. In most refineries, processes for their reduction or removal are commonplace. The sulfur

Table 3. Detailed analyses of grades 1 and 2 distillate fuel oils[a]

Hydrocarbon type, vol. %	Straight-run No. 1 furnace oils (two samples)		Hydrotreated No. 1 furnace oil	Straight-run No. 2 furnace oil	No. 2 furnace oil 10% catalytic stock	No. 2 furnace oil 50% catalytic stock
Paraffins (*n*- and *iso*-)	50.5	54.3	42.6	41.3	61.2	57.2
Monocycloparaffins	25.3	18.4	19.3	22.1	8.5	6.0
Bicycloparaffins	5.6	4.5	8.9	9.6	8.3	5.0
Tricycloparaffins	–	0.8	–	2.3	1.4	0.7
Total saturated hydrocarbons	81.4	78.0	70.9	75.3	79.4	68.9
Olefins	–	–	–	–	2.0	7.5
Alkylbenzenes	12.7	14.3	14.7	5.9	5.3	8.0
Indans/tetralins	2.9	3.8	7.5	4.1	4.3	5.4
Dinaphthenobenzenes/indenes	–	0.9	–	1.8	1.3	1.0
Naphthalenes	3.0	2.6	6.9	8.2	5.8	6.8
Biphenyls/acenaphthenes	–	0.4	–	2.6	1.1	1.6
Fluorenes/acenaphthylenes	–	–	–	1.4	0.6	0.3
Phenanthrenes	–	–	–	0.7	0.2	0.5
Total aromatic hydrocarbons	18.6	29.1	22.0	24.7	18.6	23.6

[a]Provided by the American Petroleum Institute

content of distillate fuels is limited to 0.5 wt % by ASTM D 396 and in Europe. The identities of a substantial number of these nonhydrocarbon molecules have been established. Nitrogen types include anilines, pyridines, quinolines, pyrroles, carbazoles, phenazines, benzonitriles and amides; sulfur occurs as thiols, sulfides, disulfides, thiophenes, thiaindans, benzothiophenes and dibenzothiophenes, while oxygen-containing constituents are generally acids, ethers and ketones (Jewell et al., 1965; Latham et al., 1965; Thompson et al., 1965; Green et al., 1985).

The boiling range of kerosene fuel oil (fuel oil No. 1) generally precludes the occurrence of substantial quantities of polycyclic aromatic hydrocarbons. Fuel oil No. 2, consisting predominantly of atmospheric distillate streams, contains less than 5% three- to seven-ring polycyclic aromatic hydrocarbons (as measured by the dimethyl sulfoxide extraction method of the Institute of Petroleum). If high proportions of heavy atmospheric, vacuum or light cracked distillates are present, the level may be as high as 10% (CONCAWE, 1985). Some data on the concentrations of polycyclic aromatic hydrocarbons have been reported: Gräf and Winter (1968) found 0.029 ppm benzo[a]pyrene (see IARC, 1983, 1987a) in a heating oil; Pancirov and Brown (1975) determined the concentrations of a number of three- to five-ring aromatic hydrocarbons in two fuel oils — their data for fuel oil No. 2 are shown in Table 4. The total concentration of parent hydrocarbons containing four or more rings is just over 80 ppm; the concentration of benzo[a]pyrene is 0.6 ppm.

Table 4. Polynuclear aromatic compounds in one No. 2 fuel oil sample[a]

Hydrocarbon	Molecular weight	Concentration (ppm)
Phenanthrene	178	429
2-Methylphenanthrene	192	7677
1-Methylphenanthrene	192	173
Fluoranthene	202	37
Pyrene	202	41
Benz[a]anthracene	228	1.2
Chrysene	228	2.2
Triphenylene	228	1.4
Benzo[a]pyrene	252	0.6
Benzo[e]pyrene	252	0.1

[a]From Pancirov and Brown (1975)

As mentioned in section 1.2, distillate fuels often contain additives that serve as antioxidants, dispersants and corrosion inhibitors. Antioxidants may include hindered phenols, aminophenols and phenylenediamines. Dispersants may include various detergent amines, amidazolines, succinimides and amides; while corrosion inhibitors are typically long-chain alkyl carboxylates, sulfonates and amines.

(b) Residual fuel oils

Grades No. 4 to 6 fuel oils are commonly known as 'residual oils' since they are manufactured in whole or in part from distillation residues from refinery processing. Residual fuel oils are complex mixtures of relatively high molecular weight compounds and are difficult to characterize in detail. Since they are blended from fractions with boiling-points between 350 and 650°C, the molecular weights of the constituents can span the range from about 300 to over 1000. Molecular types include asphaltenes, polar aromatics, naphthalene aromatics, aromatics, saturated hydrocarbons and heteromolecules containing sulfur, oxygen, nitrogen and metals (Jewell *et al.*, 1974; Boduszynski *et al.*, 1981; CONCAWE, 1985). Fuels that have been prepared using catalytically cracked residues or heavy catalytically cracked distillates [26] contain some high molecular weight olefins and mixed aromatic olefins. In addition, they exhibit greater concentrations of condensed aromatics than do fuels prepared entirely from uncracked residues. Neff and Anderson (1981) characterized a No. 6 fuel oil (bunker fuel) in terms of the broad compositional categories shown in Table 5.

Table 5. Gross composition of a No. 6 fuel oil[a]

Composition (wt %)		Elemental analysis (wt %)	
Saturates	21.1	Sulfur	1.46
Aromatics	34.2	Nitrogen	0.94
Polar aromatics	30.3	Nickel	89 (ppm)
Asphaltenes	14.4	Vanadium	73 (ppm)

[a]From Neff and Anderson (1981)

Appreciable concentrations of polynuclear aromatic compounds are present in residual fuels because of the common practice of using both uncracked and cracked residues in their manufacture. Most blending stocks of residual fuel oils are likely to contain 5% or more of four- to six-ring condensed aromatic hydrocarbons. Pancirov and Brown (1975) reported the concentrations of a number of three- to five-ring condensed aromatics in a No. 6 fuel oil, as shown in Table 6. The identities and concentrations of the polynuclear aromatic compounds in a particular residual fuel depend on the nature and amount of the low viscosity blending stocks and the proportions of virgin and cracked residues. If the blending stocks are predominantly atmospheric [8] or vacuum residues [21], the concentration of three- to seven-ring aromatic hydrocarbons is likely to be of the order of 6–8%; if larger quantities of heavy catalytically cracked [26, 27] or steam-cracked [34] components are used, the level may approach 20% (CONCAWE, 1985). One of the blending stocks, catalytically cracked clarified oil [27], has been reported to contain 58% three- to five-ring aromatic hydrocarbons and 22% carbazoles and benzocarbazoles (Cruzan *et al.*, 1986).

Additives to improve the combustion of residual fuel oil, when used, are mostly based on oil-soluble compounds (e.g., naphthenates) of calcium, cerium, iron or manganese. Concentrations vary with fuel type but range typically from 50 to 300 ppm weight of the active metal

Table 6. Polynuclear aromatic compounds in one sample of No. 6 fuel oil[a]

Hydrocarbon	Molecular weight	Concentration (ppm)
Phenanthrene	178	482
2-Methylphenanthrene	192	828
1-Methylphenanthrene	192	43
Fluoranthene	202	240
Pyrene	202	23
Benz[a]anthracene	228	90
Chrysene	228	196
Triphenylene	228	31
Benzo[a]pyrene	252	44
Benzo[e]pyrene	252	10
Perylene	252	22

[a]From Pancirov and Brown (1975)

ingredient. They are usually added by the customer and are not incorporated into the fuel by the oil supplier. With increasing vanadium and sodium content of residual fuels, magnesium slurries suspended in gas oil or oil-soluble magnesium components are used to prevent corrosion at high temperatures. The amounts added depend on the vanadium concentration and are determined by a magnesium:vanadium weight ratio of up to 1.25:1.0 (CONCAWE, 1988).

2. Production, Use, Occurrence and Analysis

2.1 Production and use

Production and consumption of residual fuel oils in the USA and in the 24 countries of the Organisation for Economic Cooperation and Development (OECD) combined are presented in Table 7 for 1970—85 in five-year increments (International Energy Agency, 1987).

Comparative use of distillate and residual fuels in the USA for the period 1979—83 is shown in Table 8. The data for distillates include deliveries for transportation as well as for heating uses. Consumption of both distillate and residual fuel oils declined significantly: distillates by about 20% and residual fuels by almost 50%. About 80% of the decline in distillate demand is attributable to a pronounced reduction in the use of distillates in industrial and domestic heating systems.

Use of distillate fuel oils in the USA in 1979—83 is shown in Table 9. Heating utilization of the distillate grades (i.e., fuel oils No. 1 and No. 2) has declined substantially for all of the

Table 7. Production and consumption (in thousands of tonnes) of residual fuel oils in the USA and in countries of the Organisation for Economic Cooperation and Development (OECD) for 1970–85[a]

Area	Production/ Consumption	1970	1975	1980	1985
USA	Production	38 665	88 009	101 945	57 109
	Consumption	67 083	47 978	51 372	27 396
OECD	Production	388 184	444 033	418 508	233 256
	Consumption	271 726	228 964	199 351	103 862

[a]From International Energy Agency (1987)

Table 8. Deliveries of distillate and residual fuel oils by year in the USA (thousands of barrels)[a]

Year	Distillate fuel oils	Residual fuel oils
1979	1 214 374	1 034 610
1980	1 086 709	937 466
1981	1 032 476	726 030
1982	974 864	626 510
1983	981 927	518 604

[a]From US Department of Energy (1983)

Table 9. Deliveries of distillate fuel oils by use in the USA (thousands of barrels)[a]

Year	All transportation	Heating				
		Residential	Commmercial	Industrial	Farm	Oil company and electricity utility
1979	556 402	270 306	99 723	99 583	84 926	68 622
1980	531 497	227 361	92 136	86 089	73 615	56 017
1981	538 123	197 400	78 663	80 216	69 665	47 377
1982	517 360	180 760	75 699	71 340	68 453	41 616
1983[b]	540 403	171 783	72 809	69 332	66 697	41 701

[a]From US Department of Energy (1983) Estimates
[b]Estimates

applications shown. Although fuel oil No. 1 is consumed in some residential and farm uses, it constitutes much less of the total supply of heating distillates than grade No. 2, which is the fuel most commonly used in residential heating installations and in many medium-capacity industrial burners. Residential heating constitutes the largest single nontransportation use of distillate fuels. While the intended use of these materials is as fuels, minor amounts may find their way into nonfuel uses, such as incorporation into drilling muds, herbicides and metal forming oils. The uses of kerosene range from its historical use as a lighting oil to oil for cooking and a source for fuel heating, both in furnaces and space heaters in homes and shops, and to industrial use as an aluminium roll oil.

Attempts were made to develop a carburettor that used kerosene in place of gasoline as a fuel during the early development of automobiles with an internal combustion engine. Although these efforts were abandoned, kerosene came into use as a light diesel fuel and is currently used as a diesel fuel No. 1 (see the monograph on diesel fuel), for instance, as a fuel for farm machinery. It has also had numerous other uses, e.g., as a degreasing solvent and weed killer and even in old-fashioned home remedies for treating snake bites, infections and as a deworming agent for animals and humans. It is still used in insecticides and other pesticides under regulated conditions.

Uses of residual fuel oils in the USA are shown in Table 10. Residual fuel oils are used by electric utilities, the maritime industry, industrial and commercial plants and factories, and in the petroleum industry in the production of process steam, space and water heating, and in applications such as pipeline pumping and gas compression. Electric power generation accounts for the largest percentage of US domestic consumption (~39% in 1983), followed by vessel bunkering, industrial commercial and oil company applications. Like distillates, residual fuel oils are sometimes used in nonfuel applications, such as road oils and in the manufacture of asphalt cements.

Table 10. Deliveries of residual fuel oils by use in the USA (thousands of barrels)[a]

Year	Electric utility	Vessel bunkering	Industrial	Commercial	Oil company	All other
1979	486 636	190 543	198 759	82 729	51 062	24 881
1980	390 105	213 131	163 564	98 034	59 519	13 113
1981	325 486	188 632	117 024	67 035	51 870	11 981
1982	227 419	152 586	122 619	65 781	45 319	12 783
1983	204 328	136 290	89 573[b]	46 743[b]	32 820[b]	8 940

[a]From US Department of Energy (1983)
[b]Estimates

2.2 Occurrence

(a) Occupational exposure

Potential occupational exposure to fuel oils (heating oils) has been associated with the following operations (CONCAWE, 1985): manually handled filling and discharge; tank dipping, pipeline and pump repairs, filter cleaning in refineries, distribution terminals and depots; tank inspection, cleaning and repair; servicing, testing and maintaining heating systems and equipment using heating oil; routine sampling and laboratory handling of fuel oils; and practices in which heating oils are used as cleaning agents or solvents.

Worker exposure to hydrocarbons was measured during the cleaning of ten tanks containing different types of heating oil in Sweden. The concentration of total hydrocarbons (personal sampling) was found to range from 240 mg/m^3 (time-weighted average (TWA) during 55 min) to 1615 mg/m^3 (TWA during 45 min). Hydrocarbon concentrations were higher in the cleaning of heavy oil industrial tanks than in the cleaning of home fuel oil tanks. The difference was ascribed to vaporization of heavy oil due to its handling in the heated state (Ahlström *et al.*, 1986).

Similar results were obtained in another Swedish study on tank cleaners with short-term samples ranging from 89 mg/m^3 (tank size, 3 m^3) to 1032 mg/m^3 (tank size, 150 m^3) for total hydrocarbons. Benzene (see IARC, 1982, 1987b) concentrations ranged from 4 to 8 mg/m^3. Vaporized domestic oil was found to consist of about 50% linear or branched alkanes (carbon numbers 6–14), 20% cyclopentanes and cyclohexanes and about 30% alkylbenzenes (Lillienberg, 1986; Lillienberg *et al.*, 1987).

Readings of total hydrocarbon levels taken in one emptied light-oil tank ranged from 100–300 ppm (Högstedt *et al.*, 1981). Oil tank cleaners were described as spraying white spirit and xylene onto the walls of tanks that had contained heavy oils.

The use of residual fuel oils as heating oils may result in the evolution of hydrogen sulfide gas when they are manipulated while hot (CONCAWE, 1985).

(b) Environmental occurrence

Table 11 lists some accidental releases of fuel oil that have been reported in the recent past.

2.3 Analysis

Since fuel oils are composed of a complex mixture of hydrocarbons, there are few methods for the environmental analysis of 'fuel oils' as an entity, but many methods are reported for the analysis of their component hydrocarbons. These methods are used to identify or 'fingerprint' the origin of a specific fuel oil sample on the basis of the proportions of its component hydrocarbons.

A method for the mass measurement of hydrocarbons has been applied to monitoring fuel oil vapour. It involves the collection of vapours in graphite tubes, their extraction and subsequent measurement with an infrared spectrophotometer (Ahlström *et al.*, 1986).

Table 11. Recent, selected, large accidental releases of fuel oil (heating oil)

Place	Date	Type	Quantity	Reference
West Falmouth, MA, USA	September 1969	Fuel oil No. 2 from grounding of barge, *Florida*	650 000–700 000 l	Blumer & Sass (1972); Sanders *et al.* (1980)
Chedabucto Bay, Nova Scotia, Canada	February 1970	Bunker C fuel oil from grounding of tanker, *Arrow*	108 000 barrels (1.75 million l)	Levy (1971); Keizer *et al.* (1978)
Brittany coast, France	March 1980	Bunker C fuel oil from wreck of tanker, *Tanio*	8100 tonnes	Berne & Bodennec (1984)
Yaquina Bay, OR, USA	November 1983	Bunker C fuel oil and diesel fuel from wreck of tanker, *Blue Magpie*	284 000 l	Kemp *et al.* (1986)
Stockholm, Sweden	October 1977	Fuel oil No. 5 from grounding of tanker, *Tsesis*	>1000 tonnes	Johansson *et al.* (1980)
Searsport, ME, USA	March–June 1971	Storage facility spill of fuel oil No. 2 mixed with JP-5 jet fuel	>14 tonnes	Dow *et al.* (1975)
Floreffe, PA, USA	December 1987	Rupture of fuel oil No. 2 storage tank[a]	3 million gallons (11.4 million l)	MacKerron & Kiesche (1988)

[a]See also the monograph on diesel fuel

Methods based on charcoal adsorption, carbon disulfide desorption and analysis by gas chromatography with various calibration standards have been reported and compared with the infrared spectrophotometric method (Lillienberg, 1986; Lillienberg *et al.*, 1987).

3. Biological Data Relevant to the Evaluation of Carcinogenic Risk to Humans

3.1 Carcinogenicity studies in animals

Studies on the carcinogenicity in experimental animals of straight-run kerosene [5], light [24] and heavy [26] catalytically cracked distillates, light [19] and heavy [20] vacuum distillates, catalytically cracked clarified oils [27], thermally cracked residues [31] and steam-cracked residues [34], which are components of fuel oils, are described in the monograph on occupational exposures in petroleum refining.

Skin application[1]

Mouse: Groups of 19-40 C3H mice [sex and age unspecified] received twice weekly [duration unspecified] skin applications [not otherwise specified] of 20 or 50 mg of blended fuel oils obtained by adding different amounts of residue [31] (>371°C) from thermal cracking of catalytically cracked clarified oil [the material tested was essentially thermally cracked residue [31]; the feed stream [27] is of secondary importance] to either a cracked bunker fuel (base stock A) or a West Texas uncracked residue [8 or 21] (base stock B). The benzo[*a*]pyrene content of the two blends and the incidences of skin tumours are given in Table 12. Cracked bunker fuel produced malignant and benign skin tumours at both dose levels. The addition of various amounts of cracked residue resulted in an increase in tumour frequency and a decrease in latency (Bingham *et al.*, 1980). [The Working Group noted that the original work was carried out by another investigator (Horton, 1957) in the same laboratory.]

Groups of 25 male and 25 female C3H/Bd$_f$ mice, six to eight weeks old, received thrice weekly skin applications on a 1-cm² clipped dorsal area of 50 μl undiluted, 1:1 diluted or 1:3 diluted fuel oil No. 2 (American Petroleum Institute No. 975) in acetone [duration unspecified]. Animals were killed two weeks after tumour appearance. Groups of 25 male and 25 females received thrice weekly applications of 50 μg, 25 μg or 12.5 μg benzo[*a*]pyrene dissolved in 50 μl acetone and served as positive controls. Further groups of 50 males and 50 females received 50 μl acetone thrice weekly or no treatment and served as negative controls. The fuel oil sample contained 0.04 μg/g benzo[*a*]pyrene, 0.07 μg/g five- to six-ring polycyclic aromatic hydrocarbons (1.2 wt % polyaromatic hydrocarbons). Of 150 mice treated with fuel oil No. 2, 15 developed 17 carcinomas and two papillomas of the skin. No skin tumour was observed in the acetone-treated or untreated control groups, whereas benzo[*a*]pyrene induced tumours in nearly all mice (Witschi *et al.*, 1987). [The Working Group noted that the exact distribution of tumours among the various treated groups was not reported.]

3.2 Other relevant data

(a) Experimental systems

Absorption, distribution, excretion and metabolism

(i) *Fuel oil No. 1 (Kerosene)*

Aromatic hydrocarbons were found in the blood of rats following intragastric administration of kerosene for domestic use (Gerarde, 1959, 1964).

Baboons were administered kerosene [unspecified] (15 ml/kg bw) labelled with ³H-toluéne or ¹⁴C-hexadecane by nasogastric intubation after a tracheotomy had been performed. After 6 h of exposure, ³H-toluene appeared to have been absorbed and taken up by most tissues to a greater extent than ¹⁴C-hexadecane (Mann *et al.*, 1977).

---

[1]The Working Group was aware of skin-painting studies in progress in mice using fuel oil No. 2 based on straight-run middle distillate [6] (three samples) or light catalytically cracked distillate [24] (three samples) (IARC, 1986).

Table 12. Incidences of skin tumours in C3H mice following application of blended fuel oils[a]

Base blending stock[b]	Cracked residue added (%)	Benzo[a]-pyrene content (%)	Dose (mg)	No. of mice	Final effective number[c]	No. of mice developing tumours		Average time to appearance of papillomas	
						Malignant	Benign	Weeks	SD
A	0	0.01	20	19	17	1	1	—	
			50	20	17	3	7	58.8	4.7
B	0	0	20	40	23	0	1	—	
A	5	0.05	20	30	27	15	8	41.5	3.6
			50	30	27	13	8	28.3	3.3
B	5	0.04	20	40	31	9	11	49.1	5.5
			50	48	27	9	9	36.9	3.3
A	10	0.08	20	30	26	19	7	40.4	3.2
			50	30	25	22	3	32.2	2.5
B	10	0.075	20	40	35	22	13	40.5	1.9
			50	30	30	9	18	26.7	1.6
A	20	0.16	20	25	23	12	9	25.2	2.8
B	20	0.15	20	29	28	11	16	23.4	1.7

[a]From Bingham et al. (1980)
[b] A, cracked bunker fuel; B, West Texas uncracked residue
[c]Number alive at the time of appearance of the median tumour plus the number of tumour-bearing mice that died earlier

(ii) *Fuel oil No. 2*

The accumulation and release of petroleum hydrocarbons by aquatic organisms, including selected data on fuel oil No. 2, have been reviewed (Lee, 1977; Neff & Anderson, 1981). Fuel oil No. 2 has been shown to be metabolized to conjugates of several two- and three-ring aromatic hydrocarbons in fish (Krahn & Malins, 1982; Hellou & Payne, 1987).

Toxic effects

(i) *Fuel oil No. 1 (kerosene)*

The oral LD_{50} of one brand of kerosene was 28 ml/kg bw in rabbits and 20 ml/kg bw in guinea-pigs, while 28 ml/kg bw killed four of 15 rats (Deichmann *et al.*, 1944). The LD_{50} for kerosene administered by the intratracheal route was approximately 1 ml/kg bw (Gerarde, 1959).

Air saturated at 25°C with deodorized kerosene vapours (55.2% paraffins, 40.9% naphthenes, 3.9% aromatics; 0.10 mg/l (14 ppm)) did not induce death in rats, dogs or cats following an 8-h inhalation period (Carpenter *et al.*, 1976).

In tracheotomized monkeys killed 6–8 h after administration of 45 ml/kg bw kerosene [presumably for domestic use] via a nasogastric tube, macroscopic and microscopic examination showed heavy oedematous lungs with patchy haemorrhagic areas. Similar results were observed in animals receiving 1.0 ml kerosene intravenously or 0.2 ml endotracheally (Wolfsdorf & Kundig, 1972).

The lungs of rabbits administered 25 ml/kg bw kerosene [presumably for domestic use] by stomach tube showed slight congestion and focal atelectasis but no evidence of pneumonia or bronchitis when the animals were killed seven days after dosing (Richardson & Pratt-Thomas, 1951).

Both an intravenous dose of 0.50 ml/kg bw kerosene [presumably for domestic use] and an intratracheal dose of 1.0 ml/kg bw were fatal to dogs after 8 h and 10 min, respectively. Dogs administered kerosene by stomach tube at doses of 2–30 ml/kg bw survived. In animals that were sacrificed and autopsied one to 18 days after receiving the oil, severe lung damage was seen only in animals that had vomited (Richardson & Pratt-Thomas, 1951).

Levels of haem biosynthesis enzymes (δ-aminolaevulinic acid synthetase and dehydratase) were decreased in the liver of Wistar rats 3 and 20 h after intraperitoneal administration of commercial kerosene (1.0 ml/kg bw), whereas levels of haem oxygenase (involved in haem degradation) remained unchanged (Rao & Pandya, 1980).

Rats exposed to deodorized kerosene mists at concentrations of 75 and 300 mg/m³ for 14 days developed liver steatosis characterized by an increase in free fatty acids, phospholipids and cholesterol esters and decreases in triglycerides. Various serum enzyme levels were also elevated (Starek & Kamiński, 1982).

When rats were given repeated subcutaneous administrations of commercial kerosene (0.5 ml/kg bw) on six days a week for 35 days, the weights of the liver, spleen and peripheral lymph nodes were increased and there were corresponding increases in the DNA, RNA, protein and lipid contents of liver and spleen. Histopathological effects were observed in a variety of tissues, while lymphocyte counts were lowered and neutrophil counts elevated.

The activity of liver alkaline phosphatase increased and that of benzo[*a*]pyrene hydroxylase decreased. Serum cholinesterase and carboxylesterase activities and albumin levels were reduced, while serum alkaline phosphatase activity was greatly enhanced (Rao *et al.*, 1984).

A group of 12 male and female guinea-pigs was exposed to kerosene [product obtained directly from a refinery] aerosols (ranging from 20.4 to 34 mg aerosol/l air) for 15 min daily over 21 consecutive days. Ten animals were kept in atmospheric air. Increased numbers of macrophages, neutrophils, eosinophils and lymphocytes were found in the pulmonary washings of treated animals (Noa *et al.*, 1985). Severe alterations of the ciliated epithelium of the trachea were also observed in five male guinea-pigs given a mean concentration of 32.5 mg/l (Noa & Sanabria, 1984). In 23 male guinea-pigs exposed to 20.4–34 mg/l, aortic plaques developed, with fibrous tissue, collagen and elastic fibres, and smooth-muscle cells resembling those seen in atherosclerosis (Noa & Illnait, 1987).

(ii) *Fuel oil No. 2*

The oral LD_{50}s of three No. 2 home heating oils in rats were 12.0, 15.7 and 17.5 g/kg bw. No mortality was induced in rabbits painted on the skin with the oils at 5 g/kg bw (Beck *et al.*, 1984).

The toxic effects of fuel oil No. 2 in birds and aquatic organisms have been reviewed (Rice *et al.*, 1977; Holmes *et al.*, 1978; Szaro *et al.*, 1981; Wells & Percy, 1985).

(iii) *Bunker fuel*

No adverse effect was observed in sheep fed about 100 g (10% in hay) bunker fuel per day for up to ten days (MacIntyre, 1970).

Effects on reproduction and prenatal toxicity

As reported in a review of teratology studies in rats exposed to different fuels by inhalation, exposure of animals on days 6–15 of gestation for 6 h per day to 100 and 365 ppm kerosene [unspecified] or to 85 and 410 ppm fuel oil No. 2 resulted in no teratogenic effect (Schreiner, 1984). [The Working Group noted that details were not reported.]

Several studies have shown pronounced effects of fuel oil No. 2 on the reproductive capacity of birds after application on the shell surface (decreased hatchability, deformed bills, dead embryos; Albers & Szaro, 1978; Coon *et al.*, 1979; White *et al.*, 1979; Albers & Heinz, 1983). Studies in chick embryos with fractionated fuel oil No. 2 indicated that toxicity was associated primarily with the two- to three-ring aromatic fraction (Ellenton, 1982). Bunker fuel also reduced duck egg hatchability (Szaro, 1979). [The Working Group noted that the avian system is a sensitive model for embryotoxic effects; results should be interpreted with caution with respect to possible effects in mammalian systems.]

Genetic and related effects

(i) *Fuel oil No. 1 (kerosene)*

Kerosene (boiling range, 177–271°C; 18% aromatics) was not mutagenic to *Salmonella typhimurium* TA98 or TA100 in the presence or absence of an exogenous metabolic system from rat liver, using the plate incorporation (0.001–5 μl/plate) or suspension (6.25–50 μl/ml) methods. It did not induce forward mutations in mouse lymphoma L5178Y TK$^{+/-}$ cells in the presence or absence of an exogenous metabolic system from rat or mouse liver. Kerosene did not induce chromosomal aberrations in the bone marrow of Sprague-Dawley rats killed 6 and 48 h after a single intraperitoneal injection of 0.04–0.4 ml/rat or after repeated daily intraperitoneal injections of 0.02-0.18 ml/rat for five days (Conaway et al., 1984).

(ii) *Fuel oil No. 2*

Fuel oil No. 2 gave borderline positive results for mutagenicity in *S. typhimurium* TA98 and TA100 both in the presence and absence of an exogenous metabolic system from rat liver, using the plate incorporation method (0.26–42 mg/plate), while it was clearly mutagenic to mouse lymphoma L5178Y TK$^{+/-}$ cells in forward mutation assays at a concentration of 1.2 μl/ml in the absence of an exogenous metabolic system, giving a mutation frequency 17.1 times that in solvent control cultures (Conaway et al., 1984).

Of three fractions of fuel oil No. 2 tested in *S. typhimurium* TA1535, TA1537, TA1538, TA98 and TA100, only the four- to seven-ring polycyclic aromatic hydrocarbon fraction induced a dose-dependent increase in the number of revertants in strain TA100 in the presence of an exogenous metabolic system from Aroclor 1254-induced rat liver. The same fraction and the one- to three-ring aromatic hydrocarbon fraction caused dose-dependent increases in the frequency of sister chromatid exchange, but not of chromosomal aberrations, in Chinese hamster ovary cells in the presence of an exogenous metabolic system from Aroclor 1254-induced rat liver (Ellenton & Hallett, 1981).

As reported in an abstract, home heating oil [not otherwise specified] induced transformed foci in both BALBc/3T3 and C3H/10T1/2 cells (Butala et al., 1985).

Fuel oil No. 2 induced chromosomal aberrations in the bone marrow of Sprague-Dawley rats administered 0.125–1.25 g/kg bw per day by gavage for five successive days (Conaway et al., 1984).

(iii) *Residual fuel oils*

Bunker fuel was not mutagenic to *S. typhimurium* TA1535, TA1538, TA98 or TA100 either in the presence or absence of an exogenous metabolic system from Aroclor 1254-induced rat liver (Vandermeulen et al., 1985), and did not induce forward mutation (streptomycin resistance) in *Chlamydomonas reinhardtii* (Vandermeulen & Lee, 1986). As reported in an abstract, dual-purpose and residual fuel oil were not active in *S. typhimurium* in the presence or absence of an exogenous metabolic system from Aroclor 1254-induced rat liver (Farrow et al., 1983).

B-class heavy oil (containing many polycyclic aromatic hydrocarbons and basic nitrogen-containing chemicals, such as aza-arenes) induced an increase in the frequency of chromosomal aberrations in cultured Chinese hamster lung cells (12% *versus* <5% in controls) at a concentration of 2.0 mg/ml in the presence of an exogenous metabolic system from rat liver. A fraction separated by liquid-liquid extraction, in which the basic nitrogen-containing polycyclic hydrocarbons were included, gave clearly positive results and was more active (e.g., 17% at 0.48 mg/ml; 24.0% at 0.25 mg/ml for the same fraction of another lot of B class heavy oil) than the unfractionated oil. Other similarly extracted fractions, containing high molecular weight hexane-insoluble ingredients or *n*-paraffin, *iso*-paraffin, polycyclic hydrocarbons and sulfur-containing compounds, or neutral or weakly basic nitrogen-containing compounds, did not induce chromosomal aberrations in cultured Chinese hamster lung cells even in the presence of an exogenous metabolic system (Matsuoka *et al.*, 1982).

As reported in an abstract, dual-purpose and residual fuel oils did not induce sister chromatid exchange in cultured Chinese hamster ovary cells nor mutations in cultured mouse lymphoma L5178Y $TK^{+/-}$ cells, in the presence or absence of an exogenous metabolic system from Aroclor 1254-induced rat liver (Farrow *et al.*, 1983).

(b) Humans

Absorption, distribution, excretion and metabolism

No adequate data were available to the Working Group.

Toxic effects

Series of tens to hundreds of cases of accidental ingestion of kerosene in children have been reported from Australia (Isbister, 1963), Barbados (St John, 1982), Denmark (Brunner *et al.*, 1964), India (Saksena, 1969), Indonesia (Aldy *et al.*, 1978), Iraq (Nouri & Al-Rahim, 1970), Kuwait (Majeed *et al.*, 1981), the USA (Nunn & Martin, 1934; Heacock, 1949), Zaire (Muganga *et al.*, 1986), Zimbabwe (Baldachin & Melmed, 1964) and other countries. Kerosene poisoning is a common childhood poisoning in some parts of the world; similar effects can occur in adults (Vidal & Ferrando, 1974).

Childhood kerosene poisoning (Nunn & Martin, 1934; Heacock, 1949; Isbister, 1963; Brünner *et al.*, 1964) usually occurs in children from one to three years old, most often in boys. Most cases are mild. In those more severely affected, there is initial coughing and involuntary deep respiration, followed by accelerated, rattling breathing, tachycardia and cyanosis, frequently associated with spontaneous vomiting, nausea and abdominal pain. Bronchopneumonia frequently occurs. Chest X-ray findings include multiple, small, cloudy lung infiltrations, which may coalesce to form lobular or lobar infiltrations, mostly in the lung bases. Bilateral perihilar vascular markings may also be seen. The pneumonia and X-ray changes usually resolve within several days. Complications include pleural effusion (Scott, 1944; Tal *et al.*, 1984), pneumatocele (Tal *et al.*, 1984), oedema (Lesser *et al.*, 1943) and, more rarely, mediastinal and soft-tissue emphysema (Scott, 1944; Marandian *et al.*, 1981). Central nervous system depression is seen in a minority of patients, which may progress to coma and convulsions (Nouri & Al-Rahim, 1970; Aldy *et al.*, 1978). Death occurs in up to 10% of reported cases. Individuals who die usually have rapid onset of shock and pulmonary changes, and may have convulsions. Autopsy shows generalized haemorrhagic oedema of the lungs (Baldachin & Melmed, 1964) and may show cellular degeneration in the liver (Nunn & Martin, 1934).

Subclinical small airway abnormalities and abnormal chest radiographs (residual bullae or increased markings) can be seen ten years after childhood kerosene pneumonitis; their presence is related to the severity of the acute primary pneumonia (Tal *et al.*, 1984).

Indonesian kerosene retailers who were frequently in contact with kerosene developed nocturnal itching, reddening, peeling and chapping of the skin (Suma'mur & Wenas, 1978). Irritant dermatitis has been seen in children following contact with kerosene-soaked clothing (Tagami & Ogino, 1973).

In skin patch tests of kerosene products with boiling ranges of 177–316°C, irritant reactions, sometimes of severe degree, were produced in most individuals; irritation was correlated with kerosene content. Kerosene of paraffinic origin was less irritating than that of naphthenic origin within the same boiling range (Klauder & Brill, 1947; Tagami & Ogino, 1973).

Effects on reproduction and prenatal toxicity
No data were available to the Working Group.

Genetic and related effects
A group of 16 tank cleaners were studied for cytogenetic changes; a subgroup of men who had cleaned light and heavy oil tanks was also included. Micronuclei in bone-marrow cells and chromosomal aberrations in peripheral blood lymphocytes were reported to be significantly more prevalent in the whole group than in the control group (Högstedt *et al.*, 1981). [The Working Group noted that the results were not reported separately for the different subgroups of cleaners and that the workers would have been subjected to mixed exposures.]

3.3 Epidemiological studies and case reports of carcinogenicity to humans

(*a*) *Cohort studies*

Tsuchiya (1965) conducted a large historical cohort study of some 400 000 (1 200 000 person-years) Japanese workers during the period 1957–59. Information on both exposure and disease was obtained from questionnaires distributed to health supervisors of 200 companies each employing over 1000 persons; 100% of the forms were returned. Exposure was defined either as the type of chemicals to which the worker had been exposed, listed by the health supervisor, or as the type of industry in which he was employed. No measurement of level or length of exposure was obtained. During the three-year period, 808 cancer cases were identified, 492 of which resulted in death, among workers aged 20–59 years. An excess of lung cancer (55 deaths and newly-diagnosed cases) was observed among workers described as having been exposed to kerosene, diesel oil, crude petroleum and mineral oil [estimated odds ratio, 2.7; 95% confidence interval (CI), 1.4–5.3] when considered as a group. [The Working Group noted the poor statistical analysis and the poor handling of the limited information on smoking.]

Okubo and Tsuchiya (1974) conducted a large cohort study that covered a population of about 1 200 000 employees at 515 factories in Japan. Information on exposure and on cancer deaths was obtained from questionnaires distributed to health supervisors in each factory. Exposure was assessed by industry, occupation, duration of employment and possible exposure to chemical or physical agents. During the period 1966–68, 1140 cancer deaths were identified. After controlling for age and sex, an excess of stomach cancer was observed among workers possibly exposed to kerosene, machine oil or grease. Leukaemia was reported to have occurred in excess in industries where kerosene, paraffin oil or petroleum combustibles were reported as having been used or produced.

[The Working Group noted that the results of these two studies are difficult to interpret due to the very general assessment of exposure and to the lack of information on expected numbers and on confounding variables.]

(b) Case-control studies

Using data from the Third National Cancer Survey, the National Occupational Hazard Survey and the National Health and Nutrition Examination Survey to investigate occupational health problems, Spiegelman and Wegman (1985) conducted a case-control study of 343 men diagnosed as having a colorectal cancer between 1969 and 1971 in seven US metropolitan areas and two states. Controls were 626 men with cancers other than of the digestive system, respiratory tract, urinary tract, bone, skin, mouth or pharynx or leukaemia. Exposure to 11 occupational carcinogens was assessed from occupations and industries reported to the Third National Cancer Survey. In order to control for diet as a potential confounder, a nutritional score was calculated for each subject on the basis of data from the National Health and Nutrition Examination Survey. Using logistic regression analysis, the authors observed an increased odds ratio for colorectal cancer associated with exposure to solvents (odds ratio, 1.6; 95% CI, 1.1–2.3; $p = 0.01$) and to fuel oil (odds ratio, 1.5; 1.1–2.0; $p = 0.01$), controlling for age, weight, race and diet. The increases were slightly higher for colon cancer. There was a trend with increasing exposure to solvents but not to fuel oil. [The Working Group noted that exposure to neither 'fuel oil' nor 'solvent' was defined, but the two were highly correlated.]

In a large case-control study of cancer at many sites in Montréal, Canada, which is described in detail in the monograph on gasoline (p. 185; Siematycki *et al.*, 1987), an association was observed between exposure to kerosene and stomach cancer (adjusted odds ratio, 1.7; 90% CI, 1.2–2.5) and between exposure to heating oil and rectal cancer (adjusted odds ratio, 1.4; 0.7–2.7); with 'substantial' exposure to heating oil, the odds ratio for rectal cancer was 2.6 (1.2–5.5). There was also a significant association between exposure to heating oil and oat-cell cancer of the lung (odds ratio, 1.7; 1.2–3.4). The authors noted that the association between kerosene and stomach cancer was entirely attributable to a stomach cancer risk among forestry workers.

Three case-control studies were carried out to investigate the high incidence of lung cancer in women in Hong Kong in relation to use of kerosene cooking stoves. In comparing the cooking habits of 44 women with histologically demonstrated lung cancer with those of 314 families interviewed at random in Hong Kong, Leung (1977) observed that a higher proportion of cases (91%) had used kerosene cooking stoves than controls (36%). The authors concluded that both exposure to kerosene stoves and cigarette smoking were strongly associated with lung cancer in women in Hong Kong.

In a similar study in which 189 hospitalized women with a histologically confirmed diagnosis of bronchial cancer were compared with 189 control patients from the orthopaedic wards of the same hospital, Chan *et al.* (1979) observed an odds ratio [estimated by the Working Group] for use of kerosene stoves among all women of 1.6 (95% CI, 0.99−2.6) and among nonsmoking women of 2.1 (1.1−4.1).

Koo *et al.* (1983) conducted a case-control study of 200 hospitalized women with lung cancer and 200 control women from the general population matched for age, district of residence and type of housing. Odds ratios were estimated for different types and levels of exposure after controlling for smoking. Higher risks were observed among women with more than 30 years' use of kerosene for cooking (age-adjusted odds ratio for nonsmokers, 1.4; 95% CI, 1.1−1.9; $p = 0.02$; odds ratio for smokers, 2.5; 1.2−5.4; $p = 0.02$). Controls were more likely to have used liquid petroleum gas-type fuel.

[The Working Group considered that the predominant inhalation exposure of the women in these studies would have been to the combustion products of kerosene and not to the product itself. In view of a recent study from Shanghai, China (Gao *et al.*, 1987), exposure to cooking oil may have contributed to the observed effects.]

4. Summary of Data Reported and Evaluation[1]

4.1 Exposure data

Fuel oils are complex and variable mixtures of alkanes and alkenes, cycloalkanes and aromatic hydrocarbons, containing low percentages of sulfur, nitrogen and oxygen compounds. Kerosene fuel oils are manufactured from straight-run petroleum distillates from the boiling range of kerosene [5]. Other distillate fuel oils contain straight-run middle distillate [6], often blended with straight-run gas oil [7] and light vacuum distillates [19], and light cracked distillates [24, 30]. The main components of residual fuel oils are the heavy residues from distillation and cracking operations [8, 21, 31]; various refinery by-products and heavy distillates [20, 26, 27] may be added. In fuel oils consisting mainly of atmospheric distillates, the content of three- to seven-ring polycyclic aromatic hydrocarbons is generally less than 5%. In fuel oils that contain high proportions of heavy atmospheric, vacuum and cracked distillates or atmospheric and vacuum residues, the content of three- to seven-ring polycyclic aromatic hydrocarbons may be as high as 10%; if large quantities of cracked components are incorporated, levels may approach 20%. Fuel oils are used mainly in industrial and domestic heating, as well as in the production of steam and electricity in power plants. Skin and inhalation exposures to fuel oil may occur during its production, storage, distribution and use and during maintenance of heating equipment. During the cleaning of fuel oil tanks, high, short-term exposures to total hydrocarbon vapours have been measured at levels ranging from 100−1600 mg/m^3.

---

[1]The numbers in square brackets are those assigned to the major process streams of petroleum refining in Table 2 of the monograph on occupational exposures in petroleum refining (p. 44).

4.2 Experimental data[1]

A cracked bunker fuel was tested both alone and blended with the residue from the thermal cracking of catalytically cracked clarified oil [31] by skin application to mice. When applied alone, it induced benign and malignant skin tumours; a further increase was observed when cracked residue was added to the blend.

A West Texas uncracked residue [8 or 21] was tested alone or in combination with the residue described above [31]. When tested alone, it produced one skin papilloma, but a high incidence of skin papillomas and carcinomas was observed when cracked residue was added to the blend.

One sample of fuel oil No. 2 was tested by skin application to mice and produced skin carcinomas and papillomas.

Two samples of straight-run kerosene [5], one sample of light vacuum distillate [19], several samples of heavy vacuum distillates [20] and three samples of light catalytically cracked distillates [24] produced skin tumours in mice. Several heavy catalytically cracked distillates [26], residues of catalytically cracked clarified oils [27], thermally cracked residues [31] and steam-cracked residues [34] produced high incidences of benign and malignant skin tumours in mice. (See the monograph on occupational exposures in petroleum refining.)

4.3 Human data

Two large historical cohort studies of workers were conducted in Japan. In the first, an excess of lung cancer was observed among men exposed to kerosene, diesel oil, crude petroleum and mineral oil considered as a group. In the second, an excess of stomach cancer was observed among workers possibly exposed to kerosene, machine oil or grease. Leukaemia was reported to have occurred in excess in industries where kerosene, paraffin oil or petroleum combustibles were said to have been used or produced. Since none of the exposures could be defined clearly, these results are difficult to interpret.

In a large case-control study, a significant excess of colorectal cancer was associated with estimated exposure to solvents and fuel oil. In a second, an excess of stomach cancer was associated with exposure to kerosene, and excesses of rectal cancer and oat-cell lung cancer with exposure to heating oil.

Three case-control studies found a relationship between lung cancer and use of kerosene stoves for cooking in women in Hong Kong. No distinction was made between exposure to kerosene and exposure to its combustion products.

---

[1]Subsequent to the meeting, the Secretariat became aware of one article accepted for publication in which it was reported that skin tumours developed in mice after skin application of furnace oil [probably fuel oil No. 2] in initiating/promoting studies (Gerhart *et al.*, 1988), and of another study in which it was reported that skin tumours developed in mice after skin application of several samples of commercial No. 2 heating oil [fuel oil No. 2] (Biles *et al.*, 1988).

4.4 Other relevant datas

Kerosene ingestion is a common cause of childhood poisoning and may result in lung damage.

No report specifically designed to study genetic and related effects in humans following exposure to fuel oil was available to the Working Group.

In single studies, kerosene did not induce chromosomal aberrations in rat bone marrow, nor did it induce mutation in cultured mammalian cells or in bacteria.

In single studies, fuel oil No. 2 induced chromosomal aberrations in rat bone marrow and mutation in cultured mammalian cells and in bacteria. Aromatic fractions of fuel oil No. 2 induced sister chromatid exchange, but not chromosomal aberrations, in cultured mammalian cells. One four- to seven-ring polycyclic aromatic hydrocarbon fraction of fuel oil No. 2 induced mutation in bacteria.

In single studies, a heavy fuel oil [B-class] induced chromosomal aberrations in cultured mammalian cells; bunker fuel did not induce mutation in bacteria or algae. (See Appendix 1.)

4.5 Evaluation[1]

There is *inadequate evidence* for the carcinogenicity in humans of fuel oils.

There is *sufficient evidence* for the carcinogenicity in experimental animals of residual (heavy) fuel oils.

There is *limited evidence* for the carcinogenicity in experimental animals of fuel oil No. 2.

In formulating the overall evaluation, the Working Group also took note of the following supporting evidence reported in the monograph on occupational exposures in petroleum refining. There is *sufficient evidence* for the carcinogenicity in experimental animals of light and heavy catalytically cracked distillates, of light and heavy vacuum distillates and of cracked residues derived from the refining of crude oil. There is *limited evidence* for the carcinogenicity in experimental animals of straight-run kerosene.

Overall evaluation

Residual (heavy) fuel oils *are possibly carcinogenic to humans (Group 2B)*.

Distillate (light) fuel oils *are not classifiable as to their carcinogenicity to humans (Group 3)*.

---

[1] For definitions of the italicized terms, see Preamble, pp. 24–28.

5. References

Ahlström, R., Berglund, B., Berglund, U., Lindvall, T. & Wennberg, A. (1986) Impaired odor perception in tank cleaners. *Scand. J. Work Environ. Health, 12*, 574–581

Albers, P.H. & Heinz, G.H. (1983) FLIT-MLO and no. 2 fuel oil: effects of aerosol applications to mallard eggs on hatchability and behavior of ducklings. *Environ. Res., 30*, 381–388

Albers, P.H. & Szaro, R.C. (1978) Effects of No. 2 fuel oil on common eider eggs. *Mar. Pollut. Bull., 9*, 138–139

Aldy, D., Siregar, R. & Siregar, H. (1978) Accidental poisoning in children with special reference to kerosene poisoning. *Pediatr. Indones., 18*, 45–50

American Society for Testing and Materials (1986) *Standard specifications for fuel oils (ASTM D 396-86).* In: *Annual Book of ASTM Standards*, Vol. 05.01, Philadelphia, PA, pp. 210–215

Anon. (1966) *Encyclopaedia Britannica*, Vol. 10, London, William Benton, p. 368

Baldachin, B.J. & Melmed, R.N. (1964) Clinical and therapeutic aspects of kerosene poisoning: a series of 200 cases. *Br. med. J., ii*, 28–30

Beck, L.S., Hepler, D.I. & Hansen, K.L. (1984) *The acute toxicology of selected petroleum hydrocarbons.* In: MacFarland, H.N., Holdsworth, C.E., MacGregor, J.A., Call, R.W. & Lane, M.L., eds, *Advances in Modern Environmental Toxicology*, Vol. VI, *Applied Toxicology of Petroleum Hydrocarbons*, Princeton, NJ, Princeton Scientific Publishers, pp. 1–6

Berne, S. & Bodennec, G. (1984) Evolution of hydrocarbons after the *Tanio* oil spill. A comparison with the *Amoco Cadiz* accident. *Ambio, 13*, 109–114

Biles, R.W., McKee, R.H., Lewis, S.C., Scala, R.A. & DePass, L.R. (1988) Dermal carcinogenic activity of petroleum-derived middle distillate fuels. *Toxicology, 53*, 301–314

Bingham, E., Trosset, R.P. & Warshawsky, D. (1980) Carcinogenic potential of petroleum hydrocarbons. A critical review of the literature. *J. environ. Pathol. Toxicol., 3*, 483–563

Blumer, M. & Sass, J. (1972) Oil pollution: persistence and degradation of spilled fuel oil. *Science, 176*, 1120–1122

Boduszynski, M.M., McKay, J.F. & Latham, D.R. (1981) Composition of heavy ends of a Russian petroleum. *Am. chem. Soc., 26*, 865–880

Brünner, S., Rovsing, H. & Wulf, H. (1964) Roentgenographic changes in the lungs of children with kerosene poisoning. *Am. Rev. respir. Dis., 89*, 250–254

Butala, J.H., Strother, D.E., Thilagar, A.K. & Brecher, S. (1985) Cell transformation testing of unfractionated petroleum liquids (Abstract). *Environ. Mutagenesis, 7 (Suppl. 3)*, 37–38

Carpenter, C.P., Geary, D.L., Jr, Myers, R.C., Nachreiner, D.J., Sullivan, L.J. & King, J.M. (1976) Petroleum hydrocarbon toxicity studies. XI. Animal and human response to vapors of deodorized kerosene. *Toxicol. appl. Pharmacol., 36*, 443–456

Chan, W.C., Colbourne, M.J., Fung, S.C. & Ho, H.C. (1979) Bronchial cancer in Hong Kong, 1976-1977. *Br. J. Cancer, 39*, 182–192

Conaway, C.C., Schreiner, C.A. & Cragg, S.T. (1984) *Mutagenicity evaluation of petroleum hydrocarbons.* In: MacFarland, H.N., Holdsworth, C.E., MacGregor, J.A., Call, R.W. & Lane, M.L., eds, *Advances in Modern Environmental Toxicology*, Vol. VI, *Applied Toxicology of Petroleum Hydrocarbons*, Princeton, NJ, Princeton Scientific Publishers, pp. 89-107

CONCAWE (1985) *Health Aspects of Petroleum Fuels. Potential Hazards and Precautions for Individual Classes of Fuels* (*Report No. 85/81*), The Hague, pp. 16–35

Coon, N.C., Albers, P.H. & Szaro, R.C. (1979) No. 2 fuel oil decreases embryonic survival of great black-backed gulls. *Bull. environ. Contam. Toxicol.*, *21*, 152–156

Cruzan, G., Low, L.K., Cox, G.E., Meeks, J.R., Mackerer, C.R., Craig, P.H., Singer, E.J. & Mehlman, M.A. (1986) Systemic toxicity from subchronic dermal exposure, chemical characterization, and dermal penetration of catalytically cracked clarified slurry oil. *Toxicol. ind. Health*, *2*, 429–444

Deichmann, W.B., Kitzmiller, M.D., Witherup, S. & Johansmann, R. (1944) Kerosene intoxication. *Ann. intern. Med.*, *21*, 803–823

Dow, R.L., Hurst, J.W., Jr, Mayo, D.W., Cogger, C.G., Donovan, D.J., Gambardella, R.A., Jiang, L.C., Quan, I., Barry, M. & Yevich, P.P. (1975) The ecological, chemical and histopathological evaluation of an oil spill site. *Mar. Pollut. Bull.*, *6*, 164–173

Ellenton, J.A. (1982) Teratogenic activity of aliphatic and aromatic fractions of Prudhoe Bay crude and fuel oil no. 2 in the chicken embryo. *Toxicol. appl. Pharmacol.*, *63*, 209–215

Ellenton, J.A. & Hallett, D.J. (1981) Mutagenicity and chemical analysis of aliphatic and aromatic fractions of Prudhoe Bay crude oil and fuel oil No. 2. *J. Toxicol. environ. Health*, *8*, 959–972

Farrow, M.G., McCarroll, N., Cortina, T., Draus, M., Munson, A., Steinberg, M., Kirwin, C. & Thomas, W. (1983) In vitro mutagenicity and genotoxicity of fuels and paraffinic hydrocarbons in the Ames, sister chromatid exchange, and mouse lymphoma assays (Abstract No. 144). *Toxicologist*, *3*, 36

Gao, Y.-T., Blot, W.J., Zheng, W., Ershow, A.G., Hsu, C.W., Levin, L.I., Zhang, R. & Fraumeni, J.F., Jr (1987) Lung cancer among Chinese women. *Int. J. Cancer*, *40*, 604–609

Gerarde, H.W. (1959) Toxicological studies on hydrocarbons. V. Kerosine. *Toxicol. appl. Pharmacol.*, *1*, 462–474

Gerarde, H.W. (1964) Kerosine — experimental and clinical toxicology. *Occup. Health Rev.*, *16*, 17–21

Gerhart, J.M., Hatoum, N.S., Halder, C.A., Warne, T.M. & Schmitt, S.L. (1988) Tumor initiation and promotion effects of petroleum streams in mouse skin. *Fundam. appl. Toxicol.*, *11*, 76–90

Gräf, W. & Winter, C. (1968) 3,4-Benzopyrene in petroleum (Ger.). *Arch. Hyg. Bakteriol.*, *152*, 289–293

Green, J.B., Stierwalt, B.K., Thomson, J.S. & Treese, C.A. (1985) Rapid isolation of carboxylic acids from petroleum using high-performance liquid chromatography. *Anal. Chem.*, *57*, 2207–2211

Guthrie, B.C., ed. (1960) *Petroleum Products Handbook*, New York, McGraw-Hill

Heacock, C.H. (1949) Pneumonia in children following the ingestion of petroleum products. *Radiology*, *53*, 793–797

Hellou, J. & Payne, J.F. (1987) Assessment of contamination of fish by water soluble fractions of petroleum: a role for bile metabolites. *Environ. Toxicol. Chem.*, *6*, 857–862

Hoffman, H.L. (1982) Petroleum products. In: Grayson, M., ed., *Kirk-Othmer Encyclopedia of Chemical Technology*, 3rd ed., Vol. 17, New York, John Wiley & Sons, pp. 257–271

Högstedt, B., Gullberg, B., Mark-Vendel, E., Mitelman, F. & Skerfving, S. (1981) Micronuclei and chromosome aberrations in bone marrow cells and lymphocytes of humans exposed mainly to petroleum vapors. *Hereditas*, *94*, 179–187

Holmes, W.N., Cronshaw, J. & Gorsline, J. (1978) Some effects of ingested petroleum in seawater-adapted ducks (*Anas platyrhinchos*). *Environ. Res., 17*, 177−190

Horton, A.W. (1957) *Investigation of the Relationships between the Biological and Chemical Properties of Two Series of Blended Fuel Oils*, Cincinnati, OH, University of Cincinnati, unpublished

IARC (1982) *IARC Monographs on the Evaluation of the Carcinogenic Risk of Chemicals to Humans*, Vol. 29, *Some Industrial Chemicals and Dyestuffs*, Lyon, pp. 93−148, 391−397

IARC (1983) *IARC Monographs on the Evaluation of the Carcinogenic Risk of Chemicals to Humans*, Vol. 32, *Polynuclear Aromatic Compounds, Part 1, Chemical, Environmental and Experimental Data*, Lyon, pp. 211−224

IARC (1986) *Information Bulletin on the Survey of Chemicals Being Tested for Carcinogenicity*, No. 12, Lyon, p. 286

IARC (1987a) *IARC Monographs on the Evaluation of Carcinogenic Risks to Humans*, Suppl. 7, *Overall Evaluations of Carcinogenicity: An Updating of* IARC Monographs *Volumes 1 to 42*, Lyon, pp. 120−122

IARC (1987b) *IARC Monographs on the Evaluation of Carcinogenic Risks to Humans*, Suppl. 7, *Overall Evaluations of Carcinogenicity: An Updating of IARC Monographs Volumes 1 to 42*, Lyon, p. 58

International Energy Agency (1987) *Energy Statistics 1970−1985*, Vols I and II, Paris, Organisation for Economic Cooperation and Development

Isbister, C. (1963) Poisoning in childhood, with particular reference to kerosene poisoning. *Med. J. Aust., 2*, 652−656

Jewell, D.M., Yevich, J.P. & Snyder, R.E. (1965) *Basic nitrogen compounds in petroleum*. In: *Hydrocarbon Analysis (ASTM STP 389)*, Philadelphia, American Society for Testing and Materials, pp. 363−383

Jewell, D.M., Albaugh, E.W., Davis, B.E. & Ruberto, R.G. (1974) Integration of chromatographic and spectroscopic techniques for the characterization of residual oils. *Ind. Eng. Chem. Fundam., 13*, 278−282

Johansson, S., Larsson, U. & Boehm, P. (1980) The *Tsesis* oil spill. Impact on the pelagic ecosystem. *Mar. Pollut. Bull., 11*, 284−293

Keizer, P.D., Ahern, T.P., Dale, J. & Vandermeulen, J.H. (1978) Residues of bunker C oil in Chedabucto Bay, Nova Scotia, 6 years after the *Arrow* spill. *J. Fish. Res. Board Can., 35*, 528−535

Kemp, P.F., Swartz, R.C. & Lamberson, J.O. (1986) Response of the phoxocephalid amphipod, *Rhepoxynius abronius*, to a small oil spill in Yaquina Bay, Oregon. *Estuaries, 9*, 340−347

Klauder, J.V. & Brill, F.A., Jr (1947) Correlation of boiling ranges of some petroleum solvents with irritant action on skin. *Arch. Dermatol. Syph., 56*, 197−215

Koo, L.C., Lee, N. & Ho, J.H.-C. (1983) Do cooking fuels pose a risk for lung cancer? A case-control study of women in Hong Kong. *Ecol. Dis., 2*, 255−265

Krahn, M.M. & Malins, D.C. (1982) Gas chromatographic-mass spectrometric determination of aromatic hydrocarbon metabolites from livers of fish exposed to fuel oil. *J. Chromatogr., 248*, 99−107

Latham, D.R., Okuno, I. & Haines, W.E. (1965) *Nonbasic nitrogen compounds in petroleum*. In: *Hydrocarbon Analysis (ASTM STP 389)*, Philadelphia, PA, American Society for Testing and Materials, pp. 385–397

Lee, R.F. (1977) *Accumulation and turnover of petroleum hydrocarbons in marine organisms*. In: Wolfe, D.A., ed., *Fate and Effect of Petroleum in Marine Organisms and Ecosystems*, Oxford, Pergamon Press, pp. 60–70

Lesser, L.I., Weens, H.S. & McKey, J.D. (1943) Pulmonary manifestations following the ingestion of kerosene. *J. Pediatr., 23*, 352–364

Leung, J.S.M. (1977) Cigarette smoking, the kerosene stove and lung cancer in Hong Kong. *Br. J. Dis. Chest, 71*, 273–276

Levy, E.M. (1971) The presence of petroleum residues off the east coast of Nova Scotia, in the Gulf of St Lawrence, and the St Lawrence river. *Water Res., 5*, 723–733

Lillienberg, L. (1986) *Fuel oil in tank cleaning operations* (Abstract). In: *International Congress on Industrial Hygiene, 5–9 October 1986, Rome*, Rome, Pontificia Universita Urbaniana, pp. 10–12

Lillienberg, L., Högstedt, B., Järvholm, B., Jönsson, M., Kindbom, K. & Nilson, L. (1987) *Fuel Oil in Tank Cleaning Operations (Project No. 83-0897)* (Swed.), Göteborg, Hygienic Medicine Clinic

MacIntyre, T.M. (1970) Effect of bunker 'C' oil on sheep. *Can. J. Anim. Sci., 50*, 748–749

MacKerron, C.B. & Kiesche, E.S. (1988) After the Ashland spill, more regulations? *Chem. Week, 142*, 19–20

Mair, B.J. (1964) Here's a complete, up-to-date list of the hydrocarbons isolated from petroleum. *Oil Gas J., 62*, 130–134

Majeed, H.A., Bassyouni, H., Kalaawy, M. & Farwana, S. (1981) Kerosene poisoning in children: a clinico-radiological study of 205 cases. *Ann. trop. Paediatr., 1*, 123–130

Mann, M.D., Pirie, D.J. & Wolfsdorf, J. (1977) Kerosene absorption in primates. *J. Pediatr., 91*, 495–498

Marandian, M.H., Sabouri, H., Youssefian, H., Behvad, A. & Djafarian, M. (1981) Pneumatoceles and pneumothorax following accidental hydrocarbon ingestion in children (Fr.). *Ann. Pédiatr., 28*, 687–691

Matsuoka, A., Shudo, K., Saito, Y., Sofuni, T. & Ishidate, M., Jr (1982) Clastogenic potential of heavy oil extracts and some aza-arenes in Chinese hamster cells in culture. *Mutat. Res., 102*, 275–283

Muganga, N., Mashako, M., Kanda, T. & Mulefu, K.M. (1986) Pneumopathies due to petroleum ingestion (Fr.). *Ann. Soc. belg. Méd. trop., 66*, 69–75

Neff, J.M. & Anderson, J.W. (1981) *Response of Marine Animals to Petroleum and Specific Petroleum Hydrocarbons*, London, Applied Science Publishers, pp. 10, 93–142

Noa, M. & Illnait, J. (1987) Induction of aortic plaques in guinea pigs by exposure to kerosene. *Arch. environ. Health, 42*, 31–36

Noa, M. & Sanabria, J. (1984) Tracheal ultrastructure in kerosine treated guinea pigs. A preliminary report. *Allergol. Immunopathol., 12*, 33–36

Noa, M., Illnait, J. & González, R. (1985) Cytologic and biochemical changes in pulmonary washings of guinea pigs exposed to kerosene. *Allergol. Immunopathol., 13*, 193–196

Nouri, L. & Al-Rahim, K. (1970) Kerosene poisoning in children. *Postgrad. med. J., 46*, 71–75

Nunn, J.A. & Martin, F.M. (1934) Gasoline and kerosene poisoning in children. *J. Am. med. Assoc.*, *103*, 472–474

Okubo, T. & Tsuchiya, K. (1974) An epidemiological study on the cancer mortality in various industries in Japan (Jpn). *Jpn. J. ind. Health*, *16*, 438–452

Pancirov, R.J. & Brown, R.A. (1975) *Analytical methods for polynuclear aromatic hydrocarbons in crude oils, heating oils and marine tissues.* In: *Proceedings of a Conference on Prevention and Control of Oil Pollution, San Francisco, CA*, Washington DC, American Petroleum Institute, pp. 103–113

Rao, G.S. & Pandya, K.P. (1980) Hepatic metabolism of heme in rats after exposure to benzene, gasoline and kerosene. *Arch. Toxicol.*, *46*, 313–317

Rao, G.S., Kannan, K., Goel, S.K., Pandya, K.P. & Shanker, R. (1984) Subcutaneous kerosene toxicity in albino rats. *Environ. Res.*, *35*, 516–530

Rice, S.D., Short, J.W. & Karinen, J.F. (1977) *Comparative oil toxicity and comparative animal sensitivity.* In: Wolfe, D.A., ed., *Fate and Effect of Petroleum in Marine Organisms and Ecosystems*, Oxford, Pergamon Press, pp. 78–94

Richardson, J.A. & Pratt-Thomas, H.R. (1951) Toxic effects of varying doses of kerosene administered by different routes. *Am. J. med. Sci.*, *221*, 531–536

Rossini, F.D., Bair, B.T. & Streiff, A.T. (1953) *Hydrocarbons from Petroleum*, New York, Reinhold

Royal Dutch/Shell Group of Companies (1983) *The Petroleum Handbook*, 6th ed., Amsterdam, Elsevier

Saksena, P.N. (1969) Kerosene oil poisoning in children. *J. Indian med. Assoc.*, *52*, 169–171

Sanders, H.L., Grassle, J.F., Hampson, G.R., Morse, L.S., Garner-Price, S. & Jones, C.C. (1980) Anatomy of an oil spill: long-term effects from the grounding of the barge *Florida* off West Falmouth, Massachusetts. *J. mar. Res.*, *38*, 265–380

Sax, N.I. (1984) *Dangerous Properties of Industrial Materials*, 6th ed., New York, Van Nostrand, p. 1679

Schreiner, C.A. (1984) *Petroleum and petroleum products: a brief review of studies to evaluate reproductive effects.* In: Christian, M.S., Galbraith, W.M., Voytek, P. & Mehlman, M.A., eds, *Advances in Modern Environmental Toxicology*, Vol. III, *Assessment of Reproductive and Teratogenic Hazards*, Princeton, NJ, Princeton Scientific Publishers, pp. 29–45

Scott, E.P. (1944) Pneumonia, pneumothorax, and emphysema following ingestion of kerosene. *J. Pediatr.*, *25*, 31–34

Siemiatycki, J., Dewar, R., Nadon, L., Gérin, M., Richardson, L. & Wacholder, S. (1987) Associations between several sites of cancer and twelve petroleum derived liquids. Results from a case-referent study in Montreal. *Scand. J. Work Environ. Health*, *13*, 493–504

Spiegelman, D. & Wegman, D.H. (1985) Occupation-related risks for colorectal cancer. *J. natl Cancer Inst.*, *75*, 813–821

Starek, A. & Kamiński, M. (1982) Comparative studies of the toxicity of kerosene derivatives dielectrics applied in electromachining (Pol.). *Med. Prac.*, *33*, 239–253

St John, M.A. (1982) Kerosene poisoning in children in Barbados. *Ann. trop. Pediatr.*, *2*, 37–40

Sumámur, P.K. & Wenas, S. (1978) Occupational dermatosis in kerosene retailers. *Indones. J. ind. Hyg. occup. Health Saf.*, *11*, 23–24

Szaro, R.C. (1979) Bunker C fuel oil reduces mallard egg hatchability. *Bull. environ. Contam. Toxicol.*, 22, 731–732

Szaro, R.C., Hensler, G. & Heinz, G.H. (1981) Effects of chronic ingestion of No. 2 fuel oil on mallard ducklings. *J. Toxicol. environ. Health*, 7, 789–799

Tagami, H. & Ogino, A. (1973) Kerosine dermatitis. Factors affecting skin irritability of kerosine. *Dermatologica*, 146, 123–131

Tal, A., Aviram, M., Bar-Ziv, J. & Scharf, S.M. (1984) Residual small airways lesions after kerosene pneumonitis in early childhood. *Eur. J. Pediatr.*, 142, 117–120

Thompson, C.J., Coleman, H.J., Hopkins, R.L. & Rall, H.T. (1965) *Sulfur compounds in petroleum*. In: *Hydrocarbon Analysis (ASTM STP 389)*, Philadelphia, American Society for Testing and Materials, pp. 329–360

Tsuchiya, K. (1965) The relation of occupation to cancer, especially cancer of the lung. *Cancer*, 18, 136–144

US Department of Energy (1983) *Petroleum Supply Annual*, Washington DC

Vandermeulen, J.H. & Lee, R.W. (1986) Lack of mutagenic activity of crude and refined oils in the unicellular alga *Chlamydomonas reinhardtii*. *Bull. environ. Contam. Toxicol.*, 36, 250–253

Vandermeulen, J.H., Foda, A. & Stuttard, C. (1985) Toxicity vs mutagenicity of some crude oils, distillates and their water soluble fractions. *Water Res.*, 19, 1283–1289

Vidal, B. & Ferrando, F. (1974) A case of acute pneumopathy due to ingestion of fuel oil while at work (Ital.). *Min. med.*, 65, 1898–1905

Wells, P.G. & Percy, J.A. (1985) *Effects of oil on Arctic invertebrates*. In: Engelhardt, F.R., ed., *Petroleum Effects in the Arctic Environment*, London, Elsevier, pp. 101–156

White, D.H., King, K.A. & Coon, N.C. (1979) Effects of No. 2 fuel oil on hatchability of marine and estuarine bird eggs. *Bull. environ. Contam. Toxicol.*, 21, 7–10

Witschi, H.P., Smith, L.H., Frome, E.L., Pequet-Goad, M.E., Griest, W.H., Ho, C.-H. & Guérin, M.R. (1987) Skin tumorigenic potential of crude and refined coal liquids and analogous petroleum products. *Fundam. appl. Toxicol.*, 9, 297–303

Wolfsdorf, J. & Kundig, H. (1972) Kerosene poisoning in primates. *S. Afr. med. J.*, 46, 619–621

SUMMARY OF FINAL EVALUATIONS

Agent	Degree of evidence for carcinogenicity		Overall evaluation
	Humans	Animals	
Occupational exposures in petroleum refining			2A
Working in petroleum refineries	Limited		
Light vacuum distillates		Sufficient	
Heavy vacuum distillates		Sufficient	
Light catalytically cracked distillates		Sufficient	
Heavy catalytically cracked distillates		Sufficient	
Cracked residues derived from the refining of crude oil		Sufficient	
Light straight-run naphtha		Limited	
Straight-run kerosene		Limited	
Hydrotreated kerosene		Limited	
Light catalytically cracked naphtha		Limited	
Crude oil	Inadequate	Limited	3
Gasoline[a]	Inadequate		2B
Unleaded automotive gasoline		Limited	
Jet fuel	Inadequate	Inadequate	3
Diesel fuels	Inadequate		
Distillate (light) diesel fuels			3
Marine diesel fuel[a]		Limited	2B
Fuel oils	Inadequate		
Distillate (light) fuel oils			3
Fuel oil No. 2		Limited	
Residual (heavy) fuel oils		Sufficient	2B

[a]Other relevant data described in the monographs influenced the making of the overall evaluation.

Appendix 1. Summary table of genetic and related effects of process streams and products from petroleum refining

	Nonmammalian systems				Mammalian systems			
	Prokaryotes	Lower eukaryotes	Plants	Insects	In vitro		In vivo	
					Animal cells	Human cells	Animals	Humans
	D G	D R	A D G C	R G C A	D G S M C A T I	D G S M C A T I	D G S M C DL A	D S M C A
Process streams	+							
Crude oils	∓^{b,c}				+1,^{c} −1,^{c}	−1	? −1	−1,^{a} −1,^{a}
Gasoline^d	−1,^{e}			+1,^{f}	+ ±1,^{g}	+1 −1 −1		
Jet fuel	−				+1		+1	
Diesel fuel	?^{h} −1,^{i}				−1		+1	
Fuel oils:								
Residual fuel oil	−1,^{j}					+1,^{k}		
Kerosene-type fuel oil	−1				−1		−1	
Fuel oil No. 2	+^{l}				+1 +1,^{m} −1,^{m}		+1	

^{a}Positive effects were observed in sewage-treatment workers in an oil refinery; ^{b}extracts of crude oils; ^{c}neutral aromatic fractions of crude oil; ^{d}unleaded unless otherwise specified; ^{e}DMSO extract of unleaded gasoline and residue from evaporation of unleaded gasoline; ^{f}leaded gasoline; ^{g}positive in one study using a DMSO extract and a residue from evaporation; ^{h}different results found with samples of different diesel fuels; ^{i}aliphatic and aromatic fractions; ^{j}bunker fuel; ^{k}B-class heavy oil; ^{l}including one study with an aromatic fraction; ^{m}two aromatic fractions of fuel oil No. 2

1One study

GLOSSARY

Acid and earth treatment — Refining process used for decolourizing or purifying

Acidizing — Treating production formation (limestone or dolomite) with hydrochloric, acetic or hydrofluoric acid

Additive — A substance added to e.g., *lubricating oils* to impart new or to improve existing characteristics

Aliphatic hydrocarbon — Hydrocarbon in which the carbon-hydrogen groupings are arranged in open chains which may be branched. The term includes *paraffins* and *olefins* and provides a distinction from *aromatics* and *naphthenes* which have at least some of their carbon atoms arranged in closed chains or rings

Alkane — See *Paraffin*

Alkene — See *Olefin*

Alkylation — The chemical reaction of a low molecular weight *olefin* and an isoparaffin to form multiply branched *paraffins* of high *octane rating*

Aniline point — The lowest temperature at which an oil is completely miscible with an equal volume of aniline

Antiknock — Substance added to *gasoline* to improve *octane number*, e.g., tetraethyllead

Aromatic — Compound containing one or more benzene rings that also may contain sulfur, nitrogen and oxygen

Aromatic extract — See *Extract*

Asphalt — A mixture of *bitumen* and mineral matter (sand). Note — In the USA, the term asphalt is also used for *bitumen* alone.

Asphaltene — Constituent of petroleum products with a high molecular mass and dark colour, free from wax, insoluble in *n*-heptane and soluble in hot benzene

ASTM — American Society for Testing and Materials, responsible for the issue of many of the standard methods used in the petroleum industry

Barrel — 1 barrel = 42 US gallons = 159 l; 1 metric tonne $\simeq$ 7.4 barrels (crude oil)

Batching oil — Petroleum product, e.g., heavy *gas oils* and light *lubricating oils*, used primarily in the jute industry to soften and lubricate fibres before spinning

Benzine — *Straight-run* petroleum spirit that boils within the range 80–130°C

Bitumen — A viscous liquid, semisolid or solid, consisting essentially of hydrocarbons and their derivatives, which is soluble in carbon disulfide. Bitumen is obtained from the distillation of suitable *crude oils* by treatment of the *residues* (or occasionally of the heaviest fraction). It is also a component of naturally occurring *asphalt*. According to their properties, bitumens are used for emulsions, roofing, waterproofing, insulation, road construction, binding of aggregates, etc.

Black oil — A general term applied to the heavier and darker coloured petroleum products, such as heavy *diesel fuel*, *fuel oil* and some *cylinder oils*

Blending — Intimate mixing of the various components in the preparation of a product to meet a given specification

Bottoms — Residue of petroleum distillation

Bright stock — A *lubricating oil* of high viscosity prepared from a *cylinder stock* by further *refining*, e.g., *solvent deasphalting, dewaxing, acid and earth treatment*

Bunkering — The process of refuelling, e.g., a ship, with *distillate* or *residual oil*

Bunker fuel — Heavy *residual oil*, also called bunker C, bunker C fuel oil, bunker oil

Cetane — n-Hexadecane, used as a reference fuel for rating *diesel fuel* ignition quality

Cetane number — Measure of the ignition quality of a *diesel fuel*, expressed as the percentage of *cetane* that must be mixed with liquid α-methylnaphthalene to produce the same ignition performance as the *diesel fuel* being rated, as determined by test method *ASTM* D 613. A high cetane number indicates shorter ignition lag and a cleaner burning fuel

CFR engine — A standard single-cylinder variable compression engine developed by the Co-operative Fuel Research Council to determine the *antiknock* value of motor *gasolines* or the ignition quality of *diesel fuels*

Coking — Thermal or other process yielding, e.g., *distillate, gasoline*, gas and nonvolatile *residue* (coke). Coking also occurs in *catalytic cracking*. X-ray analyses have shown coke to consist of condensed aromatic structures arranged in a disordered graphitic pattern

CONCAWE — Acronym standing for the oil companies' international study group for Conservation of Clean Air and Water – Europe

Cracking — A process whereby the relative proportion of lighter or more volatile components of an oil is increased by changing the chemical structure of the constituent hydrocarbons

Cracking, catalytic — A *cracking* process in which a catalyst is used to promote reaction

Cracking, hydro — A *cracking* process carried out at high temperature and pressure in the presence of hydrogen and in which a catalyst is used to promote reaction. The process combines *cracking* and hydrogenation.

Cracking, steam — *Thermal cracking* of, e.g., *naphtha*, at high temperatures with superheated steam injection

Cracking, thermal — A *cracking* process in which no catalyst is used to promote reaction

Crude oil — Naturally occurring mixture consisting essentially of many types of hydrocarbons, but also containing sulfur, nitrogen or oxygen derivatives. Crude oil may be of paraffinic, asphaltic or mixed base, depending on the presence of *paraffin wax, bitumen* or both *paraffin wax* and *bitumen* in the *residue* after atmospheric distillation. Crude oil composition varies according to the geological strata of its origin

Cut — The *distillate* obtained between two given temperatures during a distillation process

Cut-back (bitumen) — *Bitumen* to which a solvent has been added so it does not require heating to a high temperature before use

Cycloalkane — See *Naphthene*

Cycloparaffin — See *Naphthene*

Cylinder oil — *Lubricating oil* of high viscosity and high *flash-point* used primarily to lubricate the cylinders and valves of steam engines

Cylinder stock — Dark-coloured, *residual oil* of high viscosity used as the basis of steam *cylinder oil*

Deasphalting — The removal of asphaltic constituents from *residual* stock for *lubricating oil* manufacture. A *solvent refining* process in which the *asphalt* is precipitated, for example, by liquid propane (also called *decarbonizing*)

Decarbonizing — See *Deasphalting*

Dewaxing — The removal of waxes from *lubricating oil* stocks, now usually carried out by filtration at low temperature of a mixture of the oil and a solvent such as methyl ethyl ketone

Diesel fuel — That portion of *crude oil* that distills out within the temperature range 200–370°C. A general term covering oils used as fuel in diesel and other compression ignition engines

Diesel oil — See *Diesel fuel*

Distillate — A product obtained by condensing the vapours evolved when a liquid is boiled and collecting the condensate in a receiver which is separate from the boiling vessel

Distillation range — A single pure substance has one definite boiling-point at a given pressure. A mixture of substances, however, exhibits a range of temperatures over which boiling or distillation commences, proceeds and finishes. This range of temperatures, determined by means of standard apparatus, is termed the 'distillation' or 'boiling' range.

Doctoring — Chemical *sweetening*, used to reduce odour level of products containing mercaptans

Domestic fuel — Heating oil

Electrical oil — See *Insulating oil*

End-point — See *Final boiling-point*

Engine oil — *Lubricating oil* used in internal combustion and other types of engines

Extender oil — Diluent or carrier oil especially for rubbers and plastics

Extract — During *solvent refining* processes, other than *dewaxing* or *deasphalting*, part of the *feedstock* passes into solution in the solvent and is subsequently recovered by evaporating off the solvent. This fraction is the extract and is generally *aromatic* in character and thus referred to as an *aromatic extract*.

Feedstock — Primary material introduced into a plant for processing

Final boiling-point — Maximal temperature noted (corrected if required) during the final phase of a distillation carried out under standardized conditions

Fixed bed — Reactor used in heterogeneous catalysis when the catalyst remains in a fixed position

Flash off — To distill continuously under constant equilibrium conditions, the resulting vapour and liquid products being withdrawn continuously

Flash-point — Minimal temperature to which a product must be heated for the vapours emitted to ignite momentarily in the presence of a flame, when operating under standardized conditions

Fluid bed — Reactor used in heterogeneous catalysis, which is based on the principle of suspending finely dispersed catalyst particles in an upward flowing gas stream

Flux oil — Oil of low volatility suitable for softening *bitumen* or natural *asphalt*

Fractional distillation — See *Fractionation*

Fractionation — A distillation process in which the *distillate* is collected as a number of separate fractions each with a different boiling range

Fuel oil — A general term applied to an oil used for the production of power or heat. In a more restricted sense, it is applied to any petroleum product that is burnt under boilers or in industrial furnaces. These oils are normally *residues*, but blends of *distillates* and *residues* are also used as fuel oil. The wider term, '*liquid fuel*', is sometimes used, but the term 'fuel oil' is preferred.

Furfural extraction — A single solvent process in which furfural (the aldehyde, C_4H_3OCHO) is used to remove primarily *aromatic* but also *naphthenic*, *olefinic* and unstable hydrocarbons from a *lubricating oil* charge stock, thereby improving the *viscosity index* and stability

Gas oil — A petroleum *distillate* with a viscosity and *distillation range* intermediate between those of *kerosene* and light *lubricating oil*

Gasoline (petrol) — Refined petroleum distillate, normally boiling within the limits of 30–220°C, which, combined with certain additives, is used as fuel for spark-ignition engines. By extension, the term is also applied to other products that boil within this range

Gas turbine — Turbine driven by gas, e.g., air, that is compressed and heated by burning fuel in it

Gear oil — An oil suitable for the lubrication of gears. Gear oils vary in characteristics according to their specific application

Grease — Semisolid or solid lubricant consisting essentially of a stabilized mixture of mineral, fatty or synthetic oil with soaps or other thickeners. It may contain other ingredients.

Heating oil — *Gas oil* or *fuel oil* used for firing the boilers of central heating systems

Heat transfer oil — A medium used for the transfer of heat at temperatures above that of steam. Probably the most widely used medium is a high-boiling petroleum fraction, usually in the *gas oil* range

Heat-treating oil — An oil used for cooling metal components in hardening and tempering operations

Heavy benzine — See *Naphtha*

Heavy gasoline — See *Naphtha*

Hydraulic fluid — A fluid supplied for use in hydraulic systems. Low viscosity and low *pour-point* are desirable characteristics. Hydraulic fluids may be of petroleum or non-petroleum origin.

Hydrocracking — See *Cracking, hydro-*

Hydrodesulfurization — A desulfurization process in which the oil is treated with hydrogen

Hydrofinishing — A mild *hydrotreating* process used mainly for finishing solvent-extracted *lubricating oils*. It has largely replaced earth treating

Hydrotreatment — A general term covering treatment with hydrogen at elevated temperature and pressure, usually in the presence of a catalyst. Severity of treatment ranges from mild (*hydrofinishing*) to severe (*hydrocracking*).

Initial boiling-point — The temperature (corrected if required) at which the first drop of *distillate* falls from the condenser during a laboratory distillation carried out under standardized conditions

Insulating oil (electrical oil, transformer oil) — Oil with good dielectric properties used in electrical equipment

Institute of Petroleum — The official British organization which deals with petroleum technology and with the standardization of test methods for petroleum

Isomerization — Process for converting compounds into structural or geometric isomers (molecules composed of the same type and number of atoms)

Jet fuel — *Kerosene* or *gasoline/kerosene* mixture for fuelling aircraft *gas turbine* engines

Kerosene — A refined petroleum *distillate* intermediate in volatility between *gasoline* and *gas oil*. Its *distillation range* generally falls within the limits of 150 and 300°C. Its main uses are as a jet engine fuel, an illuminant, for heating purposes and as a fuel for certain types of internal combustion engines

Kerosine — European term for *kerosene*

Light distillate — A term lacking precise meaning, but commonly applied to *distillates*, the *final boiling-point* of which does not exceed 300°C

Liquefied natural gas — Oilfield or naturally occurring gas, chiefly methane, liquefied for transport purposes

Liquefied petroleum gas — Light hydrocarbon material, gaseous at atmospheric temperature and pressure, held in the liquid state by pressure to facilitate storage, transport and handling. Commercial liquefied gas consists essentially of either propane or butane, or mixtures thereof.

Liquid fuel — See *Fuel oil*

Loading, bottom — The filling of the compartments of a road tanker vehicle from the bottom up via the manifold or delivery hose connection point

Loading, top — The filling of the compartments of a road tanker vehicle from the top, i.e., through the manholes

Long residue — The residual fraction from the atmospheric pressure distillation of *crude oil*

Lubricating oil — Oil, usually refined, primarily intended to reduce friction between moving surfaces

Lubricating oil distillate — A *vacuum distillation* cut with a *distillation range* and viscosity such that, after refining, it yields *lubricating oil*

Machine oil — Oil with a viscosity of about 11 cSt at 100°C used for the lubrication of the moving parts of lightly loaded machines operating at moderate temperatures. Historically, an unrefined or mildly refined *distillate*, but not commonly applied to oils of the relevant viscosity

Maintenance staff — Within the context of this volume, those persons who carry out repair work on and scheduled overhauls of *refinery* equipment

Microcrystalline wax — Product consisting predominantly of a mixture of non-normal saturated hydrocarbons, solid at ordinary temperatures, with a finer crystalline structure than *paraffin wax*. It is manufactured from *bright stock slack wax.*

Middle distillate — One of the *distillates* obtained between *kerosene* and *lubricating oil* fractions in the *refining* processes. These include light *fuel oils* and *diesel fuels.*

Mould oil — A lubricant used to ensure easy parting of ceramic, glass, concrete or other material from the mould in which it is cast

Moving bed — Reactor used in heterogeneous catalysis in which the catalyst is constantly recycled through the reactor and a *regenerator*

Naphtha — *Straight-run* gasoline fractions boiling below *kerosene* and frequently used as a *feedstock* for *reforming* processes. Also known as *heavy benzine* or *heavy gasoline*

Naphthene — Petroleum industry term for a *cycloparaffin* (*cycloalkane*)

Naphthenic oil — A petroleum oil derived from *crude oil* containing little or no wax

Octane number — See *Octane rating*

Octane rating (of gasoline) — The percentage by volume of iso-octane in a mixture of iso-octane and *n*-heptane which is found to have the same knocking tendency as the gasoline under test in a *CFR engine* operated under standard conditions (also called *octane number*)

Oil mist — Suspended liquid droplets of oil which are produced when there is condensation of the oil from the gaseous to the liquid state; alternatively, a mist can be produced by dispersion of liquid oil

Olefin — Synonymous with *alkene*

Operator — Within the context of this volume, one of the employees who actually runs (operates) the various units, plant and equipment that make up a *refinery*

Pale — Term of US origin used to describe a lightly refined, low *viscosity index naphthenic oil*

Paraffinic oil — A petroleum oil derived from a *crude oil* with a substantial wax content

Paraffin (alkane) — One of a series of saturated aliphatic hydrocarbons, the lowest numbers of which are methane, ethane and propane. The higher homologues are solid waxes.

Paraffin wax — Product obtained from petroleum *distillates* consisting essentially of a mixture of saturated hydrocarbons, solid at ordinary temperatures. Fully-refined paraffin wax has a low oil content and a rather marked crystalline structure

Petrol — See *Gasoline*

Platforming — A refining process using a platinum-containing catalyst which includes 0.1-8.0% fluorine or chlorine on an alumina base

Pour-point — The lowest temperature at which a petroleum oil will pour or flow when it is chilled without disturbance under prescribed conditions

Preflash tower — Type of *refinery* distillation unit

Preservative oil — Oil used to coat metal parts temporarily in order to protect them against corrosion; usually contains additives

Process oil — Oil used as a processing aid or ingredient of a formulation not destined for use as a lubricant, e.g., jute batching oil, concrete *mould oil, rubber extender oil*

Raffinate — Refined product resulting from a *solvent refining* process, i.e., that portion of the *feedstock* not soluble in the solvent

Reduced crude — Term of US origin. The product obtained after removal, by atmospheric distillation, of the light components of *crude oil*

Refinery — A plant, together with all its equipment, for the manufacture of finished or semifinished products from *crude oil*

Refining — The separation of *crude oil* into its component parts and the manufacture therefrom of products. Important processes in *lubricating oil* refining are distillation, *hydrotreatment* and *solvent extraction*

Reforming — A process for treating light petroleum fractions to yield *gasoline* with a higher *aromatic* content and a higher *octane number* than the *feedstock*

Reforming, catalytic — *Reforming* in which reaction is promoted by a catalyst

Reforming, thermal — *Reforming* without the use of a catalyst

Regenerator — That part of a *catalytic cracking* unit in which the coke that deposits on the catalyst during cracking is burnt off

Residual oil — Grade No. 4 to grade No. 6 *fuel oils*

Residue (residuum) — The heavy fraction or *bottoms* remaining undistilled after volatilization of all lower-boiling constituents

Riser — Vertical pipe

Rolling oil (slurry oil) — The bottom, i.e., heaviest, product from a *catalytic cracking* unit (also known as *roll oil*)

Roll oil — See *Rolling oil*

Rubber extender oil (extending oil, extenders) — Highly aromatic petroleum oils, usually *aromatic extracts* containing 80–90% aromatics, added to latex in large quantities (up to 50% in rubber) to extend the bulk of the rubber

Rubber processing oils — Mineral oils such as light *naphthenic oils* containing up to about 40% *aromatics*, added in relatively small quantities during the milling of polymerized rubber to improve properties

Short residue — The residual fraction from the *vacuum distillation* of long residue

Slack wax — Crude petroleum wax obtained by *dewaxing* a *distillate*; it contains a high proportion of liquid hydrocarbons

Slurry oil — See *Rolling oil*

Soluble oil — Oil containing emulsifiers and capable of forming stable emulsions or colloidal suspensions in water, used particularly for lubrication and cooling in metal working

Solutizer — Solubility promoter, e.g., for mercaptans in a *sweetening* process

Solvent deasphalting — A process for removing *asphaltic* and resinous materials from reduced *crude oil* residues, *lubricating oil* stocks, *gas oils* or *middle distillates* by the extraction or precipitant action of solvents in which *asphalt* is soluble. The principal *deasphalting* solvents are low molecular weight hydrocarbons, particularly liquid propane, and oxygenated compounds, such as alcohols and esters

Solvent dewaxing — A process for removing wax from oils by means of suitable solvents

Solvent extraction — Processes in which solvents are used to dissolve out undesirable constituents, e.g., the removal of *aromatics* from *kerosene* by extraction with liquid sulfur dioxide

Solvent refining — Processes in which solvents are used to eliminate undesirable constituents, either by dissolving them out, i.e., *solvent extraction*, or by precipitating them, as in *solvent dewaxing* and *solvent deasphalting*

Sour — Acidic and malodorous

Standpipe — Pipe rising vertically from the ground

Steam cylinder oil — Oil used to lubricate cylinders of steam engines. Usually dark, viscous petroleum oils of high *flash-point*, sometimes compounded with fatty oil

Steam turbine oil — Highly-refined petroleum oil usually containing additives, used for the lubrication of steam turbines and with the property of resisting the formation of stable emulsions with water

Straight-run product — A product of the primary distillation of *crude oil*

Stream (refinery) — *Refinery* intermediate; product or by-product from a treating or distillation unit

Stripping (in catalytic cracking) — Process whereby spent catalyst from a *catalytic cracking* unit comes into contact at an elevated temperature with steam, with the aim of desorbing adsorbed hydrocarbons

Sweating — Separation of liquid hydrocarbons from certain *slack waxes* by the action of slow progressive heating

Sweetening — Removal or conversion of undesirably acidic and malodorous constituents present in *sour feedstock* or *refinery stream*, e.g., conversion of mercaptans to disulfides

Topping — Distillation to remove light fractions only

Transformer oil — A well-refined, pale petroleum oil of low viscosity, resistant to oxidation under conditions of use. Used in transformers for cooling and for electrical insulation

Transmission lubricant — An oil or other fluid used to lubricate the transmission of an automobile

Treatments — Somewhat loosely used to cover all those *refining* operations in which small proportions of undesirable constituents are removed from products by chemical or physical means, e.g., *acid and earth treatment* and *sweetening*

Turbine oil — A well-refined, selected petroleum distillate, or mixture of such with a *bright stock*, used for lubricating steam turbines. These oils show high resistance to emulsification with water and to oxidation under conditions of use

Vacuum distillation — Distillation under reduced, as opposed to atmospheric, pressure, e.g., *fractional distillation* of *short residue* to produce *distillates* for *lubricating oil* manufacture

Visbreaking — Viscosity breaking; lowering or 'breaking' the viscosity of a *residue* by *thermal cracking*

Viscosity index — An arbitrary number used to characterize the rate at which the viscosity of a *lubricating oil* changes with changing temperature. Oils of high viscosity index exhibit relatively small change of viscosity with changing temperature and *vice versa*.

Waxy distillate — Distillation *cut* containing a relatively large amount of *paraffin wax*

Wide-cut — Wide boiling range

SUPPLEMENTARY CORRIGENDA TO VOLUMES 1–44

Corrigenda to Volumes 1–42 are listed in Volume 42, pp. 251-264 and in Volume 43, p. 261.

Volume 41

Methyl bromide
  p. 198   para 2 lines 3–4   *replace* 50–10 400 mmol/l (4.75–9874 mg/m³) *by* 50–10 400 nmol/l (4.75–987.4 mg/m³)

Supplement 7

Asbestos
  p. 109   para 3 line 12   *replace* Chrysolite induced unscheduled DNA synthesis in rat hepatocytes. *by* Chrysolite did not induce unscheduled DNA synthesis in rat hepatocytes.

Nickel and nickel compounds
  p. 267   reference 20   *replace* Goldbold *by* Godbold

Volume 43

Man-made mineral fibres and Radon
  pp. 152 and 241   footnote   *replace* see Preamble, pp. 28–34 *by* see Preamble, pp. 27–30

CUMULATIVE CROSS INDEX TO IARC MONOGRAPHS ON THE EVALUATION OF CARCINOGENIC RISKS TO HUMANS

The volume, page and year are given. References to corrigenda are given in parentheses.

A

A-α-C	40, 245 (1986)
	Suppl. 7, 56 (1987)
Acetaldehyde	36, 101 (1985) (corr. 42, 263)
	Suppl. 7, 77 (1987)
Acetaldehyde formylmethylhydrazone (see Gyromitrin)	
Acetamide	7, 197 (1974)
	Suppl. 7, 389 (1987)
Acridine orange	16, 145 (1978)
	Suppl. 7, 56 (1987)
Acriflavinium chloride	13, 31 (1977)
	Suppl. 7, 56 (1987)
Acrolein	19, 479 (1979)
	36, 133 (1985)
	Suppl. 7, 78 (1987)
Acrylamide	39, 41 (1986)
	Suppl. 7, 56 (1987)
Acrylic acid	19, 47 (1979)
	Suppl. 7, 56 (1987)
Acrylic fibres	19, 86 (1979)
	Suppl. 7, 56 (1987)
Acrylonitrile	19, 73 (1979)
	Suppl. 7, 79 (1987)
Acrylonitrile-butadiene-styrene copolymers	19, 9 (1979)
	Suppl. 7, 56 (1987)
Actinolite (see Asbestos)	
Actinomycins	10, 29 (1976) (corr. 42, 255)
	Suppl. 7, 80 (1987)
Adriamycin	10, 43 (1976)
	Suppl. 7, 81 (1987)

AF-2	*31*, 47 (1983)
	Suppl. 7, 56 (1987)
Aflatoxins	*1*, 145 (1972) (*corr. 42*, 251)
	10, 51 (1976)
	Suppl. 7, 82 (1987)

Aflatoxin B$_1$ (*see* Aflatoxins)
Aflatoxin B$_2$ (*see* Aflatoxins)
Aflatoxin G$_1$ (*see* Aflatoxins)
Aflatoxin G$_2$ (*see* Aflatoxins)
Aflatoxin M$_1$ (*see* Aflatoxins)

Agaritine	*31*, 63 (1983)
	Suppl. 7, 56 (1987)
Alcohol drinking	*44*
Aldrin	*5*, 25 (1974)
	Suppl. 7, 88 (1987)
Allyl chloride	*36*, 39 (1985)
	Suppl. 7, 56 (1987)
Allyl isothiocyanate	*36*, 55 (1985)
	Suppl. 7, 56 (1987)
Allyl isovalerate	*36*, 69 (1985)
	Suppl. 7, 56 (1987)
Aluminium production	*34*, 37 (1984)
	Suppl. 7, 89 (1987)
Amaranth	*8*, 41 (1975)
	Suppl. 7, 56 (1987)
5-Aminoacenaphthene	*16*, 243 (1978)
	Suppl. 7, 56 (1987)
2-Aminoanthraquinone	*27*, 191 (1982)
	Suppl. 7, 56 (1987)
para-Aminoazobenzene	*8*, 53 (1975)
	Suppl. 7, 390 (1987)
ortho-Aminoazotoluene	*8*, 61 (1975) (*corr. 42*, 254)
	Suppl. 7, 56 (1987)
para-Aminobenzoic acid	*16*, 249 (1978)
	Suppl. 7, 56 (1987)
4-Aminobiphenyl	*1*, 74 (1972) (*corr. 42*, 251)
	Suppl. 7, 91 (1987)

2-Amino-3,4-dimethylimidazo[4,5-*f*]quinoline (*see* MeIQ)
2-Amino-3,8-dimethylimidazo[4,5-*f*]quinoxaline (*see* MeIQx)
3-Amino-1,4-dimethyl-5*H*-pyrido[4,3-*b*]indole (*see* Trp-P-1)
2-Aminodipyrido[1,2-*a*:3',2'-*d*]imidazole (*see* Glu-P-2)

1-Amino-2-methylanthraquinone	*27*, 199 (1982)
	Suppl. 7, 57 (1987)

2-Amino-3-methylimidazo[4,5-*f*]quinoline (*see* IQ)
2-Amino-6-methyldipyrido[1,2-*a*:3',2'-*d*]-imidazole (*see* Glu-P-1)
2-Amino-3-methyl-9*H*-pyrido[2,3-*b*]indole (*see* MeA-α-C)
3-Amino-1-methyl-5*H*-pyrido[4,3-*b*]indole (*see* Trp-P-2)

2-Amino-5-(5-nitro-2-furyl)-1,3,4-thiadiazole	7, 143 (1974)
	Suppl. 7, 57 (1987)
4-Amino-2-nitrophenol	16, 43 (1978)
	Suppl. 7, 57 (1987)
2-Amino-5-nitrothiazole	31, 71 (1983)
	Suppl. 7, 57 (1987)
2-Amino-9H-pyrido[2,3-b]indole (see A-α-C)	
11-Aminoundecanoic acid	39, 239 (1986)
	Suppl. 7, 57 (1987)
Amitrole	7, 31 (1974)
	41, 293 (1986)
	Suppl. 7, 92 (1987)
Ammonium potassium selenide (see Selenium and selenium compounds)	
Amorphous silica (see also Silica)	Suppl. 7, 341 (1987)
Amosite (see Asbestos)	
Anabolic steroids (see Androgenic (anabolic) steroids)	
Anaesthetics, volatile	11, 285 (1976)
	Suppl. 7, 93 (1987)
Analgesic mixtures containing phenacetin (see also Phenacetin)	Suppl. 7, 310 (1987)
Androgenic (anabolic) steroids	Suppl. 7, 96 (1987)
Angelicin and some synthetic derivatives (see also Angelicins)	40, 291 (1986)
Angelicin plus ultraviolet radiation (see also Angelicin and some synthetic derivatives)	Suppl. 7, 57 (1987)
Angelicins	Suppl. 7, 57 (1987)
Aniline	4, 27 (1974) (corr. 42, 252)
	27, 39 (1982)
	Suppl. 7, 99 (1987)
ortho-Anisidine	27, 63 (1982)
	Suppl. 7, 57 (1987)
para-Anisidine	27, 65 (1982)
	Suppl. 7, 57 (1987)
Anthanthrene	32, 95 (1983)
	Suppl. 7, 57 (1987)
Anthophyllite (see Asbestos)	
Anthracene	32, 105 (1983)
	Suppl. 7, 57 (1987)
Anthranilic acid	16, 265 (1978)
	Suppl. 7, 57 (1987)
ANTU (see 1-Naphthylthiourea)	
Apholate	9, 31 (1975)
	Suppl. 7, 57 (1987)
Aramite®	5, 39 (1974)
	Suppl. 7, 57 (1987)
Areca nut (see Betel quid)	
Arsanilic acid (see Arsenic and arsenic compounds)	

Arsenic and arsenic compounds	*1*, 41 (1972)
	2, 48 (1973)
	23, 39 (1980)
	Suppl. 7, 100 (1987)
Arsenic pentoxide (*see* Arsenic and arsenic compounds)	
Arsenic sulphide (*see* Arsenic and arsenic compounds)	
Arsenic trioxide (*see* Arsenic and arsenic compounds)	
Arsine (*see* Arsenic and arsenic compounds)	
Asbestos	*2*, 17 (1973) (*corr. 42*, 252)
	14 (1977) (*corr. 42*, 256)
	Suppl. 7, 106 (1987) (*corr. 45*, 283)
Attapulgite	*42*, 159 (1987)
	Suppl. 7, 117 (1987)
Auramine (technical-grade)	*1*, 69 (1972) (*corr. 42*, 251)
	Suppl. 7, 118 (1987)
Auramine, manufacture of (*see also* Auramine, technical-grade)	Suppl. 7, 118 (1987)
Aurothioglucose	*13*, 39 (1977)
	Suppl. 7, 57 (1987)
5-Azacytidine	*26*, 37 (1981)
	Suppl. 7, 57 (1987)
Azaserine	*10*, 73 (1976) (*corr. 42*, 255)
	Suppl. 7, 57 (1987)
Azathioprine	*26*, 47 (1981)
	Suppl. 7, 119 (1987)
Aziridine	*9*, 37 (1975)
	Suppl. 7, 58 (1987)
2-(1-Aziridinyl)ethanol	*9*, 47 (1975)
	Suppl. 7, 58 (1987)
Aziridyl benzoquinone	*9*, 51 (1975)
	Suppl. 7, 58 (1987)
Azobenzene	*8*, 75 (1975)
	Suppl. 7, 58 (1987)

B

Barium chromate (*see* Chromium and chromium compounds)	
Basic chromic sulphate (*see* Chromium and chromium compounds)	
BCNU (*see* Bischloroethyl nitrosourea)	
Benz[*a*]acridine	*32*, 123 (1983)
	Suppl. 7, 58 (1987)
Benz[*c*]acridine	*3*, 241 (1973)
	32, 129 (1983)
	Suppl. 7, 58 (1987)
Benzal chloride (*see also* α-Chlorinated toluenes)	*29*, 65 (1982)
	Suppl. 7, 148 (1987)
Benz[*a*]anthracene	*3*, 45 (1973)
	32, 135 (1983)
	Suppl. 7, 58 (1987)

Benzene	7, 203 (1974) (corr. 42, 254)
	29, 93, 391 (1982)
	Suppl. 7, 120 (1987)
Benzidine	1, 80 (1972)
	29, 149, 391 (1982)
	Suppl. 7, 123 (1987)
Benzidine-based dyes	Suppl. 7, 125 (1987)
Benzo[b]fluoranthene	3, 69 (1973)
	32, 147 (1983)
	Suppl. 7, 58 (1987)
Benzo[j]fluoranthene	3, 82 (1973)
	32, 155 (1983)
	Suppl. 7, 58 (1987)
Benzo[k]fluoranthene	32, 163 (1983)
	Suppl. 7, 58 (1987)
Benzo[ghi]fluoranthene	32, 171 (1983)
	Suppl. 7, 58 (1987)
Benzo[a]fluorene	32, 177 (1983)
	Suppl. 7, 58 (1987)
Benzo[b]fluorene	32, 183 (1983)
	Suppl. 7, 58 (1987)
Benzo[c]fluorene	32, 189 (1983)
	Suppl. 7, 58 (1987)
Benzo[ghi]perylene	32, 195 (1983)
	Suppl. 7, 58 (1987)
Benzo[c]phenanthrene	32, 205 (1983)
	Suppl. 7, 58 (1987)
Benzo[a]pyrene	3, 91 (1973)
	32, 211 (1983)
	Suppl. 7, 58 (1987)
Benzo[e]pyrene	3, 137 (1973)
	32, 225 (1983)
	Suppl. 7, 58 (1987)
para-Benzoquinone dioxime	29, 185 (1982)
	Suppl. 7, 58 (1987)
Benzotrichloride (see also α-Chlorinated toluenes)	29, 73 (1982)
	Suppl. 7, 148 (1987)
Benzoyl chloride	29, 83 (1982) (corr. 42, 261)
	Suppl. 7, 126 (1987)
Benzoyl peroxide	36, 267 (1985)
	Suppl. 7, 58 (1987)
Benzyl acetate	40, 109 (1986)
	Suppl. 7, 58 (1987)
Benzyl chloride (see also α-Chlorinated toluenes)	11, 217 (1976) (corr. 42, 256)
	29, 49 (1982)
	Suppl. 7, 148 (1987)
Benzyl violet 4B	16, 153 (1978)
	Suppl. 7, 58 (1987)
Bertrandite (see Beryllium and beryllium compounds)	

Beryllium and beryllium compounds	*1*, 17 (1972)
	23, 143 (1980) (*corr. 42*, 260)
	Suppl. 7, 127 (1987)

Beryllium acetate (*see* Beryllium and beryllium compounds)
Beryllium acetate, basic (*see* Beryllium and beryllium compounds)
Beryllium-aluminium alloy (*see* Beryllium and beryllium compounds)
Beryllium carbonate (*see* Beryllium and beryllium compounds)
Beryllium chloride (*see* Beryllium and beryllium compounds)
Beryllium-copper alloy (*see* Beryllium and beryllium compounds)
Beryllium-copper-cobalt alloy (*see* Beryllium and beryllium compounds)
Beryllium fluoride (*see* Beryllium and beryllium compounds)
Beryllium hydroxide (*see* Beryllium and beryllium compounds)
Beryllium-nickel alloy (*see* Beryllium and beryllium compounds)
Beryllium oxide (*see* Beryllium and beryllium compounds)
Beryllium phosphate (*see* Beryllium and beryllium compounds)
Beryllium silicate (*see* Beryllium and beryllium compounds)
Beryllium sulphate (*see* Beryllium and beryllium compounds)
Beryl ore (*see* Beryllium and beryllium compounds)

Betel quid	*37*, 141 (1985)
	Suppl. 7, 128 (1987)

Betel-quid chewing (*see* Betel quid)
BHA (*see* Butylated hydroxyanisole)
BHT (*see* Butylated hydroxytoluene)

Bis(1-aziridinyl)morpholinophosphine sulphide	*9*, 55 (1975)
	Suppl. 7, 58 (1987)
Bis(2-chloroethyl)ether	*9*, 117 (1975)
	Suppl. 7, 58 (1987)
N,N-Bis(2-chloroethyl)-2-naphthylamine	*4*, 119 (1974) (*corr. 42*, 253)
	Suppl. 7, 130 (1987)
Bischloroethyl nitrosourea (*see also* Chloroethyl nitrosoureas)	*26*, 79 (1981)
	Suppl. 7, 150 (1987)
1,2-Bis(chloromethoxy)ethane	*15*, 31 (1977)
	Suppl. 7, 58 (1987)
1,4-Bis(chloromethoxymethyl)benzene	*15*, 37 (1977)
	Suppl. 7, 58 (1987)
Bis(chloromethyl)ether	*4*, 231 (1974) (*corr. 42*, 253)
	Suppl. 7, 131 (1987)
Bis(2-chloro-1-methylethyl)ether	*41*, 149 (1986)
	Suppl. 7, 59 (1987)
Bitumens	*35*, 39 (1985)
	Suppl. 7, 133 (1987)
Bleomycins	*26*, 97 (1981)
	Suppl. 7, 134 (1987)
Blue VRS	*16*, 163 (1978)
	Suppl. 7, 59 (1987)

Boot and shoe manufacture and repair	*25*, 249 (1981)
	Suppl. 7, 232 (1987)
Bracken fern	*40*, 47 (1986)
	Suppl. 7, 135 (1987)
Brilliant Blue FCF	*16*, 171 (1978) (*corr. 42*, 257)
	Suppl. 7, 59 (1987)
1,3-Butadiene	*39*, 155 (1986) (*corr. 42*, 264)
	Suppl. 7, 136 (1987)
1,4-Butanediol dimethanesulphonate	*4*, 247 (1974)
	Suppl. 7, 137 (1987)
n-Butyl acrylate	*39*, 67 (1986)
	Suppl. 7, 59 (1987)
Butylated hydroxyanisole	*40*, 123 (1986)
	Suppl. 7, 59 (1987)
Butylated hydroxytoluene	*40*, 161 (1986)
	Suppl. 7, 59 (1987)
Butyl benzyl phthalate	*29*, 193 (1982) (*corr. 42*, 261)
	Suppl. 7, 59 (1987)
β-Butyrolactone	*11*, 225 (1976)
	Suppl. 7, 59 (1987)
γ-Butyrolactone	*11*, 231 (1976)
	Suppl. 7, 59 (1987)

C

Cabinet-making (*see* Furniture and cabinet-making)	
Cadmium acetate (*see* Cadmium and cadmium compounds)	
Cadmium and cadmium compounds	*2*, 74 (1973)
	11, 39 (1976) (*corr. 42*, 255)
	Suppl. 7, 139 (1987)
Cadmium chloride (*see* Cadmium and cadmium compounds)	
Cadmium oxide (*see* Cadmium and cadmium compounds)	
Cadmium sulphate (*see* Cadmium and cadmium compounds)	
Cadmium sulphide (*see* Cadmium and cadmium compounds)	
Calcium arsenate (*see* Arsenic and arsenic compounds)	
Calcium chromate (*see* Chromium and chromium compounds)	
Calcium cyclamate (*see* Cyclamates)	
Calcium saccharin (*see* Saccharin)	
Cantharidin	*10*, 79 (1976)
	Suppl. 7, 59 (1987)
Caprolactam	*19*, 115 (1979) (*corr. 42*, 258)
	39, 247 (1986) (*corr. 42*, 264)
	Suppl. 7, 390 (1987)
Captan	*30*, 295 (1983)
	Suppl. 7, 59 (1987)
Carbaryl	*12*, 37 (1976)
	Suppl. 7, 59 (1987)

Carbazole	*32*, 239 (1983)
	Suppl. 7, 59 (1987)
3-Carbethoxypsoralen	*40*, 317 (1986)
	Suppl. 7, 59 (1987)
Carbon blacks	*3*, 22 (1973)
	33, 35 (1984)
	Suppl. 7, 142 (1987)
Carbon tetrachloride	*1*, 53 (1972)
	20, 371 (1979)
	Suppl. 7, 143 (1987)
Carmoisine	*8*, 83 (1975)
	Suppl. 7, 59 (1987)
Carpentry and joinery	*25*, 139 (1981)
	Suppl. 7, 378 (1987)
Carrageenan	*10*, 181 (1976) (*corr. 42*, 255)
	31, 79 (1983)
	Suppl. 7, 59 (1987)
Catechol	*15*, 155 (1977)
	Suppl. 7, 59 (1987)
CCNU (*see* 1-(2-Chloroethyl)-3-cyclohexyl-1-nitrosourea)	
Ceramic fibres (*see* Man-made mineral fibres)	
Chemotherapy, combined, including alkylating agents (*see* MOPP and other combined chemotherapy including alkylating agents)	
Chlorambucil	*9*, 125 (1975)
	26, 115 (1981)
	Suppl. 7, 144 (1987)
Chloramphenicol	*10*, 85 (1976)
	Suppl. 7, 145 (1987)
Chlordane (*see also* Chlordane/Heptachlor)	*20*, 45 (1979) (*corr. 42*, 258)
Chlordane/Heptachlor	*Suppl. 7*, 146 (1987)
Chlordecone	*20*, 67 (1979)
	Suppl. 7, 59 (1987)
Chlordimeform	*30*, 61 (1983)
	Suppl. 7, 59 (1987)
Chlorinated dibenzodioxins (other than TCDD)	*15*, 41 (1977)
	Suppl. 7, 59 (1987)
α-Chlorinated toluenes	*Suppl. 7*, 148 (1987)
Chlormadinone acetate (*see also* Progestins; Combined oral contraceptives)	*6*, 149 (1974)
	21, 365 (1979)
Chlornaphazine (*see* N,N-Bis(2-chloroethyl)-2-naphthylamine)	
Chlorobenzilate	*5*, 75 (1974)
	30, 73 (1983)
	Suppl. 7, 60 (1987)
Chlorodifluoromethane	*41*, 237 (1986)
	Suppl. 7, 149 (1987)
1-(2-Chloroethyl)-3-cyclohexyl-1-nitrosourea (*see also* Chloroethyl nitrosoureas)	*26*, 173 (1981) (*corr. 42*, 260)
	Suppl. 7, 150 (1987)

1-(2-Chloroethyl)-3-(4-methylcyclohexyl)-1-nitrosourea (see also Chloroethyl nitrosoureas)	Suppl. 7, 150 (1987)
Chloroethyl nitrosoureas	Suppl. 7, 150 (1987)
Chlorofluoromethane	41, 229 (1986)
	Suppl. 7, 60 (1987)
Chloroform	1, 61 (1972)
	20, 401 (1979)
	Suppl. 7, 152 (1987)
Chloromethyl methyl ether (technical-grade) (see also Bis(chloromethyl) ether)	4, 239 (1974)
(4-Chloro-2-methylphenoxy)-acetic acid (see MCPA)	
Chlorophenols	Suppl. 7, 154 (1987)
Chlorophenols (occupational exposures to)	41, 319 (1986)
Chlorophenoxy herbicides	Suppl. 7, 156 (1987)
Chlorophenoxy herbicides (occupational exposures to)	41, 357 (1986)
4-Chloro-*ortho*-phenylenediamine	27, 81 (1982)
	Suppl. 7, 60 (1987)
4-Chloro-*meta*-phenylenediamine	27, 82 (1982)
	Suppl. 7, 60 (1987)
Chloroprene	19, 131 (1979)
	Suppl. 7, 160 (1987)
Chloropropham	12, 55 (1976)
	Suppl. 7, 60 (1987)
Chloroquine	13, 47 (1977)
	Suppl. 7, 60 (1987)
Chlorothalonil	30, 319 (1983)
	Suppl. 7, 60 (1987)
para-Chloro-*ortho*-toluidine (see also Chlordimeform)	16, 277 (1978)
	30, 65 (1983)
	Suppl. 7, 60 (1987)
Chlorotrianisene (see also Nonsteroidal oestrogens)	21, 139 (1979)
2-Chloro-1,1,1-trifluoroethane	41, 253 (1986)
	Suppl. 7, 60 (1987)
Cholesterol	10, 99 (1976)
	31, 95 (1983)
	Suppl. 7, 161 (1987)
Chromic acetate (see Chromium and chromium compounds)	
Chromic chloride (see Chromium and chromium compounds)	
Chromic oxide (see Chromium and chromium compounds	
Chromic phosphate (see Chromium and chromium compounds)	
Chromite ore (see Chromium and chromium compounds)	
Chromium and chromium compounds	2, 100 (1973)
	23, 205 (1980)
	Suppl. 7, 165 (1987)
Chromium carbonyl (see Chromium and chromium compounds)	
Chromium potassium sulphate (see Chromium and chromium compounds)	
Chromium sulphate (see Chromium and chromium compounds)	

Chromium trioxide (*see* Chromium and chromium compounds)
Chrysene   *3*, 159 (1973)
                                                              32, 247 (1983)
                                                              Suppl. 7, 60 (1987)
Chrysoidine   *8*, 91 (1975)
                                                              Suppl. 7, 169 (1987)
Chrysotile (*see* Asbestos)
CI Disperse Yellow 3   *8*, 97 (1975)
                                                              Suppl. 7, 60 (1987)
Cinnamyl anthranilate   *16*, 287 (1978)
                                                              31, 133 (1983)
                                                              Suppl. 7, 60 (1987)
Cisplatin   *26*, 151 (1981)
                                                              Suppl. 7, 170 (1987)
Citrinin   *40*, 67 (1986)
                                                              Suppl. 7, 60 (1987)
Citrus Red No. 2   *8*, 101 (1975) (*corr. 42*, 254)
                                                              Suppl. 7, 60 (1987)
Clofibrate   *24*, 39 (1980)
                                                              Suppl. 7, 171 (1987)
Clomiphene citrate   *21*, 551 (1979)
                                                              Suppl. 7, 172 (1987)
Coal gasification   *34*, 65 (1984)
                                                              Suppl. 7, 173 (1987)
Coal-tar pitches (*see also* Coal-tars)   *Suppl. 7*, 174 (1987)
Coal-tars   *35*, 83 (1985)
                                                              Suppl. 7, 175 (1987)
Cobalt-chromium alloy (*see* Chromium and chromium
    compounds)
Coke production   *34*, 101 (1984)
                                                              Suppl. 7, 176 (1987)
Combined oral contraceptives (*see also* Oestrogens, progestins   *Suppl. 7*, 297 (1987)
    and combinations)
Conjugated oestrogens (*see also* Steroidal oestrogens)   *21*, 147 (1979)
Contraceptives, oral (*see* Combined oral contraceptives;
    Sequential oral contraceptives)
Copper 8-hydroxyquinoline   *15*, 103 (1977)
                                                              Suppl. 7, 61 (1987)
Coronene   *32*, 263 (1983)
                                                              Suppl. 7, 61 (1987)
Coumarin   *10*, 113 (1976)
                                                              Suppl. 7, 61 (1987)
Creosotes (*see also* Coal-tars)   *Suppl. 7*, 177 (1987)
meta-Cresidine   *27*, 91 (1982)
                                                              Suppl. 7, 61 (1987)
para-Cresidine   *27*, 92 (1982)
                                                              Suppl. 7, 61 (1987)

Crocidolite (*see* Asbestos)	
Crude oil	*45*, 119 (1989)
Crystalline silica (*see also* Silica)	*Suppl. 7*, 341 (1987)
Cycasin	*1*, 157 (1972) (*corr. 42*, 251)
	10, 121 (1976)
	Suppl. 7, 61 (1987)
Cyclamates	*22*, 55 (1980)
	Suppl. 7, 178 (1987)
Cyclamic acid (*see* Cyclamates)	
Cyclochlorotine	*10*, 139 (1976)
	Suppl. 7, 61 (1987)
Cyclohexylamine (*see* Cyclamates)	
Cyclopenta[*cd*]pyrene	*32*, 269 (1983)
	Suppl. 7, 61 (1987)
Cyclopropane (*see* Anaesthetics, volatile)	
Cyclophosphamide	*9*, 135 (1975)
	26, 165 (1981)
	Suppl. 7, 182 (1987)

D

2,4-D (*see also* Chlorophenoxy herbicides; Chlorophenoxy herbicides, occupational exposures to)	*15*, 111 (1977)
Dacarbazine	*26*, 203 (1981)
	Suppl. 7, 184 (1987)
D & C Red No. 9	*8*, 107 (1975)
	Suppl. 7, 61 (1987)
Dapsone	*24*, 59 (1980)
	Suppl. 7, 185 (1987)
Daunomycin	*10*, 145 (1976)
	Suppl. 7, 61 (1987)
DDD (*see* DDT)	
DDE (*see* DDT)	
DDT	*5*, 83 (1974) (*corr. 42*, 253)
	Suppl. 7, 186 (1987)
Diacetylaminoazotoluene	*8*, 113 (1975)
	Suppl. 7, 61 (1987)
N,N'-Diacetylbenzidine	*16*, 293 (1978)
	Suppl. 7, 61 (1987)
Diallate	*12*, 69 (1976)
	30, 235 (1983)
	Suppl. 7, 61 (1987)
2,4-Diaminoanisole	*16*, 51 (1978)
	27, 103 (1982)
	Suppl. 7, 61 (1987)

4,4'-Diaminodiphenyl ether	*16*, 301 (1978);
	29, 203 (1982)
Suppl. 7, 61 (1987)	
1,2-Diamino-4-nitrobenzene	*16*, 63 (1978)
	Suppl. 7, 61 (1987)
1,4-Diamino-2-nitrobenzene	*16*, 73 (1978)
	Suppl. 7, 61 (1987)
2,6-Diamino-3-(phenylazo)pyridine (*see* Phenazopyridine hydrochloride)	
2,4-Diaminotoluene (*see also* Toluene diisocyanates)	*16*, 83 (1978)
	Suppl. 7, 61 (1987)
2,5-Diaminotoluene (*see also* Toluene diisocyanates)	*16*, 97 (1978)
	Suppl. 7, 61 (1987)
ortho-Dianisidine (*see* 3,3'-Dimethoxybenzidine)	
Diazepam	*13*, 57 (1977)
	Suppl. 7, 189 (1987)
Diazomethane	*7*, 223 (1974)
	Suppl. 7, 61 (1987)
Dibenz[*a,h*]acridine	*3*, 247 (1973)
	32, 277 (1983)
	Suppl. 7, 61 (1987)
Dibenz[*a,j*]acridine	*3*, 254 (1973)
	32, 283 (1983)
	Suppl. 7, 61 (1987)
Dibenz[*a,c*]anthracene	*32*, 289 (1983) (*corr. 42*, 262)
	Suppl. 7, 61 (1987)
Dibenz[*a,h*]anthracene	*3*, 178 (1973) (*corr. 43*, 261)
	32, 299 (1983)
	Suppl. 7, 61 (1987)
Dibenz[*a,j*]anthracene	*32*, 309 (1983)
	Suppl. 7, 61 (1987)
7*H*-Dibenzo[*c,g*]carbazole	*3*, 260 (1973)
	32, 315 (1983)
	Suppl. 7, 61 (1987)
Dibenzodioxins, chlorinated (other than TCDD) [*see* Chlorinated dibenzodioxins (other than TCDD)]	
Dibenzo[*a,e*]fluoranthene	*32*, 321 (1983)
	Suppl. 7, 61 (1987)
Dibenzo[*h,rst*]pentaphene	*3*, 197 (1973)
	Suppl. 7, 62 (1987)
Dibenzo[*a,e*]pyrene	*3*, 201 (1973)
	32, 327 (1983)
	Suppl. 7, 62 (1987)
Dibenzo[*a,h*]pyrene	*3*, 207 (1973)
	32, 331 (1983)
	Suppl. 7, 62 (1987)

Dibenzo[*a,i*]pyrene	*3*, 215 (1973)
	32, 337 (1983)
	Suppl. 7, 62 (1987)
Dibenzo[*a,l*]pyrene	*3*, 224 (1973)
	32, 343 (1983)
	Suppl. 7, 62 (1987)
1,2-Dibromo-3-chloropropane	*15*, 139 (1977)
	20, 83 (1979)
	Suppl. 7, 191 (1987)
Dichloroacetylene	*39*, 369 (1986)
	Suppl. 7, 62 (1987)
ortho-Dichlorobenzene	*7*, 231 (1974)
	29, 213 (1982)
	Suppl. 7, 192 (1987)
para-Dichlorobenzene	*7*, 231 (1974)
	29, 215 (1982)
	Suppl. 7, 192 (1987)
3,3'-Dichlorobenzidine	*4*, 49 (1974)
	29, 239 (1982)
	Suppl. 7, 193 (1987)
trans-1,4-Dichlorobutene	*15*, 149 (1977)
	Suppl. 7, 62 (1987)
3,3'-Dichloro-4,4'-diaminodiphenyl ether	*16*, 309 (1978)
	Suppl. 7, 62 (1987)
1,2-Dichloroethane	*20*, 429 (1979)
	Suppl. 7, 62 (1987)
Dichloromethane	*20*, 449 (1979)
	41, 43 (1986)
	Suppl. 7, 194 (1987)
2,4-Dichlorophenol (*see* Chlorophenols; Chlorophenols, occupational exposures to)	
(2,4-Dichlorophenoxy)acetic acid (*see* 2,4-D)	
2,6-Dichloro-*para*-phenylenediamine	*39*, 325 (1986)
	Suppl. 7, 62 (1987)
1,2-Dichloropropane	*41*, 131 (1986)
	Suppl. 7, 62 (1987)
1,3-Dichloropropene (technical-grade)	*41*, 113 (1986)
	Suppl. 7, 195 (1987)
Dichlorvos	*20*, 97 (1979)
	Suppl. 7, 62 (1987)
Dicofol	*30*, 87 (1983)
	Suppl. 7, 62 (1987)
Dicyclohexylamine (*see* Cyclamates)	
Dieldrin	*5*, 125 (1974)
	Suppl. 7, 196 (1987)
Dienoestrol (*see also* Nonsteroidal oestrogens)	*21*, 161 (1979)

Diepoxybutane	*11*, 115 (1976) (*corr. 42*, 255)
	Suppl. 7, 62 (1987)
Diesel fuels	*45*, 219 (1989)
Diethyl ether (*see* Anaesthetics, volatile)	
Di(2-ethylhexyl)adipate	*29*, 257 (1982)
	Suppl. 7, 62 (1987)
Di(2-ethylhexyl)phthalate	*29*, 269 (1982) (*corr. 42*, 261)
	Suppl. 7, 62 (1987)
1,2-Diethylhydrazine	*4*, 153 (1974)
	Suppl. 7, 62 (1987)
Diethylstilboestrol	*6*, 55 (1974)
	21, 172 (1979) (*corr. 42*, 259)
	Suppl. 7, 273 (1987)
Diethylstilboestrol dipropionate (*see* Diethylstilboestrol)	
Diethyl sulphate	*4*, 277 (1974)
	Suppl. 7, 198 (1987)
Diglycidyl resorcinol ether	*11*, 125 (1976)
	36, 181 (1985)
	Suppl. 7, 62 (1987)
Dihydrosafrole	*1*, 170 (1972)
	10, 233 (1976)
	Suppl. 7, 62 (1987)
Dihydroxybenzenes (*see* Catechol; Hydroquinone; Resorcinol)	
Dihydroxymethylfuratrizine	*24*, 77 (1980)
	Suppl. 7, 62 (1987)
Dimethisterone (*see also* Progestins; Sequential oral contraceptives)	*6*, 167 (1974)
	21, 377 (1979)
Dimethoxane	*15*, 177 (1977)
	Suppl. 7, 62 (1987)
3,3'-Dimethoxybenzidine	*4*, 41 (1974)
	Suppl. 7, 198 (1987)
3,3'-Dimethoxybenzidine-4,4'-diisocyanate	*39*, 279 (1986)
	Suppl. 7, 62 (1987)
para-Dimethylaminoazobenzene	*8*, 125 (1975)
	Suppl. 7, 62 (1987)
para-Dimethylaminoazobenzenediazo sodium sulphonate	*8*, 147 (1975)
	Suppl. 7, 62 (1987)
trans-2-[(Dimethylamino)methylimino]-5-[2-(5-nitro-2-furyl)-vinyl]-1,3,4-oxadiazole	*7*, 147 (1974) (*corr. 42*, 253)
	Suppl. 7, 62 (1987)
4,4'-Dimethylangelicin plus ultraviolet radiation (*see also* Angelicin and some synthetic derivatives)	*Suppl. 7*, 57 (1987)
4,5'-Dimethylangelicin plus ultraviolet radiation (*see also* Angelicin and some synthetic derivatives)	*Suppl. 7*, 57 (1987)
Dimethylarsinic acid (*see* Arsenic and arsenic compounds)	
3,3'-Dimethylbenzidine	*1*, 87 (1972)
	Suppl. 7, 62 (1987)

Dimethylcarbamoyl chloride	*12*, 77 (1976)
	Suppl. 7, 199 (1987)
1,1-Dimethylhydrazine	*4*, 137 (1974)
	Suppl. 7, 62 (1987)
1,2-Dimethylhydrazine	*4*, 145 (1974) (*corr. 42*, 253)
	Suppl. 7, 62 (1987)
1,4-Dimethylphenanthrene	*32*, 349 (1983)
	Suppl. 7, 62 (1987)
Dimethyl sulphate	*4*, 271 (1974)
	Suppl. 7, 200 (1987)
1,8-Dinitropyrene	*33*, 171 (1984)
	Suppl. 7, 63 (1987)
Dinitrosopentamethylenetetramine	*11*, 241 (1976)
	Suppl. 7, 63 (1987)
1,4-Dioxane	*11*, 247 (1976)
	Suppl. 7, 201 (1987)
2,4'-Diphenyldiamine	*16*, 313 (1978)
	Suppl. 7, 63 (1987)
Direct Black 38 (*see also* Benzidine-based dyes)	*29*, 295 (1982) (*corr. 42*, 261)
Direct Blue 6 (*see also* Benzidine-based dyes)	*29*, 311 (1982)
Direct Brown 95 (*see also* Benzidine-based dyes)	*29*, 321 (1982)
Disulfiram	*12*, 85 (1976)
	Suppl. 7, 63 (1987)
Dithranol	*13*, 75 (1977)
	Suppl. 7, 63 (1987)
Divinyl ether (*see* Anaesthetics, volatile)	
Dulcin	*12*, 97 (1976)
	Suppl. 7, 63 (1987)

E

Endrin	*5*, 157 (1974)
	Suppl. 7, 63 (1987)
Enflurane (*see* Anaesthetics, volatile)	
Eosin	*15*, 183 (1977)
	Suppl. 7, 63 (1987)
Epichlorohydrin	*11*, 131 (1976) (*corr. 42*, 256)
	Suppl. 7, 202 (1987)
1-Epoxyethyl-3,4-epoxycyclohexane	*11*, 141 (1976)
	Suppl. 7, 63 (1987)
3,4-Epoxy-6-methylcyclohexylmethyl-3,4-epoxy-6-methyl-cyclohexane carboxylate	*11*, 147 (1976)
	Suppl. 7, 63 (1987)
cis-9,10-Epoxystearic acid	*11*, 153 (1976)
	Suppl. 7, 63 (1987)
Erionite	*42*, 225 (1987)
	Suppl. 7, 203 (1987)

Ethinyloestradiol (see also Steroidal oestrogens)	6, 77 (1974)
	21, 233 (1979)
Ethionamide	13, 83 (1977)
	Suppl. 7, 63 (1987)
Ethyl acrylate	19, 57 (1979)
	39, 81 (1986)
	Suppl. 7, 63 (1987)
Ethylene	19, 157 (1979)
	Suppl. 7, 63 (1987)
Ethylene dibromide	15, 195 (1977)
	Suppl. 7, 204 (1987)
Ethylene oxide	11, 157 (1976)
	36, 189 (1985) (corr. 42, 263)
	Suppl. 7, 205 (1987)
Ethylene sulphide	11, 257 (1976)
	Suppl. 7, 63 (1987)
Ethylene thiourea	7, 45 (1974)
	Suppl. 7, 207 (1987)
Ethyl methanesulphonate	7, 245 (1974)
	Suppl. 7, 63 (1987)
N-Ethyl-N-nitrosourea	1, 135 (1972)
	17, 191 (1978)
	Suppl. 7, 63 (1987)
Ethyl selenac (see also Selenium and selenium compounds)	12, 107 (1976)
	Suppl. 7, 63 (1987)
Ethyl tellurac	12, 115 (1976)
	Suppl. 7, 63 (1987)
Ethynodiol diacetate (see also Progestins; Combined oral contraceptives)	6 173 (1974)
	21, 387 (1979)
Eugenol	36, 75 (1985)
	Suppl. 7, 63 (1987)
Evans blue	8, 151 (1975)
	Suppl. 7, 63 (1987)

F

Fast Green FCF	16, 187 (1978)
	Suppl. 7, 63 (1987)
Ferbam	12, 121 (1976) (corr. 42, 256)
	Suppl. 7, 63 (1987)
Ferric oxide	1, 29 (1972)
	Suppl. 7, 216 (1987)
Ferrochromium (see Chromium and chromium compounds)	
Fluometuron	30, 245 (1983)
	Suppl. 7, 63 (1987)
Fluoranthene	32, 355 (1983)
	Suppl. 7, 63 (1987)

Fluorene	*32*, 365 (1983)
	Suppl. 7, 63 (1987)
Fluorides (inorganic, used in drinking-water)	*27*, 237 (1982)
	Suppl. 7, 208 (1987)
5-Fluorouracil	*26*, 217 (1981)
	Suppl. 7, 210 (1987)
Fluorspar (*see* Fluorides)	
Fluosilicic acid (*see* Fluorides)	
Fluroxene (*see* Anaesthetics, volatile)	
Formaldehyde	*29*, 345 (1982)
	Suppl. 7, 211 (1987)
2-(2-Formylhydrazino)-4-(5-nitro-2-furyl)thiazole	*7*, 151 (1974) (*corr. 42*, 253)
	Suppl. 7, 63 (1987)
Fuel oils (heating oils)	*45*, 239 (1989)
Furazolidone	*31*, 141 (1983)
	Suppl. 7, 63 (1987)
Furniture and cabinet-making	*25*, 99 (1981)
	Suppl. 7, 380 (1987)
2-(2-Furyl)-3-(5-nitro-2-furyl)acrylamide (*see* AF-2)	
Fusarenon-X	*11*, 169 (1976)
	31, 153 (1983)
	Suppl. 7, 64 (1987)

G

Gasoline	*45*, 159 (1989)
Glass fibres (*see* Man-made mineral fibres)	
Glasswool (*see* Man-made mineral fibres)	
Glass filaments (*see* Man-made mineral fibres)	
Glu-P-1	*40*, 223 (1986)
	Suppl. 7, 64 (1987)
Glu-P-2	*40*, 235 (1986)
	Suppl. 7, 64 (1987)
L-Glutamic acid, 5-[2-(4-hydroxymethyl)phenylhydrazide] (*see* Agaratine)	
Glycidaldehyde	*11*, 175 (1976)
	Suppl. 7, 64 (1987)
Glycidyl oleate	*11*, 183 (1976)
	Suppl. 7, 64 (1987)
Glycidyl stearate	*11*, 187 (1976)
	Suppl. 7, 64 (1987)
Griseofulvin	*10*, 153 (1976)
	Suppl. 7, 391 (1987)
Guinea Green B	*16*, 199 (1978)
	Suppl. 7, 64 (1987)
Gyromitrin	*31*, 163 (1983)
	Suppl. 7, 391 (1987)

H

Haematite	*1*, 29 (1972)
	Suppl. 7, 216 (1987)
Haematite and ferric oxide	*Suppl. 7*, 216 (1987)
Haematite mining, underground, with exposure to radon	*1*, 29 (1972)
	Suppl. 7, 216 (1987)
Hair dyes, epidemiology of	*16*, 29 (1978)
	27, 307 (1982)
Halothane (*see* Anaesthetics, volatile)	
α-HCH (*see* Hexachlorocyclohexanes)	
β-HCH (*see* Hexachlorocyclohexanes)	
γ-HCH (*see* Hexachlorocyclohexanes)	
Heating oils (*see* Fuel oils)	
Heptachlor (*see also* Chlordane/Heptachlor)	*5*, 173 (1974)
	20, 129 (1979)
Hexachlorobenzene	*20*, 155 (1979)
	Suppl. 7, 219 (1987)
Hexachlorobutadiene	*20*, 179 (1979)
	Suppl. 7, 64 (1987)
Hexachlorocyclohexanes	*5*, 47 (1974)
	20, 195 (1979) (*corr. 42*, 258)
	Suppl. 7, 220 (1987)
Hexachlorocyclohexane, technical-grade (*see* Hexachlorocyclohexanes)	
Hexachloroethane	*20*, 467 (1979)
	Suppl. 7, 64 (1987)
Hexachlorophene	*20*, 241 (1979)
	Suppl. 7, 64 (1987)
Hexamethylphosphoramide	*15*, 211 (1977)
	Suppl. 7, 64 (1987)
Hexoestrol (*see* Nonsteroidal oestrogens)	
Hycanthone mesylate	*13*, 91 (1977)
	Suppl. 7, 64 (1987)
Hydralazine	*24*, 85 (1980)
	Suppl. 7, 222 (1987)
Hydrazine	*4*, 127 (1974)
	Suppl. 7, 223 (1987)
Hydrogen peroxide	*36*, 285 (1985)
	Suppl. 7, 64 (1987)
Hydroquinone	*15*, 155 (1977)
	Suppl. 7, 64 (1987)
4-Hydroxyazobenzene	*8*, 157 (1975)
	Suppl. 7, 64 (1987)
17α-Hydroxyprogesterone caproate (*see also* Progestins)	*21*, 399 (1979) (*corr. 42*, 259)
8-Hydroxyquinoline	*13*, 101 (1977)
	Suppl. 7, 64 (1987)
8-Hydroxysenkirkine	*10*, 265 (1976)
	Suppl. 7, 64 (1987)

I

Indeno[1,2,3-*cd*]pyrene	*3*, 229 (1973)
	32, 373 (1983)
	Suppl. 7, 64 (1987)
IQ	*40*, 261 (1986)
	Suppl. 7, 64 (1987)
Iron and steel founding	*34*, 133 (1984)
	Suppl. 7, 224 (1987)
Iron-dextran complex	*2*, 161 (1973)
	Suppl. 7, 226 (1987)
Iron-dextrin complex	*2*, 161 (1973) (*corr. 42*, 252)
	Suppl. 7, 64 (1987)
Iron oxide (*see* Ferric oxide)	
Iron oxide, saccharated (*see* Saccharated iron oxide)	
Iron sorbitol-citric acid complex	*2*, 161 (1973)
	Suppl. 7, 64 (1987)
Isatidine	*10*, 269 (1976)
	Suppl. 7, 65 (1987)
Isoflurane (*see* Anaesthetics, volatile)	
Isoniazid (*see* Isonicotinic acid hydrazide)	
Isonicotinic acid hydrazide	*4*, 159 (1974)
	Suppl. 7, 227 (1987)
Isophosphamide	*26*, 237 (1981)
	Suppl. 7, 65 (1987)
Isopropyl alcohol	*15*, 223 (1977)
	Suppl. 7, 229 (1987)
Isopropyl alcohol manufacture (strong-acid process) (*see also* Isopropyl alcohol)	*Suppl. 7*, 229 (1987)
Isopropyl oils	*15*, 223 (1977)
	Suppl. 7, 229 (1987)
Isosafrole	*1*, 169 (1972)
	10, 232 (1976)
	Suppl. 7, 65 (1987)

J

Jacobine	*10*, 275 (1976)
	Suppl. 7, 65 (1987)
Jet fuel	*45*, 203 (1989)
Joinery (*see* Carpentry and joinery)	

K

Kaempferol	*31*, 171 (1983)
	Suppl. 7, 65 (1987)
Kepone (*see* Chlordecone)	

L

Lasiocarpine	*10*, 281 (1976)
	Suppl. 7, 65 (1987)
Lauroyl peroxide	*36*, 315 (1985)
	Suppl. 7, 65 (1987)
Lead acetate (*see* Lead and lead compounds)	
Lead and lead compounds	*1*, 40 (1972) (*corr. 42*, 251)
	2, 52, 150 (1973)
	12, 131 (1976)
	23, 40, 208, 209, 325 (1980)
	Suppl. 7, 230 (1987)
Lead arsenate (*see* Arsenic and arsenic compounds)	
Lead carbonate (*see* Lead and lead compounds)	
Lead chloride (*see* Lead and lead compounds)	
Lead chromate (*see* Chromium and chromium compounds)	
Lead chromate oxide (*see* Chromium and chromium compounds)	
Lead naphthenate (*see* Lead and lead compounds)	
Lead nitrate (*see* Lead and lead compounds)	
Lead oxide (*see* Lead and lead compounds)	
Lead phosphate (*see* Lead and lead compounds)	
Lead subacetate (*see* Lead and lead compounds)	
Lead tetroxide (*see* Lead and lead compounds)	
Leather goods manufacture	*25*, 279 (1981)
	Suppl. 7, 235 (1987)
Leather industries	*25*, 199 (1981)
	Suppl. 7, 232 (1987)
Leather tanning and processing	*25*, 201 (1981)
	Suppl. 7, 236 (1987)
Ledate (*see also* Lead and lead compounds)	*12*, 131 (1976)
Light Green SF	*16*, 209 (1978)
	Suppl. 7, 65 (1987)
Lindane (*see* Hexachlorocyclohexanes)	
The lumber and sawmill industries (including logging)	*25*, 49 (1981)
	Suppl. 7, 383 (1987)
Luteoskyrin	*10*, 163 (1976)
	Suppl. 7, 65 (1987)
Lynoestrenol (*see also* Progestins; Combined oral contraceptives)	*21*, 407 (1979)

M

Magenta	*4*, 57 (1974) (*corr. 42*, 252)
	Suppl. 7, 238 (1987)
Magenta, manufacture of (*see also* Magenta)	*Suppl. 7*, 238 (1987)
Malathion	*30*, 103 (1983)
	Suppl. 7, 65 (1987)
Maleic hydrazide	*4*, 173 (1974) (*corr. 42*, 253)
	Suppl. 7, 65 (1987)

Malonaldehyde	*36*, 163 (1985)
	Suppl. 7, 65 (1987)
Maneb	*12*, 137 (1976)
	Suppl. 7, 65 (1987)
Man-made mineral fibres	*43*, 39 (1988)
Mannomustine	*9*, 157 (1975)
	Suppl. 7, 65 (1987)
MCPA (*see also* Chlorophenoxy herbicides; Chlorophenoxy herbicides, occupational exposures)	*30*, 255 (1983)
MeA-α-C	*40*, 253 (1986)
	Suppl. 7, 65 (1987)
Medphalan	*9*, 168 (1975)
	Suppl. 7, 65 (1987)
Medroxyprogesterone acetate	*6*, 157 (1974)
	21, 417 (1979) (*corr. 42*, 259)
	Suppl. 7, 289 (1987)
Megestrol acetate (*see* also Progestins; Combined oral contraceptives)	*21*, 431 (1979)
MeIQ	*40*, 275 (1986)
	Suppl. 7, 65 (1987)
MeIQx	*40*, 283 (1986)
	Suppl. 7, 65 (1987)
Melamine	*39*, 333 (1986)
	Suppl. 7, 65 (1987)
Melphalan	*9*, 167 (1975)
	Suppl. 7, 239 (1987)
6-Mercaptopurine	*26*, 249 (1981)
	Suppl. 7, 240 (1987)
Merphalan	*9*, 169 (1975)
	Suppl. 7, 65 (1987)
Mestranol (*see also* Steroidal oestrogens)	*6*, 87 (1974)
	21, 257 (1979) (*corr. 42*, 259)
Methanearsonic acid, disodium salt (*see* Arsenic and arsenic compounds)	
Methanearsonic acid, monosodium salt (*see* Arsenic and arsenic compounds)	
Methotrexate	*26*, 267 (1981)
	Suppl. 7, 241 (1987)
Methoxsalen (*see* 8-Methoxypsoralen)	
Methoxychlor	*5*, 193 (1974)
	20, 259 (1979)
	Suppl. 7, 66 (1987)
Methoxyflurane (*see* Anaesthetics, volatile)	
5-Methoxypsoralen	*40*, 327 (1986)
	Suppl. 7, 242 (1987)
8-Methoxypsoralen (*see also* 8-Methoxypsoralen plus ultraviolet radiation)	*24*, 101 (1980)
8-Methoxypsoralen plus ultraviolet radiation	*Suppl. 7*, 243 (1987)

Methyl acrylate	*19*, 52 (1979)
	39, 99 (1986)
	Suppl. 7, 66 (1987)
5-Methylangelicin plus ultraviolet radiation (*see also* Angelicin and some synthetic derivatives)	*Suppl. 7*, 57 (1987)
2-Methylaziridine	*9*, 61 (1975)
	Suppl. 7, 66 (1987)
Methylazoxymethanol acetate	*1*, 164 (1972)
	10, 121 (1976)
	Suppl. 7, 66 (1987)
Methyl bromide	*41*, 187 (1986) (*corr. 45*, 283)
	Suppl. 7, 245 (1987)
Methyl carbamate	*12*, 151 (1976)
	Suppl. 7, 66 (1987)
Methyl-CCNU [*see* 1-(2-Chloroethyl)-3-(4-methyl-cyclohexyl)-1-nitrosourea]	
Methyl chloride	*41*, 161 (1986)
	Suppl. 7, 246 (1987)
1-, 2-, 3-, 4-, 5- and 6-Methylchrysenes	*32*, 379 (1983)
	Suppl. 7, 66 (1987)
N-Methyl-*N*,4-dinitrosoaniline	*1*, 141 (1972)
	Suppl. 7, 66 (1987)
4,4'-Methylene bis(2-chloroaniline)	*4*, 65 (1974) (*corr. 42*, 252)
	Suppl. 7, 246 (1987)
4,4'-Methylene bis(*N*,*N*-dimethyl)benzenamine	*27*, 119 (1982)
	Suppl. 7, 66 (1987)
4,4'-Methylene bis(2-methylaniline)	*4*, 73 (1974)
	Suppl. 7, 248 (1987)
4,4'-Methylenedianiline	*4*, 79 (1974) (*corr. 42*, 252)
	39, 347 (1986)
	Suppl. 7, 66 (1987)
4,4'-Methylenediphenyl diisocyanate	*19*, 314 (1979)
	Suppl. 7, 66 (1987)
2-Methylfluoranthene	*32*, 399 (1983)
	Suppl. 7, 66 (1987)
3-Methylfluoranthene	*32*, 399 (1983)
	Suppl. 7, 66 (1987)
Methyl iodide	*15*, 245 (1977)
	41, 213 (1986)
	Suppl. 7, 66 (1987)
Methyl methacrylate	*19*, 187 (1979)
	Suppl. 7, 66 (1987)
Methyl methanesulphonate	*7*, 253 (1974)
	Suppl. 7, 66 (1987)
2-Methyl-1-nitroanthraquinone	*27*, 205 (1982)
	Suppl. 7, 66 (1987)

N-Methyl-N'-nitro-N-nitrosoguanidine	4, 183 (1974)
	Suppl. 7, 248 (1987)
3-Methylnitrosaminopropionaldehyde (see 3-(N-Nitroso-methylamino)propionaldehyde)	
3-Methylnitrosaminopropionitrile (see 3-(N-Nitrosomethyl-amino)propionitrile)	
4-(Methylnitrosamino)-4-(3-pyridyl)-1-butanal (see 4-(N-Nitrosomethylamino)-4-(3-pyridyl)-1-butanal)	
4-(Methylnitrosamino)-1-(3-pyridyl)-1-butanone (see 4-(N-Nitrosomethylamino)-1-(3-pyridyl)-1-butanone)	
N-Methyl-N-nitrosourea	1, 125 (1972)
	17, 227 (1978)
	Suppl. 7, 66 (1987)
N-Methyl-N-nitrosourethane	4, 211 (1974)
	Suppl. 7, 66 (1987)
Methyl parathion	30, 131 (1983)
	Suppl. 7, 392 (1987)
1-Methylphenanthrene	32, 405 (1983)
	Suppl. 7, 66 (1987)
7-Methylpyrido[3,4-c]psoralen	40, 349 (1986)
	Suppl. 7, 71 (1987)
Methyl red	8, 161 (1975)
	Suppl. 7, 66 (1987)
Methyl selenac (see also Selenium and selenium compounds)	12, 161 (1976)
	Suppl. 7, 66 (1987)
Methylthiouracil	7, 53 (1974)
	Suppl. 7, 66 (1987)
Metronidazole	13, 113 (1977)
	Suppl. 7, 250 (1987)
Mineral oils	3, 30 (1973)
	33, 87 (1984) (corr. 42, 262)
	Suppl. 7, 252 (1987)
Mirex	5, 203 (1974)
	20, 283 (1979) (corr. 42, 258)
	Suppl. 7, 66 (1987)
Mitomycin C	10, 171 (1976)
	Suppl. 7, 67 (1987)
MNNG (see N-Methyl-N'-nitro-N-nitrosoguanidine)	
MOCA (see 4,4'-Methylene bis(2-chloroaniline))	
Modacrylic fibres	19, 86 (1979)
	Suppl. 7, 67 (1987)
Monocrotaline	10, 291 (1976)
	Suppl. 7, 67 (1987)
Monuron	12, 167 (1976)
	Suppl. 7, 67 (1987)
MOPP and other combined chemotherapy including alkylating agents	Suppl. 7, 254 (1987)

5-(Morpholinomethyl)-3-[(5-nitrofurfurylidene)amino]-2-oxazolidinone   7, 161 (1974)
Suppl. 7, 67 (1987)
Mustard gas   9. 181 (1975) (*corr. 42*, 254)
Suppl. 7, 259 (1987)

Myleran (*see* 1,4-Butanediol dimethanesulphonate)

N

Nafenopin   *24*, 125 (1980)
Suppl. 7, 67 (1987)

1,5-Naphthalenediamine   *27*, 127 (1982)
Suppl. 7, 67 (1987)

1,5-Naphthalene diisocyanate   *19*, 311 (1979)
Suppl. 7, 67 (1987)

1-Naphthylamine   *4*, 87 (1974) (*corr. 42*, 253)
Suppl. 7, 260 (1987)

2-Naphthylamine   *4*, 97 (1974)
Suppl. 7, 261 (1987)

1-Naphthylthiourea   *30*, 347 (1983)
Suppl. 7, 263 (1987)

Nickel acetate (*see* Nickel and nickel compounds)
Nickel ammonium sulphate (*see* Nickel and nickel compounds)
Nickel and nickel compounds   *2*, 126 (1973) (*corr. 42*, 252)
11, 75 (1976)
Suppl. 7, 264 (1987)
(*corr. 45*, 283)

Nickel carbonate (*see* Nickel and nickel compounds)
Nickel carbonyl (*see* Nickel and nickel compounds)
Nickel chloride (*see* Nickel and nickel compounds)
Nickel-gallium alloy (*see* Nickel and nickel compounds)
Nickel hydroxide (*see* Nickel and nickel compounds)
Nickelocene (*see* Nickel and nickel compounds)
Nickel oxide (*see* Nickel and nickel compounds)
Nickel subsulphide (*see* Nickel and nickel compounds)
Nickel sulphate (*see* Nickel and nickel compounds)
Niridazole   *13*, 123 (1977)
Suppl. 7, 67 (1987)

Nithiazide   *31*, 179 (1983)
Suppl. 7, 67 (1987)

5-Nitroacenaphthene   *16*, 319 (1978)
Suppl. 7, 67 (1987)

5-Nitro-*ortho*-anisidine   *27*, 133 (1982)
Suppl. 7, 67 (1987)

9-Nitroanthracene   *33*, 179 (1984)
Suppl. 7, 67 (1987)

6-Nitrobenzo[*a*]pyrene   *33*, 187 (1984)
Suppl. 7, 67 (1987)

4-Nitrobiphenyl   *4*, 113 (1974)
Suppl. 7, 67 (1987)

6-Nitrochrysene	*33*, 195 (1984)
	Suppl. 7, 67 (1987)
Nitrofen (technical-grade)	*30*, 271 (1983)
	Suppl. 7, 67 (1987)
3-Nitrofluoranthene	*33*, 201 (1984)
	Suppl. 7, 67 (1987)
5-Nitro-2-furaldehyde semicarbazone	*7*, 171 (1974)
	Suppl. 7, 67 (1987)
1-[(5-Nitrofurfurylidene)amino]-2-imidazolidinone	*7*, 181 (1974)
	Suppl. 7, 67 (1987)
N-[4-(5-Nitro-2-furyl)-2-thiazolyl]acetamide	*1*, 181 (1972)
	7, 185 (1974)
	Suppl. 7, 67 (1987)
Nitrogen mustard	*9*, 193 (1975)
	Suppl. 7, 269 (1987)
Nitrogen mustard N-oxide	*9*, 209 (1975)
	Suppl. 7, 67 (1987)
2-Nitropropane	*29*, 331 (1982)
	Suppl. 7, 67 (1987)
1-Nitropyrene	*33*, 209 (1984)
	Suppl. 7, 67 (1987)
N-Nitrosatable drugs	*24*, 297 (1980) (*corr. 42*, 260)
N-Nitrosatable pesticides	*30*, 359 (1983)
N'-Nitrosoanabasine	*37*, 225 (1985)
	Suppl. 7, 67 (1987)
N'-Nitrosoanatabine	*37*, 233 (1985)
	Suppl. 7, 67 (1987)
N-Nitrosodi-n-butylamine	*4*, 197 (1974)
	17, 51 (1978)
	Suppl. 7, 67 (1987)
N-Nitrosodiethanolamine	*17*, 77 (1978)
	Suppl. 7, 67 (1987)
N-Nitrosodiethylamine	*1*, 107 (1972) (*corr. 42*, 251)
	17, 83 (1978) (*corr. 42*, 257)
	Suppl. 7, 67 (1987)
N-Nitrosodimethylamine	*1*, 95 (1972)
	17, 125 (1978) (*corr. 42*, 257)
	Suppl. 7, 67 (1987)
N-Nitrosodiphenylamine	*27*, 213 (1982)
	Suppl. 7, 67 (1987)
para-Nitrosodiphenylamine	*27*, 227 (1982) (*corr. 42*, 261)
	Suppl. 7, 68 (1987)
N-Nitrosodi-n-propylamine	*17*, 177 (1978)
	Suppl. 7, 68 (1987)
N-Nitroso-N-ethylurea (*see* N-Ethyl-N-nitrosourea)	
N-Nitrosofolic acid	*17*, 217 (1978)
	Suppl. 7, 68 (1987)

N-Nitrosoguvacine	37, 263 (1985)
	Suppl. 7, 68 (1987)
N-Nitrosoguvacoline	37, 263 (1985)
	Suppl. 7, 68 (1987)
N-Nitrosohydroxyproline	17, 304 (1978)
	Suppl. 7, 68 (1987)
3-(*N*-Nitrosomethylamino)propionaldehyde	37, 263 (1985)
	Suppl. 7, 68 (1987)
3-(*N*-Nitrosomethylamino)propionitrile	37, 263 (1985)
	Suppl. 7, 68 (1987)
4-(*N*-Nitrosomethylamino)-4-(3-pyridyl)-1-butanal	37, 205 (1985)
	Suppl. 7, 68 (1987)
4-(*N*-Nitrosomethylamino)-1-(3-pyridyl)-1-butanone	37, 209 (1985)
	Suppl. 7, 68 (1987)
N-Nitrosomethylethylamine	17, 221 (1978)
	Suppl. 7, 68 (1987)
N-Nitroso-*N*-methylurea (see *N*-Methyl-*N*-nitrosourea)	
N-Nitroso-*N*-methylurethane (see *N*-Methyl-*N*-nitrosourethane)	
N-Nitrosomethylvinylamine	17, 257 (1978)
	Suppl. 7, 68 (1987)
N-Nitrosomorpholine	17, 263 (1978)
	Suppl. 7, 68 (1987)
N'-Nitrosonornicotine	17, 281 (1978)
	37, 241 (1985)
	Suppl. 7, 68 (1987)
N-Nitrosopiperidine	17, 287 (1978)
	Suppl. 7, 68 (1987)
N-Nitrosoproline	17, 303 (1978)
	Suppl. 7, 68 (1987)
N-Nitrosopyrrolidine	17, 313 (1978)
	Suppl. 7, 68 (1987)
N-Nitrososarcosine	17, 327 (1978)
	Suppl. 7, 68 (1987)
Nitrosoureas, chloroethyl (see Chloroethyl nitrosoureas)	
Nitrous oxide (see Anaesthetics, volatile)	
Nitrovin	31, 185 (1983)
	Suppl. 7, 68 (1987)
NNA (see 4-(*N*-Nitrosomethylamino)-4-(3-pyridyl)-1-butanal)	
NNK (see 4-(*N*-Nitrosomethylamino)-1-(3-pyridyl)-1-butanone)	
Nonsteroidal oestrogens (see also Oestrogens, progestins and combinations)	Suppl. 7, 272 (1987)
Noresthisterone (see also Progestins; Combined oral contraceptives)	6, 179 (1974)
	21, 441 (1979)
Norethynodrel (see also Progestins; Combined oral contraceptives)	6, 191 (1974)
	21, 46 (1979) (corr. 42, 259)

Norgestrel (*see also* Progestins; Combined oral contraceptives)	*6*, 201 (1974)
	21, 479 (1979)
Nylon 6	*19*, 120 (1979)
	Suppl. 7, 68 (1987)

O

Ochratoxin A	*10*, 191 (1976)
	31, 191 (1983) (*corr. 42*, 262)
	Suppl. 7, 271 (1987)
Oestradiol-17β (*see also* Steroidal oestrogens)	*6*, 99 (1974)
	21, 279 (1979)
Oestradiol 3-benzoate (*see* Oestradiol-17β)	
Oestradiol dipropionate (*see* Oestradiol-17β)	
Oestradiol mustard	*9*, 217 (1975)
Oestradiol-17β-valerate (*see* Oestradiol-17β)	
Oestriol (*see also* Steroidal oestrogens)	*6*, 117 (1974)
	21, 327 (1979)
Oestrogen-progestin combinations (*see* Oestrogens, progestins and combinations)	
Oestrogen-progestin replacement therapy (*see also* Oestrogens, progestins and combinations)	*Suppl. 7*, 308 (1987)
Oestrogen replacement therapy (*see also* Oestrogens, progestins and combinations)	*Suppl. 7*, 280 (1987)
Oestrogens (*see* Oestrogens, progestins and combinations)	
Oestrogens, conjugated (*see* Conjugated oestrogens)	
Oestrogens, nonsteroidal (*see* Nonsteroidal oestrogens)	
Oestrogens, progestins and combinations	*6* (1974)
	21 (1979)
	Suppl. 7, 272 (1987)
Oestrogens, steroidal (*see* Steroidal oestrogens)	
Oestrone (*see also* Steroidal oestrogens)	*6*, 123 (1974)
	21, 343 (1979) (*corr. 42*, 259)
Oestrone benzoate (*see* Oestrone)	
Oil Orange SS	*8*, 165 (1975)
	Suppl. 7, 69 (1987)
Oral contraceptives, combined (*see* Combined oral contraceptives)	
Oral contraceptives, investigational (*see* Combined oral contraceptives)	
Oral contraceptives, sequential (*see* Sequential oral contraceptives)	
Orange I	*8*, 173 (1975)
	Suppl. 7, 69 (1987)
Orange G	*8*, 181 (1975)
	Suppl. 7, 69 (1987)
Organolead compounds (*see also* Lead and lead compounds)	*Suppl. 7*, 230 (1987)
Oxazepam	*13*, 58 (1977)
	Suppl. 7, 69 (1987)

Oxymetholone (*see also* Androgenic (anabolic) steroids)   *13*, 131 (1977)
Oxyphenbutazone   *13*, 185 (1977)
    Suppl. 7, 69 (1987)

P

Panfuran S (*see also* Dihydroxymethylfuratrizine)   *24*, 77 (1980)
    Suppl. 7, 69 (1987)
Paper manufacture (*see* Pulp and paper manufacture)
Parasorbic acid   *10*, 199 (1976) (*corr. 42*, 255)
    Suppl. 7, 69 (1987)
Parathion   *30*, 153 (1983)
    Suppl. 7, 69 (1987)
Patulin   *10*, 205 (1976)
    40, 83 (1986)
    Suppl. 7, 69 (1987)
Penicillic acid   *10*, 211 (1976)
    Suppl. 7, 69 (1987)
Pentachloroethane   *41*, 99 (1986)
    Suppl. 7, 69 (1987)
Pentachloronitrobenzene (*see* Quintozene)
Pentachlorophenol (*see also* Chlorophenols; Chlorophenols,   *20*, 303 (1979)
    occupational exposures to)
Perylene   *32*, 411 (1983)
    Suppl. 7, 69 (1987)
Petasitenine   *31*, 207 (1983)
    Suppl. 7, 69 (1987)
Petasites japonicus (*see* Pyrrolizidine alkaloids)
Petroleum refining (occupational exposures in)   *45*, 39 (1989)
Phenacetin   *3*, 141 (1973)
    24, 135 (1980)
    Suppl. 7, 310 (1987)
Phenanthrene   *32*, 419 (1983)
    Suppl. 7, 69 (1987)
Phenazopyridine hydrochloride   *8*, 117 (1975)
    24, 163 (1980) (*corr. 42*, 260)
    Suppl. 7, 312 (1987)
Phenelzine sulphate   *24*, 175 (1980)
    Suppl. 7, 312 (1987)
Phenicarbazide   *12*, 177 (1976)
    Suppl. 7, 70 (1987)
Phenobarbital   *13*, 157 (1977)
    Suppl. 7, 313 (1987)
Phenoxyacetic acid herbicides (*see* Chlorophenoxy herbicides)
Phenoxybenzamine hydrochloride   *9*, 223 (1975)
    24, 185 (1980)
    Suppl. 7, 70 (1987)

Phenylbutazone	*13*, 183 (1977)
	Suppl. 7, 316 (1987)
meta-Phenylenediamine	*16*, 111 (1978)
	Suppl. 7, 70 (1987)
para-Phenylenediamine	*16*, 125 (1978)
	Suppl. 7, 70 (1987)
N-Phenyl-2-naphthylamine	*16*, 325 (1978) (*corr. 42*, 257)
	Suppl. 7, 318 (1987)
ortho-Phenylphenol	*30*, 329 (1983)
	Suppl. 7, 70 (1987)
Phenytoin	*13*, 201 (1977)
	Suppl. 7, 319 (1987)
Piperazine oestrone sulphate (*see* Conjugated oestrogens)	
Piperonyl butoxide	*30*, 183 (1983)
	Suppl. 7, 70 (1987)
Pitches, coal-tar (*see* Coal-tar pitches)	
Polyacrylic acid	*19*, 62 (1979)
	Suppl. 7, 70 (1987)
Polybrominated biphenyls	*18*, 107 (1978)
	41, 261 (1986)
	Suppl. 7, 321 (1987)
Polychlorinated biphenyls	*7*, 261 (1974)
	18, 43 (1978) (*corr. 42*, 258)
	Suppl. 7, 322 (1987)
Polychlorinated camphenes (*see* Toxaphene)	
Polychloroprene	*19*, 141 (1979)
	Suppl. 7, 70 (1987)
Polyethylene	*19*, 164 (1979)
	Suppl. 7, 70 (1987)
Polymethylene polyphenyl isocyanate	*19*, 314 (1979)
	Suppl. 7, 70 (1987)
Polymethyl methacrylate	*19*, 195 (1979)
	Suppl. 7, 70 (1987)
Polyoestradiol phosphate (*see* Oestradiol-17β)	
Polypropylene	*19*, 218 (1979)
	Suppl. 7, 70 (1987)
Polystyrene	*19*, 245 (1979)
	Suppl. 7, 70 (1987)
Polytetrafluoroethylene	*19*, 288 (1979)
	Suppl. 7, 70 (1987)
Polyurethane foams	*19*, 320 (1979)
	Suppl. 7, 70 (1987)
Polyvinyl acetate	*19*, 346 (1979)
	Suppl. 7, 70 (1987)
Polyvinyl alcohol	*19*, 351 (1979)
	Suppl. 7, 70 (1987)

Polyvinyl chloride	7, 306 (1974)
	19, 402 (1979)
	Suppl. 7, 70 (1987)
Polyvinyl pyrrolidone	19, 463 (1979)
	Suppl. 7, 70 (1987)
Ponceau MX	8, 189 (1975)
	Suppl. 7, 70 (1987)
Ponceau 3R	8, 199 (1975)
	Suppl. 7, 70 (1987)
Ponceau SX	8, 207 (1975)
	Suppl. 7, 70 (1987)
Potassium arsenate (see Arsenic and arsenic compounds)	
Potassium arsenite (see Arsenic and arsenic compounds)	
Potassium bis(2-hydroxyethyl)dithiocarbamate	12, 183 (1976)
	Suppl. 7, 70 (1987)
Potassium bromate	40, 207 (1986)
	Suppl. 7, 70 (1987)
Potassium chromate (see Chromium and chromium compounds)	
Potassium dichromate (see Chromium and chromium compounds)	
Prednisone	26, 293 (1981)
	Suppl. 7, 326 (1987)
Procarbazine hydrochloride	26, 311 (1981)
	Suppl. 7, 327 (1987)
Proflavine salts	24, 195 (1980)
	Suppl. 7, 70 (1987)
Progesterone (see also Progestins; Combined oral contraceptives	6, 135 (1974)
	21, 49 (1979) (corr. 42, 259)
Progestins (see also Oestrogens, progestins and combinations)	Suppl. 7, 289 (1987)
Pronetalol hydrochloride	13, 227 (1977) (corr. 42, 256)
	Suppl. 7, 70 (1987)
1,3-Propane sultone	4, 253 (1974) (corr. 42, 253)
	Suppl. 7, 70 (1987)
Propham	12, 189 (1976)
	Suppl. 7, 70 (1987)
β-Propiolactone	4, 259 (1974) (corr. 42, 253)
	Suppl. 7, 70 (1987)
n-Propyl carbamate	12, 201 (1976)
	Suppl. 7, 70 (1987)
Propylene	19, 213 (1979)
	Suppl. 7, 71 (1987)
Propylene oxide	11, 191 (1976)
	36, 227 (1985) (corr. 42, 263)
	Suppl. 7, 328 (1987)
Propylthiouracil	7, 67 (1974)
	Suppl. 7, 329 (1987)
Ptaquiloside (see also Bracken fern)	40, 55 (1986)
	Suppl. 7, 71 (1987)

Pulp and paper manufacture	*25*, 157 (1981)
	Suppl. 7, 385 (1987)
Pyrene	*32*, 431 (1983)
	Suppl. 7, 71 (1987)
Pyrido[3,4-*c*]psoralen	*40*, 349 (1986)
	Suppl. 7, 71 (1987)
Pyrimethamine	*13*, 233 (1977)
	Suppl. 7, 71 (1987)
Pyrrolizidine alkaloids (*see also* Hydroxysenkirkine; Isatidine; Jacobine; Lasiocarpine; Monocrotaline; Retrorsine; Riddelline; Seneciphylline; Senkirkine)	*10*, 333 (1976)

Q

Quercetin (*see also* Bracken fern)	*31*, 213 (1983)
	Suppl. 7, 71 (1987)
para-Quinone	*15*, 255 (1977)
	Suppl. 7, 71 (1987)
Quintozene	*5*, 211 (1974)
	Suppl. 7, 71 (1987)

R

Radon	*43*, 173 (1988) (*corr. 45*, 283)
Reserpine	*10*, 217 (1976)
	24, 211 (1980) (*corr. 42*, 260)
	Suppl. 7, 330 (1987)
Resorcinol	*15*, 155 (1977)
	Suppl. 7, 71 (1987)
Retrorsine	*10*, 303 (1976)
	Suppl. 7, 71 (1987)
Rhodamine B	*16*, 221 (1978)
	Suppl. 7, 71 (1987)
Rhodamine 6G	*16*, 233 (1978)
	Suppl. 7, 71 (1987)
Riddelliine	*10*, 313 (1976)
	Suppl. 7, 71 (1987)
Rifampicin	*24*, 243 (1980)
	Suppl. 7, 71 (1987)
Rockwool (*see* Man-made mineral fibres)	
The rubber industry	*28* (1982) (*corr. 42*, 261)
	Suppl. 7, 332 (1987)
Rugulosin	*40*, 99 (1986)
	Suppl. 7, 71 (1987)

S

Saccharated iron oxide	*2*, 161 (1973)
	Suppl. 7, 71 (1987)

Saccharin	*22*, 111 (1980) (*corr. 42*, 259)
	Suppl. 7, 334 (1987)
Safrole	*1*, 169 (1972)
	10, 231 (1976)
	Suppl. 7, 71 (1987)
The sawmill industry (including logging) (*see* The lumber and sawmill industry (including logging))	
Scarlet Red	*8*, 217 (1975)
	Suppl. 7, 71 (1987)
Selenium and selenium compounds	*9*, 245 (1975) (*corr. 42*, 255)
	Suppl. 7, 71 (1987)
Selenium dioxide (*see* Selenium and selenium compounds)	
Selenium oxide (*see* Selenium and selenium compounds)	
Semicarbazide hydrochloride	*12*, 209 (1976) (*corr. 42*, 256)
	Suppl. 7, 71 (1987)
Senecio jacobaea L. (*see* Pyrrolizidine alkaloids)	
Senecio longilobus (*see* Pyrrolizidine alkaloids)	
Seneciphylline	*10*, 319, 335 (1976)
	Suppl. 7, 71 (1987)
Senkirkine	*10*, 327 (1976)
	31, 231 (1983)
	Suppl. 7, 71 (1987)
Sepiolite	*42*, 175 (1987)
	Suppl. 7, 71 (1987)
Sequential oral contraceptives (*see also* Oestrogens, progestins and combinations)	*Suppl. 7*, 296 (1987)
Shale-oils	*35*, 161 (1985)
	Suppl. 7, 339 (1987)
Shikimic acid (*see also* Bracken fern)	*40*, 55 (1986)
	Suppl. 7, 71 (1987)
Shoe manufacture and repair (*see* Boot and shoe manufacture and repair)	
Silica (*see also* Amorphous silica; Crystalline silica)	*42*, 39 (1987)
Slagwool (*see* Man-made mineral fibres)	
Sodium arsenate (*see* Arsenic and arsenic compounds)	
Sodium arsenite (*see* Arsenic and arsenic compounds)	
Sodium cacodylate (*see* Arsenic and arsenic compounds)	
Sodium chromate (*see* Chromium and chromium compounds)	
Sodium cyclamate (*see* Cyclamates)	
Sodium dichromate (*see* Chromium and chromium compounds)	
Sodium diethyldithiocarbamate	*12*, 217 (1976)
	Suppl. 7, 71 (1987)
Sodium equilin sulphate (*see* Conjugated oestrogens)	
Sodium fluoride (*see* Fluorides)	
Sodium monofluorophosphate (*see* Fluorides)	
Sodium oestrone sulphate (*see* Conjugated oestrogens)	
Sodium *ortho*-phenylphenate (*see also ortho*-Phenylphenol)	*30*, 329 (1983)
	Suppl. 7, 392 (1987)

Sodium saccharin (*see* Saccharin)	
Sodium selenate (*see* Selenium and selenium compounds)	
Sodium selenite (*see* Selenium and selenium compounds)	
Sodium silicofluoride (*see* Fluorides)	
Soots	*3*, 22 (1973)
	35, 219 (1985)
	Suppl. 7, 343 (1987)
Spironolactone	*24*, 259 (1980)
	Suppl. 7, 344 (1987)
Stannous fluoride (*see* Fluorides)	
Steel founding (*see* Iron and steel founding)	
Sterigmatocystin	*1*, 175 (1972)
	10, 245 (1976)
	Suppl. 7, 72 (1987)
Steroidal oestrogens (*see also* Oestrogens, progestins and combinations)	*Suppl. 7*, 280 (1987)
Streptozotocin	*4*, 221 (1974)
	17, 337 (1978)
	Suppl. 7, 72 (1987)
Strobane® (*see* Terpene polychlorinates)	
Strontium chromate (*see* Chromium and chromium compounds)	
Styrene	*19*, 231 (1979) (*corr. 42*, 258)
	Suppl. 7, 345 (1987)
Styrene-acrylonitrile copolymers	*19*, 97 (1979)
	Suppl. 7, 72 (1987)
Styrene-butadiene copolymers	*19*, 252 (1979)
	Suppl. 7, 72 (1987)
Styrene oxide	*11*, 201 (1976)
	19, 275 (1979)
	36, 245 (1985)
	Suppl. 7, 72 (1987)
Succinic anhydride	*15*, 265 (1977)
	Suppl. 7, 72 (1987)
Sudan I	*8*, 225 (1975)
	Suppl. 7, 72 (1987)
Sudan II	*8*, 233 (1975)
	Suppl. 7, 72 (1987)
Sudan III	*8*, 241 (1975)
	Suppl. 7, 72 (1987)
Sudan Brown RR	*8*, 249 (1975)
	Suppl. 7, 72 (1987)
Sudan Red 7B	*8*, 253 (1975)
	Suppl. 7, 72 (1987)
Sulfafurazole	*24*, 275 (1980)
	Suppl. 7, 347 (1987)
Sulfallate	*30*, 283 (1983)
	Suppl. 7, 72 (1987)

Sulfamethoxazole	*24*, 285 (1980)
	Suppl. 7, 348 (1987)
Sulphisoxazole (*see* Sulfafurazole)	
Sulphur mustard (*see* Mustard gas)	
Sunset Yellow FCF	*8*, 257 (1975)
	Suppl. 7, 72 (1987)
Symphytine	*31*, 239 (1983)
	Suppl. 7, 72 (1987)

T

2,4,5-T (*see also* Chlorophenoxy herbicides; Chlorophenoxy herbicides, occupational exposures to)	*15*, 273 (1977)
Talc	*42*, 185 (1987)
	Suppl. 7, 349 (1987)
Tannic acid	*10*, 253 (1976) (*corr. 42*, 255)
	Suppl. 7, 72 (1987)
Tannins (*see also* Tannic acid)	*10*, 254 (1976)
	Suppl. 7, 72 (1987)
TCDD (*see* 2,3,7,8-Tetrachlorodibenzo-*para*-dioxin)	
TDE (*see* DDT)	
Terpene polychlorinates	*5*, 219 (1974)
	Suppl. 7, 72 (1987)
Testosterone (*see also* Androgenic (anabolic) steroids)	*6*, 209 (1974)
	21, 519 (1979)
Testosterone oenanthate (*see* Testosterone)	
Testosterone propionate (*see* Testosterone)	
2,2′,5,5′-Tetrachlorobenzidine	*27*, 141 (1982)
	Suppl. 7, 72 (1987)
2,3,7,8-Tetrachlorodibenzo-*para*-dioxin	*15*, 41 (1977)
	Suppl. 7, 350 (1987)
1,1,1,2-Tetrachloroethane	*41*, 87 (1986)
	Suppl. 7, 72 (1987)
1,1,2,2-Tetrachloroethane	*20*, 477 (1979)
	Suppl. 7, 354 (1987)
Tetrachloroethylene	*20*, 491 (1979)
	Suppl. 7, 355 (1987)
2,3,4,6-Tetrachlorophenol (*see* Chlorophenols; Chlorophenols, occupational exposure to)	
Tetrachlorvinphos	*30*, 197 (1983)
	Suppl. 7, 72 (1987)
Tetraethyllead (*see* Lead and lead compounds)	
Tetrafluoroethylene	*19*, 285 (1979)
	Suppl. 7, 72 (1987)
Tetramethyllead (*see* Lead and lead compounds)	
Thioacetamide	*7*, 77 (1974)
	Suppl. 7, 72 (1987)

4,4'-Thiodianiline	*16*, 343 (1978)
	27, 147 (1982)
	Suppl. 7, 72 (1987)
Thiotepa (*see* Tris(1-aziridinyl)phosphine sulphide)	
Thiouracil	*7*, 85 (1974)
	Suppl. 7, 72 (1987)
Thiourea	*7*, 95 (1974)
	Suppl. 7, 72 (1987)
Thiram	*12*, 225 (1976)
	Suppl. 7, 72 (1987)
Tobacco habits other than smoking (*see* Tobacco products, smokeless)	
Tobacco products, smokeless	*37* (1985) (*corr. 42*, 263)
	Suppl. 7, 357 (1987)
Tobacco smoke	*38* (1986) (*corr. 42*, 263)
	Suppl. 7, 357 (1987)
Tobacco smoking (*see* Tobacco smoke)	
ortho-Tolidine (*see* 3,3'-Dimethylbenzidine)	
2,4-Toluene diisocyanate (*see also* Toluene diisocyanates)	*19*, 303 (1979)
	39, 287 (1986)
2,6-Toluene diisocyanate (*see also* Toluene diisocyanates)	*19*, 303 (1979)
	39, 289 (1986)
Toluene diisocyanates	*39*, 287 (1986) (*corr. 42*, 264)
	Suppl. 7, 72 (1987)
Toluenes, α-chlorinated (*see* α-Chlorinated toluenes)	
ortho-Toluenesulphonamide (*see* Saccharin)	
ortho-Toluidine	*16*, 349 (1978)
	27, 155 (1982)
	Suppl. 7, 362 (1987)
Toxaphene	*20*, 327 (1979)
	Suppl. 7, 72 (1987)
Tremolite (*see* Asbestos)	
Treosulphan	*26*, 341 (1981)
	Suppl. 7, 363 (1987)
Triaziquone (see Tris(aziridinyl)-*para*-benzoquinone))	
Trichlorfon	*30*, 207 (1983)
	Suppl. 7, 73 (1987)
1,1,1-Trichloroethane	*20*, 515 (1979)
	Suppl. 7, 73 (1987)
1,1,2-Trichloroethane	*20*, 533 (1979)
	Suppl. 7, 73 (1987)
Trichloroethylene	*11*, 263 (1976)
	20, 545 (1979)
	Suppl. 7, 364 (1987)
2,4,5-Trichlorophenol (*see also* Chlorophenols; Chlorophenols, occupational exposure to)	*20*, 349 (1979)

2,4,6-Trichlorophenol (see also Chlorophenols; Chlorophenols, occupational exposures to)   20, 349 (1979)

(2,4,5-Trichlorophenoxy)acetic acid (see 2,4,5-T)

Trichlorotriethylamine hydrochloride   9, 229 (1975)
Suppl. 7, 73 (1987)

T_2-Trichothecene   31, 265 (1983)
Suppl. 7, 73 (1987)

Triethylene glycol diglycidyl ether   11, 209 (1976)
Suppl. 7, 73 (1987)

4,4',6-Trimethylangelicin plus ultraviolet radiation (see also Angelicin and some synthetic derivatives)   Suppl. 7, 57 (1987)

2,4,5-Trimethylaniline   27, 177 (1982)
Suppl. 7, 73 (1987)

2,4,6-Trimethylaniline   27, 178 (1982)
Suppl. 7, 73 (1987)

4,5',8-Trimethylpsoralen   40, 357 (1986)
Suppl. 7, 366 (1987)

Triphenylene   32, 447 (1983)
Suppl. 7, 73 (1987)

Tris(aziridinyl)-para-benzoquinone   9, 67 (1975)
Suppl. 7, 367 (1987)

Tris(1-aziridinyl)phosphine oxide   9, 75 (1975)
Suppl. 7, 73 (1987)

Tris(1-aziridinyl)phosphine sulphide   9, 85 (1975)
Suppl. 7, 368 (1987)

2,4,6-Tris(1-aziridinyl)-s-triazine   9, 95 (1975)
Suppl. 7, 73 (1987)

1,2,3-Tris(chloromethoxy)propane   15, 301 (1977)
Suppl. 7, 73 (1987)

Tris(2,3-dibromopropyl) phosphate   20, 575 (1979)
Suppl. 7, 369 (1987)

Tris(2-methyl-1-aziridinyl)phosphine oxide   9, 107 (1975)
Suppl. 7, 73 (1987)

Trp-P-1   31, 247 (1983)
Suppl. 7, 73 (1987)

Trp-P-2   31, 255 (1983)
Suppl. 7, 73 (1987)

Trypan blue   8, 267 (1975)
Suppl. 7, 73 (1987)

Tussilago farfara L. (see Pyrrolizidine alkaloids)

U

Ultraviolet radiation   40, 379 (1986)

Underground haematite mining with exposure to radon   1, 29 (1972)
Suppl. 7, 216 (1987)

Uracil mustard   9, 235 (1975)
Suppl. 7, 370 (1987)

Urethane	7, 111 (1974)
	Suppl. 7, 73 (1987)
V	
Vinblastine sulphate	26, 349 (1981) (*corr. 42*, 261)
	Suppl. 7, 371 (1987)
Vincristine sulphate	26, 365 (1981)
	Suppl. 7, 372 (1987)
Vinyl acetate	19, 341 (1979)
	39, 113 (1986)
	Suppl. 7, 73 (1987)
Vinyl bromide	19, 367 (1979)
	39, 133 (1986)
	Suppl. 7, 73 (1987)
Vinyl chloride	7, 291 (1974)
	19, 377 (1979) (*corr. 42*, 258)
	Suppl. 7, 373 (1987)
Vinyl chloride-vinyl acetate copolymers	7, 311 (1976)
	19, 412 (1979) (*corr. 42*, 258)
	Suppl. 7, 73 (1987)
4-Vinylcyclohexene	11, 277 (1976)
	39, 181 (1986)
	Suppl. 7, 73 (1987)
Vinyl fluoride	39, 147 (1986)
	Suppl. 7, 73 (1987)
Vinylidene chloride	19, 439 (1979)
	39, 195 (1986)
	Suppl. 7, 376 (1987)
Vinylidene chloride-vinyl chloride copolymers	19, 448 (1979) (*corr. 42*, 258)
	Suppl. 7, 73 (1987)
Vinylidene fluoride	39, 227 (1986)
	Suppl. 7, 73 (1987)
N-Vinyl-2-pyrrolidine	19, 461 (1979)
	Suppl. 7, 73 (1987)
W	
Wollastonite	42, 145 (1987)
	Suppl. 7, 377 (1987)
Wood industries	25 (1981)
	Suppl. 7, 378 (1987)
X	
2,4-Xylidine	16, 367 (1978)
	Suppl. 7, 74 (1987)
2,5-Xylidine	16, 377 (1978)
	Suppl. 7, 74 (1987)

Y

Yellow AB   8, 279 (1975)
                                       Suppl. 7, 74 (1987)
Yellow OB   8, 287 (1975)
                                       Suppl. 7, 74 (1987)

Z

Zearalenone   31, 279 (1983)
                                       Suppl. 7, 74 (1987)
Zectran   12, 237 (1976)
                                       Suppl. 7, 74 (1987)
Zinc beryllium silicate (see Beryllium and beryllium compounds)
Zinc chromate (see Chromium and chromium compounds)
Zinc chromate hydroxide (see Chromium and chromium compounds)
Zinc potassium chromate (see Chromium and chromium compounds)
Zinc yellow (see Chromium and chromium compounds)
Zineb   12, 245 (1976)
                                       Suppl. 7, 74 (1987)
Ziram   12, 259 (1976)
                                       Suppl. 7, 74 (1987)

PUBLICATIONS OF THE INTERNATIONAL AGENCY FOR RESEARCH ON CANCER
SCIENTIFIC PUBLICATIONS SERIES

(Available from Oxford University Press)
through local bookshops

No. 1 LIVER CANCER
1971; 176 pages; out of print

No. 2 ONCOGENESIS AND HERPESVIRUSES
Edited by P.M. Biggs, G. de-Thé & L.N. Payne
1972; 515 pages; out of print

No. 3 N-NITROSO COMPOUNDS: ANALYSIS AND FORMATION
Edited by P. Bogovski, R. Preussmann & E. A. Walker
1972; 140 pages; out of print

No. 4 TRANSPLACENTAL CARCINOGENESIS
Edited by L. Tomatis & U. Mohr
1973; 181 pages; out of print

*No. 5 PATHOLOGY OF TUMOURS IN LABORATORY ANIMALS. VOLUME 1. TUMOURS OF THE RAT. PART 1
Editor-in-Chief V.S. Turusov
1973; 214 pages

*No. 6 PATHOLOGY OF TUMOURS IN LABORATORY ANIMALS. VOLUME 1. TUMOURS OF THE RAT. PART 2
Editor-in-Chief V.S. Turusov
1976; 319 pages
*reprinted in one volume, Price £50.00

No. 7 HOST ENVIRONMENT INTERACTIONS IN THE ETIOLOGY OF CANCER IN MAN
Edited by R. Doll & I. Vodopija
1973; 464 pages; £32.50

No. 8 BIOLOGICAL EFFECTS OF ASBESTOS
Edited by P. Bogovski, J.C. Gilson, V. Timbrell & J.C. Wagner
1973; 346 pages; out of print

No. 9 N-NITROSO COMPOUNDS IN THE ENVIRONMENT
Edited by P. Bogovski & E. A. Walker
1974; 243 pages; £16.50

No. 10 CHEMICAL CARCINOGENESIS ESSAYS
Edited by R. Montesano & L. Tomatis
1974; 230 pages; out of print

No. 11 ONCOGENESIS AND HERPESVIRUSES II
Edited by G. de-Thé, M.A. Epstein & H. zur Hausen
1975; Part 1, 511 pages; Part 2, 403 pages; £65.-

No. 12 SCREENING TESTS IN CHEMICAL CARCINOGENESIS
Edited by R. Montesano, H. Bartsch & L. Tomatis
1976; 666 pages; £12.-

No. 13 ENVIRONMENTAL POLLUTION AND CARCINOGENIC RISKS
Edited by C. Rosenfeld & W. Davis
1976; 454 pages; out of print

No. 14 ENVIRONMENTAL N-NITROSO COMPOUNDS: ANALYSIS AND FORMATION
Edited by E.A. Walker, P. Bogovski & L. Griciute
1976; 512 pages; £37.50

No. 15 CANCER INCIDENCE IN FIVE CONTINENTS. VOLUME III
Edited by J. Waterhouse, C. Muir, P. Correa & J. Powell
1976; 584 pages; out of print

No. 16 AIR POLLUTION AND CANCER IN MAN
Edited by U. Mohr, D. Schmähl & L. Tomatis
1977; 311 pages; out of print

No. 17 DIRECTORY OF ON-GOING RESEARCH IN CANCER EPIDEMIOLOGY 1977
Edited by C.S. Muir & G. Wagner
1977; 599 pages; out of print

No. 18 ENVIRONMENTAL CARCINOGENS: SELECTED METHODS OF ANALYSIS
Edited-in-Chief H. Egan
VOLUME 1. ANALYSIS OF VOLATILE NITROSAMINES IN FOOD
Edited by R. Preussmann, M. Castegnaro, E.A. Walker & A.E. Wassermann
1978; 212 pages; out of print

No. 19 ENVIRONMENTAL ASPECTS OF N-NITROSO COMPOUNDS
Edited by E.A. Walker, M. Castegnaro, L. Griciute & R.E. Lyle
1978; 566 pages; out of print

No. 20 NASOPHARYNGEAL CARCINOMA: ETIOLOGY AND CONTROL
Edited by G. de-Thé & Y. Ito
1978; 610 pages; out of print

No. 21 CANCER REGISTRATION AND ITS TECHNIQUES
Edited by R. MacLennan, C. Muir, R. Steinitz & A. Winkler
1978; 235 pages; £35.-

Prices, valid for October 1988, are subject to change without notice

SCIENTIFIC PUBLICATIONS SERIES

No. 22 ENVIRONMENTAL CARCINOGENS: SELECTED METHODS OF ANALYSIS
Editor-in-Chief H. Egan
VOLUME 2. METHODS FOR THE MEASUREMENT OF VINYL CHLORIDE IN POLY(VINYL CHLORIDE), AIR, WATER AND FOODSTUFFS
Edited by D.C.M. Squirrell & W. Thain
1978; 142 pages; out of print

No. 23 PATHOLOGY OF TUMOURS IN LABORATORY ANIMALS. VOLUME II. TUMOURS OF THE MOUSE
Editor-in-Chief V.S. Turusov
1979; 669 pages; out of print

No. 24 ONCOGENESIS AND HERPESVIRUSES III
Edited by G. de-Thé, W. Henle & F. Rapp
1978; Part 1, 580 pages; Part 2, 522 pages; out of print

No. 25 CARCINOGENIC RISKS: STRATEGIES FOR INTERVENTION
Edited by W. Davis & C. Rosenfeld
1979; 283 pages; out of print

No. 26 DIRECTORY OF ON-GOING RESEARCH IN CANCER EPIDEMIOLOGY 1978
Edited by C.S. Muir & G. Wagner,
1978; 550 pages; out of print

No. 27 MOLECULAR AND CELLULAR ASPECTS OF CARCINOGEN SCREENING TESTS
Edited by R. Montesano, H. Bartsch & L. Tomatis
1980; 371 pages; £22.50

No. 28 DIRECTORY OF ON-GOING RESEARCH IN CANCER EPIDEMIOLOGY 1979
Edited by C.S. Muir & G. Wagner
1979; 672 pages; out of print

No. 29 ENVIRONMENTAL CARCINOGENS: SELECTED METHODS OF ANALYSIS
Editor-in-Chief H. Egan
VOLUME 3. ANALYSIS OF POLYCYCLIC AROMATIC HYDROCARBONS IN ENVIRONMENTAL SAMPLES
Edited by M. Castegnaro, P. Bogovski, H. Kunte & E.A. Walker
1979; 240 pages; out of print

No. 30 BIOLOGICAL EFFECTS OF MINERAL FIBRES
Editor-in-Chief J.C. Wagner
1980; Volume 1, 494 pages; Volume 2, 513 pages; £55.-

No. 31 N-NITROSO COMPOUNDS: ANALYSIS, FORMATION AND OCCURRENCE
Edited by E.A. Walker, L. Griciute, M. Castegnaro & M. Börzsönyi
1980; 841 pages; out of print

No. 32 STATISTICAL METHODS IN CANCER RESEARCH. VOLUME 1. THE ANALYSIS OF CASE-CONTROL STUDIES
By N.E. Breslow & N.E. Day
1980; 338 pages; £20.-

No. 33 HANDLING CHEMICAL CARCINOGENS IN THE LABORATORY: PROBLEMS OF SAFETY
Edited by R. Montesano, H. Bartsch, E. Boyland, G. Della Porta, L. Fishbein, R.A. Griesemer, A.B. Swan & L. Tomatis
1979; 32 pages; out of print

No. 34 PATHOLOGY OF TUMOURS IN LABORATORY ANIMALS. VOLUME III. TUMOURS OF THE HAMSTER
Editor-in-Chief V.S. Turusov
1982; 461 pages; £32.50

No. 35 DIRECTORY OF ON-GOING RESEARCH IN CANCER EPIDEMIOLOGY 1980
Edited by C.S. Muir & G. Wagner
1980; 660 pages; out of print

No. 36 CANCER MORTALITY BY OCCUPATION AND SOCIAL CLASS 1851-1971
By W.P.D. Logan
1982; 253 pages; £22.50

No. 37 LABORATORY DECONTAMINATION AND DESTRUCTION OF AFLATOXINS B_1, B_2, G_1, G_2 IN LABORATORY WASTES
Edited by M. Castegnaro, D.C. Hunt, E.B. Sansone, P.L. Schuller, M.G. Siriwardana, G.M. Telling, H.P. Van Egmond & E.A. Walker
1980; 59 pages; £6.50

No. 38 DIRECTORY OF ON-GOING RESEARCH IN CANCER EPIDEMIOLOGY 1981
Edited by C.S. Muir & G. Wagner
1981; 696 pages; out of print

No. 39 HOST FACTORS IN HUMAN CARCINOGENESIS
Edited by H. Bartsch & B. Armstrong
1982; 583 pages; £37.50

No. 40 ENVIRONMENTAL CARCINOGENS: SELECTED METHODS OF ANALYSIS
Edited-in-Chief H. Egan
VOLUME 4. SOME AROMATIC AMINES AND AZO DYES IN THE GENERAL AND INDUSTRIAL ENVIRONMENT
Edited by L. Fishbein, M. Castegnaro, I.K. O'Neill & H. Bartsch
1981; 347 pages; £22.50

No. 41 N-NITROSO COMPOUNDS: OCCURRENCE AND BIOLOGICAL EFFECTS
Edited by H. Bartsch, I.K. O'Neill, M. Castegnaro & M. Okada
1982; 755 pages; £37.50

No. 42 CANCER INCIDENCE IN FIVE CONTINENTS. VOLUME IV
Edited by J. Waterhouse, C. Muir, K. Shanmugaratnam & J. Powell
1982; 811 pages; £37.50

SCIENTIFIC PUBLICATIONS SERIES

No. 43 LABORATORY DECONTAMINATION
AND DESTRUCTION OF CARCINOGENS IN
LABORATORY WASTES: SOME N-NITROSAMINES
Edited by M. Castegnaro, G. Eisenbrand, G. Ellen,
L. Keefer, D. Klein, E.B. Sansone, D. Spincer,
G. Telling & K. Webb
1982; 73 pages; £7.50

No. 44 ENVIRONMENTAL CARCINOGENS:
SELECTED METHODS OF ANALYSIS
Editor-in-Chief H. Egan
VOLUME 5. SOME MYCOTOXINS
Edited by L. Stoloff, M. Castegnaro, P. Scott,
I.K. O'Neill & H. Bartsch
1983; 455 pages; £22.50

No. 45 ENVIRONMENTAL CARCINOGENS:
SELECTED METHODS OF ANALYSIS
Editor-in-Chief H. Egan
VOLUME 6. N-NITROSO COMPOUNDS
Edited by R. Preussmann, I.K. O'Neill, G. Eisenbrand,
B. Spiegelhalder & H. Bartsch
1983; 508 pages; £22.50

No. 46 DIRECTORY OF ON-GOING RESEARCH
IN CANCER EPIDEMIOLOGY 1982
Edited by C.S. Muir & G. Wagner
1982; 722 pages; out of print

No. 47 CANCER INCIDENCE IN SINGAPORE
1968-1977
Edited by K. Shanmugaratnam, H.P. Lee & N.E. Day
1982; 171 pages; out of print

No. 48 CANCER INCIDENCE IN THE USSR
Second Revised Edition
Edited by N.P. Napalkov, G.F. Tserkovny,
V.M. Merabishvili, D.M. Parkin, M. Smans & C.S. Muir,
1983; 75 pages; £12.-

No. 49 LABORATORY DECONTAMINATION AND
DESTRUCTION OF CARCINOGENS IN
LABORATORY WASTES: SOME POLYCYCLIC
AROMATIC HYDROCARBONS
Edited by M. Castegnaro, G. Grimmer, O. Hutzinger,
W. Karcher, H. Kunte, M. Lafontaine, E.B. Sansone,
G. Telling & S.P. Tucker
1983; 81 pages; £9.-

No. 50 DIRECTORY OF ON-GOING RESEARCH
IN CANCER EPIDEMIOLOGY 1983
Edited by C.S. Muir & G. Wagner
1983; 740 pages; out of print

No. 51 MODULATORS OF EXPERIMENTAL
CARCINOGENESIS
Edited by V. Turusov & R. Montesano
1983; 307 pages; £22.50

No. 52 SECOND CANCER IN RELATION TO
RADIATION TREATMENT FOR CERVICAL
CANCER
Edited by N.E. Day & J.D. Boice, Jr
1984; 207 pages; £20.-

No. 53 NICKEL IN THE HUMAN ENVIRONMENT
Editor-in-Chief F.W. Sunderman, Jr
1984: 530 pages; £32.50

No. 54 LABORATORY DECONTAMINATION
AND DESTRUCTION OF CARCINOGENS IN
LABORATORY WASTES: SOME HYDRAZINES
Edited by M. Castegnaro, G. Ellen, M. Lafontaine,
H.C. van der Plas, E.B. Sansone & S.P. Tucker
1983; 87 pages; £9.-

No. 55 LABORATORY DECONTAMINATION
AND DESTRUCTION OF CARCINOGENS IN
LABORATORY WASTES: SOME N-NITROSAMIDES
Edited by M. Castegnaro, M. Benard,
L.W. van Broekhoven, D. Fine, R. Massey,
E.B. Sansone, P.L.R. Smith, B. Spiegelhalder,
A. Stacchini, G. Telling & J.J. Vallon
1984; 65 pages; £7.50

No. 56 MODELS, MECHANISMS AND ETIOLOGY
OF TUMOUR PROMOTION
Edited by M. Börszönyi, N.E. Day, K. Lapis
& H. Yamasaki
1984; 532 pages; £32.50

No. 57 N-NITROSO COMPOUNDS:
OCCURRENCE, BIOLOGICAL EFFECTS
AND RELEVANCE TO HUMAN CANCER
Edited by I.K. O'Neill, R.C. von Borstel, C.T. Miller,
J. Long & H. Bartsch
1984; 1011 pages; £80.-

No. 58 AGE-RELATED FACTORS IN
CARCINOGENESIS
Edited by A. Likhachev, V. Anisimov & R. Montesano
1985; 288 pages; £20.-

No. 59 MONITORING HUMAN EXPOSURE TO
CARCINOGENIC AND MUTAGENIC AGENTS
Edited by A. Berlin, M. Draper, K. Hemminki
& H. Vainio
1984; 457 pages; £27.50

No. 60 BURKITT'S LYMPHOMA: A HUMAN
CANCER MODEL
Edited by G. Lenoir, G. O'Conor & C.L.M. Olweny
1985; 484 pages; £22.50

No. 61 LABORATORY DECONTAMINATION
AND DESTRUCTION OF CARCINOGENS IN
LABORATORY WASTES: SOME HALOETHERS
Edited by M. Castegnaro, M. Alvarez, M. Iovu,
E.B. Sansone, G.M. Telling & D.T. Williams
1984; 53 pages; £7.50

No. 62 DIRECTORY OF ON-GOING RESEARCH
IN CANCER EPIDEMIOLOGY 1984
Edited by C.S. Muir & G.Wagner
1984; 728 pages; £26.-

No. 63 VIRUS-ASSOCIATED CANCERS IN AFRICA
Edited by A.O. Williams, G.T. O'Conor, G.B. de-Thé
& C.A. Johnson
1984; 774 pages; £22.-

SCIENTIFIC PUBLICATIONS SERIES

No. 64 LABORATORY DECONTAMINATION AND DESTRUCTION OF CARCINOGENS IN LABORATORY WASTES: SOME AROMATIC AMINES AND 4-NITROBIPHENYL
Edited by M. Castegnaro, J. Barek, J. Dennis, G. Ellen, M. Klibanov, M. Lafontaine, R. Mitchum, P. Van Roosmalen, E.B. Sansone, L.A. Sternson & M. Vahl
1985; 85 pages; £6.95

No. 65 INTERPRETATION OF NEGATIVE EPIDEMIOLOGICAL EVIDENCE FOR CARCINOGENICITY
Edited by N.J. Wald & R. Doll
1985; 232 pages; £20.-

No. 66 THE ROLE OF THE REGISTRY IN CANCER CONTROL
Edited by D.M. Parkin, G. Wagner & C. Muir
1985; 155 pages; £10.-

No. 67 TRANSFORMATION ASSAY OF ESTABLISHED CELL LINES: MECHANISMS AND APPLICATION
Edited by T. Kakunaga & H. Yamasaki
1985; 225 pages; £20.-

No. 68 ENVIRONMENTAL CARCINOGENS: SELECTED METHODS OF ANALYSIS VOLUME 7. SOME VOLATILE HALOGENATED HYDROCARBONS
Edited by L. Fishbein & I.K. O'Neill
1985; 479 pages; £20.-

No. 69 DIRECTORY OF ON-GOING RESEARCH IN CANCER EPIDEMIOLOGY 1985
Edited by C.S. Muir & G. Wagner
1985; 756 pages; £22.

No. 70 THE ROLE OF CYCLIC NUCLEIC ACID ADDUCTS IN CARCINOGENESIS AND MUTAGENESIS
Edited by B. Singer & H. Bartsch
1986; 467 pages; £40.-

No. 71 ENVIRONMENTAL CARCINOGENS: SELECTED METHODS OF ANALYSIS VOLUME 8. SOME METALS: As, Be, Cd, Cr, Ni, Pb, Se, Zn
Edited by I.K. O'Neill, P. Schuller & L. Fishbein
1986; 485 pages; £20.

No. 72 ATLAS OF CANCER IN SCOTLAND 1975-1980: INCIDENCE AND EPIDEMIOLOGICAL PERSPECTIVE
Edited by I. Kemp, P. Boyle, M. Smans & C. Muir
1985; 282 pages; £35.-

No. 73 LABORATORY DECONTAMINATION AND DESTRUCTION OF CARCINOGENS IN LABORATORY WASTES: SOME ANTINEOPLASTIC AGENTS
Edited by M. Castegnaro, J. Adams, M. Armour, J. Barek, J. Benvenuto, C. Confalonieri, U. Goff, S. Ludeman, D. Reed, E.B. Sansone & G. Telling
1985; 163 pages; £10.-

No. 74 TOBACCO: A MAJOR INTERNATIONAL HEALTH HAZARD
Edited by D. Zaridze & R. Peto
1986; 324 pages; £20.-

No. 75 CANCER OCCURRENCE IN DEVELOPING COUNTRIES
Edited by D.M. Parkin
1986; 339 pages; £20.-

No. 76 SCREENING FOR CANCER OF THE UTERINE CERVIX
Edited by M. Hakama, A.B. Miller & N.E. Day
1986; 315 pages; £25.-

No. 77 HEXACHLOROBENZENE: PROCEEDINGS OF AN INTERNATIONAL SYMPOSIUM
Edited by C.R. Morris & J.R.P. Cabral
1986; 668 pages; £50.-

No. 78 CARCINOGENICITY OF ALKYLATING CYTOSTATIC DRUGS
Edited by D. Schmähl & J. M. Kaldor
1986; 338 pages; £25.-

No. 79 STATISTICAL METHODS IN CANCER RESEARCH. VOLUME III. THE DESIGN AND ANALYSIS OF LONG-TERM ANIMAL EXPERIMENTS
By J.J. Gart, D. Krewski, P.N. Lee, R.E. Tarone & J. Wahrendorf
1986; 219 pages; £20.-

No. 80 DIRECTORY OF ON-GOING RESEARCH IN CANCER EPIDEMIOLOGY 1986
Edited by C.S. Muir & G. Wagner
1986; 805 pages; £22.-

No. 81 ENVIRONMENTAL CARCINOGENS: METHODS OF ANALYSIS AND EXPOSURE MEASUREMENT. VOLUME 9. PASSIVE SMOKING
Edited by I.K. O'Neill, K.D. Brunnemann, B. Dodet & D. Hoffmann
1987; 379 pages; £30.-

No. 82 STATISTICAL METHODS IN CANCER RESEARCH. VOLUME II. THE DESIGN AND ANALYSIS OF COHORT STUDIES
By N.E. Breslow & N.E. Day
1987; 404 pages; £30.-

No. 83 LONG-TERM AND SHORT-TERM ASSAYS FOR CARCINOGENS: A CRITICAL APPRAISAL
Edited by R. Montesano, H. Bartsch, H. Vainio, J. Wilbourn & H. Yamasaki
1986; 575 pages; £32.50

No. 84 THE RELEVANCE OF N-NITROSO COMPOUNDS TO HUMAN CANCER: EXPOSURES AND MECHANISMS
Edited by H. Bartsch, I.K. O'Neill & R. Schulte-Hermann
1987; 671 pages; £50.-

SCIENTIFIC PUBLICATIONS SERIES

No. 85 ENVIRONMENTAL CARCINOGENS: METHODS OF ANALYSIS AND EXPOSURE MEASUREMENT. VOLUME 10. BENZENE AND ALKYLATED BENZENES
Edited by L. Fishbein & I.K. O'Neill
1988; 318 pages; £35.-

No. 86 DIRECTORY OF ON-GOING RESEARCH IN CANCER EPIDEMIOLOGY 1987
Edited by D.M. Parkin & J. Wahrendorf
1987; 685 pages; £22.-

No. 87 INTERNATIONAL INCIDENCE OF CHILDHOOD CANCER
Edited by D.M. Parkin, C.A. Stiller, G.J. Draper, C.A. Bieber, B. Terracini & J.L. Young
1988; 402 pages; £35.-

No. 88 CANCER INCIDENCE IN FIVE CONTINENTS. VOLUME V
Edited by C. Muir, J. Waterhouse, T. Mack, J. Powell & S. Whelan
1988; 1004 pages; £50.-

No. 89 METHODS FOR DETECTING DNA DAMAGING AGENTS IN HUMANS: APPLICATIONS IN CANCER EPIDEMIOLOGY AND PREVENTION
Edited by H. Bartsch, K. Hemminki & I.K. O'Neill
1988; 518 pages; £45.-

No. 90 NON-OCCUPATIONAL EXPOSURE TO MINERAL FIBRES
Edited by J. Bignon, J. Peto & R. Saracci
1988; 530 pages; £45.-

No. 91 TRENDS IN CANCER INCIDENCE IN SINGAPORE 1968-1982
Edited by H.P. Lee, N.E. Day & K. Shanmugaratnam
1988; 160 pages; £25.-

No. 92 CELL DIFFERENTIATION, GENES AND CANCER
Edited by T. Kakunaga, T. Sugimura, L. Tomatis and H. Yamasaki
1988; 204 pages; £25.-

No. 93 DIRECTORY OF ON-GOING RESEARCH IN CANCER EPIDEMIOLOGY 1988
Edited by M. Coleman & J. Wahrendorf
1988; 662 pages; £26.-

No. 94 HUMAN PAPILLOMAVIRUS AND CERVICAL CANCER
Edited by N. Muñoz, F.X Bosch & O.M. Jensen.
1989; 154 pages; £18.-

No. 95 CANCER REGISTRATION: PRINCIPLES AND METHODS
Edited by D.M. Parkin & O.M. Jensen
c. 200 pages (in press)

No. 96 PERINATAL AND MULTIGENERATION CARCINOGENESIS
Edited by N.P. Napalkov, J.M. Rice, L. Tomatis & H. Yamasaki
c. 400 pages (in press)

No. 97 OCCUPATIONAL EXPOSURE TO SILICA AND CANCER RISK
Edited by L. Simonato, A.C. Fletcher, R. Saracci & T. Thomas
c. 160 pages (in press)

IARC MONOGRAPHS ON THE EVALUATION OF CARCINOGENIC RISKS TO HUMANS
(English editions only)

(Available from booksellers through the network of WHO Sales Agents*)

Volume 1
Some inorganic substances, chlorinated hydrocarbons, aromatic amines, N-nitroso compounds, and natural products
1972; 184 pages; out of print

Volume 2
Some inorganic and organometallic compounds
1973; 181 pages; out of print

Volume 3
Certain polycyclic aromatic hydrocarbons and heterocyclic compounds
1973; 271 pages; out of print

Volume 4
Some aromatic amines, hydrazine and related substances, N-nitroso compounds and miscellaneous alkylating agents
1974; 286 pages; Sw. fr. 18.-

Volume 5
Some organochlorine pesticides
1974; 241 pages; out of print

Volume 6
Sex hormones
1974; 243 pages; out of print

Volume 7
Some anti-thyroid and related substances, nitrofurans and industrial chemicals
1974; 326 pages; out of print

Volume 8
Some aromatic azo compounds
1975; 357 pages; Sw.fr. 36.-

Volume 9
Some aziridines, N-, S- and O-mustards and selenium
1975; 268 pages; Sw. fr. 27.-

Volume 10
Some naturally occurring substances
1976; 353 pages; out of print

Volume 11
Cadmium, nickel, some epoxides, miscellaneous industrial chemicals and general considerations on volatile anaesthetics
1976; 306 pages; out of print

Volume 12
Some carbamates, thiocarbamates and carbazides
1976; 282 pages; Sw. fr. 34.-

Volume 13
Some miscellaneous pharmaceutical substances
1977; 255 pages; Sw. fr. 30.-

Volume 14
Asbestos
1977; 106 pages; out of print

Volume 15
Some fumigants, the herbicides 2,4-D and 2,4,5-T, chlorinated dibenzodioxins and miscellaneous industrial chemicals
1977; 354 pages; Sw. fr. 50.-

Volume 16
Some aromatic amines and related nitro compounds — hair dyes, colouring agents and miscellaneous industrial chemicals
1978; 400 pages; Sw. fr. 50.-

Volume 17
Some N-nitroso compounds
1978; 365 pages; Sw. fr. 50.

Volume 18
Polychlorinated biphenyls and polybrominated biphenyls
1978; 140 pages; Sw. fr. 20.-

Volume 19
Some monomers, plastics and synthetic elastomers, and acrolein
1979; 513 pages; Sw. fr. 60.-

Volume 20
Some halogenated hydrocarbons
1979; 609 pages; Sw. fr. 60.-

Volume 21
Sex hormones (II)
1979; 583 pages; Sw. fr. 60.-

Volume 22
Some non-nutritive sweetening agents
1980; 208 pages; Sw. fr. 25.-

Volume 23
Some metals and metallic compounds
1980; 438 pages; Sw. fr. 50.-

Volume 24
Some pharmaceutical drugs
1980; 337 pages; Sw. fr. 40.-

Volume 25
Wood, leather and some associated industries
1981; 412 pages; Sw. fr. 60.-

Volume 26
Some antineoplastic and immunosuppressive agents
1981; 411 pages; Sw. fr. 62.-

*A list of these Agents may be obtained by writing to the World Health Organization, Distribution and Sales Service, 1211 Geneva 27, Switzerland

IARC MONOGRAPHS SERIES

Volume 27
Some aromatic amines, anthraquinones and nitroso compounds, and inorganic fluorides used in drinking-water and dental preparations
1982; 341 pages; Sw. fr. 40.-

Volume 28
The rubber industry
1982; 486 pages; Sw. fr. 70.-

Volume 29
Some industrial chemicals and dyestuffs
1982; 416 pages; Sw. fr. 60.-

Volume 30
Miscellaneous pesticides
1983; 424 pages; Sw. fr. 60.-

Volume 31
Some food additives, feed additives and naturally occurring substances
1983; 14 pages; Sw. fr. 60.-

Volume 32
Polynuclear aromatic compounds, Part 1, Chemical, environmental and experimental data
1984; 477 pages; Sw. fr. 60.-

Volume 33
Polynuclear aromatic compounds, Part 2, Carbon blacks, mineral oils and some nitroarenes
1984; 245 pages; Sw. fr. 50.-

Volume 34
Polynuclear aromatic compounds, Part 3, Industrial exposures in aluminium production, coal gasification, coke production, and iron and steel founding
1984; 219 pages; Sw. fr. 48.-

Volume 35
Polynuclear aromatic compounds, Part 4, Bitumens, coal-tars and derived products, shale-oils and soots
1985; 271 pages; Sw. fr.70.-

Volume 36
Allyl compounds, aldehydes, epoxides and peroxides
1985; 369 pages; Sw. fr. 70.-

Volume 37
Tobacco habits other than smoking; betel-quid and areca-nut chewing; and some related nitrosamines
1985; 291 pages; Sw. fr. 70.-

Volume 38
Tobacco smoking
1986; 421 pages; Sw. fr. 75.-

Volume 39
Some chemicals used in plastics and elastomers
1986; 403 pages; Sw. fr. 60.-

Volume 40
Some naturally occurring and synthetic food components, furocoumarins and ultraviolet radiation
1986; 444 pages; Sw. fr. 65.-

Volume 41
Some halogenated hydrocarbons and pesticide exposures
1986; 434 pages; Sw. fr. 65.-

Volume 42
Silica and some silicates
1987; 289 pages; Sw. fr. 65.-

*Volume 43
Man-made mineral fibres and radon
1988; 300 pages; Sw. fr. 65.-

Volume 44
Alcohol drinking
1988; 416 pages; Sw. fr. 65.-

Volume 45
Occupational exposures in petroleum refining; crude oil and major petroleum fuels
1989; 322 pages; Sw. fr. 65.-

Supplement No. 1
Chemicals and industrial processes associated with cancer in humans (IARC Monographs, Volumes 1 to 20)
1979; 71 pages; out of print

Supplement No. 2
Long-term and short-term screening assays for carcinogens: a critical appraisal
1980; 426 pages; Sw. fr. 40.-

Supplement No. 3
Cross index of synonyms and trade names in Volumes 1 to 26
1982; 199 pages; Sw. fr. 60.-

Supplement No. 4
Chemicals, industrial processes and industries associated with cancer in humans (IARC Monographs, Volumes 1 to 29)
1982; 292 pages; Sw. fr. 60.-

Supplement No. 5
Cross index of synonyms and trade names in Volumes 1 to 36
1985; 259 pages; Sw. fr. 60.-

*Supplement No. 6
Genetic and related effects: An updating of selected IARC Monographs from Volumes 1-42
1987; 730 pages; Sw. fr. 80.-

Supplement No. 7
Overall evaluations of carcinogenicity: An updating of IARC Monographs Volumes 1-42
1987; 440 pages; Sw. fr. 65.-

*From Volume 43 and Supplement No. 6 onwards, the series title was changed to IARC MONOGRAPHS ON THE EVALUATION OF CARCINOGENIC RISKS TO HUMANS from IARC MONOGRAPHS ON THE EVALUATION OF THE CARCINOGENIC RISK OF CHEMICALS TO HUMANS

INFORMATION BULLETINS ON THE SURVEY OF CHEMICALS BEING TESTED FOR CARCINOGENICITY*

No. 8 (1979)
Edited by M.-J. Ghess, H. Bartsch
& L. Tomatis
604 pages; Sw. fr. 40.-

No. 9 (1981)
Edited by M.-J. Ghess, J.D. Wilbourn,
H. Bartsch & L. Tomatis
294 pages; Sw. fr. 41.-

No. 10 (1982)
Edited by M.-J. Ghess, J.D. Wilbourn
& H. Bartsch
362 pages; Sw. fr. 42.-

No. 11 (1984)
Edited by M.-J. Ghess, J.D. Wilbourn,
H. Vainio & H. Bartsch
362 pages; Sw. fr. 50.-

No. 12 (1986)
Edited by M.-J. Ghess, J.D. Wilbourn,
A. Tossavainen & H. Vainio
385 pages; Sw. fr. 50.-

No. 13 (1988)
Edited by M.-J. Ghess, J.D. Wilbourn
& A. Aitio
404 pages; Sw. fr. 43.-

*Available from IARC; or the World Health Organization Distribution and Sales Services, 1211 Geneva 27, Switzerland or WHO Sales Agents.

NON-SERIAL PUBLICATIONS

(Available from IARC)

ALCOOL ET CANCER
By A. Tuyns (in French only)
1978; 42 pages; Fr. fr. 35.-

CANCER MORBIDITY AND CAUSES OF
DEATH AMONG DANISH BREWERY
WORKERS
By O.M. Jensen
1980; 143 pages; Fr. fr. 75.-

DIRECTORY OF COMPUTER SYSTEMS
USED IN CANCER REGISTRIES
By H.R. Menck & D.M. Parkin
1986; 236 pages; Fr. fr. 50.-

**IARC Monographs are distributed
by the
World Health Organization,
Distribution and Sales Service,
1211 Geneva 27, Switzerland
and are available from booksellers
through the network of WHO Sales Agents.**

A list of these Agents may be obtained
by writing to the above address.

www.ingramcontent.com/pod-product-compliance
Ingram Content Group UK Ltd.
Pitfield, Milton Keynes, MK11 3LW, UK
UKHW051258180426
11947UKWH00020B/1787

9 789283 212454